Subcortical Functions
in Language and Memory

Subcortical Functions in Language and Memory

B R U C E   C R O S S O N,   P H. D.

THE GUILFORD PRESS
New York   London

Printed in the United States of America

This book is printed on acid-free paper.

Last digit is print number: 9 8 7 6 5 4 3 2 1

Library of Congress Cataloging-in-Publication Data

Crosson, Bruce A.
    Subcortical functions in language and memory / Bruce A. Crosson.
        p.   cm.
    Includes bibliographical references and index.
    ISBN 0-89862-790-7
    1. Neurolinguistics.   2. Memory   3. Thalamus   4. Prosencepha-
lon   5. Basal ganglia.   I. Title.
    [DNLM: 1. Basal Ganglia—physiology.   2. Cerebral Cortex—
physiology.   3. Language.   4. Memory—Physiology.   WL 340
C951s]
QP399.C76   1992
153.6—dc20
DNLM/DLC
for Library of Congress   91-42906
                                                                                   CIP

To Susan, Brent, and Courtney,
without whose support
this work would have been impossible

Acknowledgments

The author would like to thank the following persons: Carroll W. Hughes, Ph.D., and Russell M. Bauer, Ph.D., for their helpful comments on the manuscript; Randi K. Lincoln and David J. Williamson for their assistance in proofreading; Louis Clark for his work on the drawings in Chapters 1 and 5; Sharon Panulla, Susan Marples, Anna Brackett, Curt Tow, and the staff of Guilford Publications for their time, patience, and assistance in the various stages of this project.

Contents

Introduction

Until the 1970s, it was generally accepted that the basal ganglia were part of the extrapyramidal motor system controlling motor tone and that the thalamus was a relay station passing information from lower centers to the cortex. The cerebral cortex was considered to be the seat of cognition. Subcortical structures were thought to affect cognition only through generalized effects on the cortex, such as the arousal of the cortex (e.g., see Luria, 1973, 1977). Of course, notable exceptions to these prevailing notions could be found. Wallesch and Papagno (1988) noted that in 1908, Moutier, a student of Pierre Marie, described three cases of nonfluent aphasia in which the lesions were purely subcortical. Even earlier, in 1872, Broadbent had assumed that the striatum generated words as motor acts. In more recent times, Penfield and Roberts (1959) described a case of aphasia after thalamic lesion, and they speculated that the thalamus played an integrative role in language. A similar assumption was made by Schuell, Jenkins, and Jimenez-Pabon (1965). Numerous studies of lesion and electrical stimulation of subcortical structures during the 1960s hinted at a role for these entities in language (e.g., Allen, Turner, & Gadea-Ciria, 1966; Asso, Crown, Russell, & Logue, 1969; Bell, 1968; Cooper et al., 1968; Hermann, Turner, Gillingham, & Gaze, 1966; Ojemann & Fedio, 1968; Ojemann, Fedio, & Van Buren, 1968; Riklan, Levita, Zimmerman, & Cooper, 1969; Samra et al., 1969; Schaltenbrand, 1965; Selby, 1967; Svennilson, Torvik, Lowe, & Leksell, 1960; Van Buren, 1963, 1966; Van Buren, Li, & Ojemann, 1966).

However, the generally held beliefs about the basal ganglia and thalamus were not widely challenged until computerized tomography became widely used as a diagnostic tool in the 1970s. X-ray computed tomography, for the first time, made it possible to visualize naturally occurring vascular lesions that were primarily confined to the thalamus, basal ganglia, and/or the surrounding white matter pathways. Inevitably, reports emerged in which impaired cognition was correlated with subcortical lesion. Some reports are now beginning to appear that also use magnetic resonance imaging for similar purposes (e.g., Puel, Demonet, Cardebat, Berry, & Celsis, 1989), and single photon emission computed tomography and positron emission tomography are being used to explore subcortical participation in normal (Wallesch, Henriksen, Kornhuber, & Paulson, 1985) and abnormal language (Baron et al., 1986; Demonet et al., 1989; Fasanaro et al., 1987; Metter et al., 1983, 1984, 1986, 1988, 1989; Olsen, Bruhn, & Oberg, 1986; Puel et al., 1989).

Unavoidably, as a consequence of these data, a number of viewpoints regarding the participation of subcortical structures in language have been set forth. With respect to language, some investigators have denied a role for subcortical structures beyond affecting the arousal of cortical structures involved in language (e.g., Luria, 1977). Some have suggested a specific role for the thalamus and basal ganglia in language (e.g., Crosson, 1985; Wallesch & Papagno, 1988), while others have proposed that the basal ganglia are not directly involved in language, though the thalamus might be (e.g., Alexander, Naeser, & Palumbo, 1987).

The story is rather different for memory. Gamper (1928) had suggested that the mammillary bodies are involved in memory, and this viewpoint appeared frequently in the literature until challenged by Victor, Adams, and Collins (1971). On the basis of their autopsies of alcoholic Korsakoff's patients, the latter investigators concluded that the dorsal medial thalamus was the diencephalic structure involved in memory. Although there is some general agreement that the diencephalon is involved in memory, some disagreement continues concerning whether the mammillary bodies, the dorsal medial thalamus, the anterior thalamus, or all these structures are involved in memory. One fundamental difference between the language and memory literatures is the development of animal models for memory, and the work of Mishkin and his colleagues has shed some light on the matter of diencephalic participation in memory (e.g., Aggleton, 1986; Bachevalier, Parkinson, & Mishkin, 1985; Mishkin, 1982). More recent works have also suggested participation of the basal forebrain (e.g., Butters, 1985; Damasio, Eslinger, Damasio, Van Hoesen, & Cornell, 1985; Damasio, Graff-Radford, Eslinger, Damasio, & Kassell, 1985; Phillips, Sangalang, & Sterns, 1987) and basal ganglia (e.g., Butters,

Wolfe, Granholm, & Martone, 1986; Butters, Wolfe, Martone, Granholm, & Cermak, 1985; Martone, Butters, Payne, Becker, & Sax, 1984; Shimamura, Salmon, Squire, & Butters, 1987; Smith, Butters, White, Lyon, & Granholm, 1988) in memory.

Others have emphasized the necessity not only of considering grey matter structures involved in memory, but also of looking at the subcortical pathways between the various cortical and subcortical centers involved in memory (Cramon, Hebel, & Schuri, 1985, 1986, 1988; Crosson, 1986; Graff-Radford, Tranel, Van Hoesen, & Brandt, 1990). Awareness of the nature and location of pathways between grey matter structures is particularly important in considering lesion data because white matter as well as grey matter is damaged in most lesions. If we restrict our interest only to the grey matter, we are more likely to draw erroneous conclusions regarding which structures are involved in a particular cognitive function (Cramon, 1989).

Ultimately, understanding structures such as the thalamus, basal ganglia, and basal forebrain will bring us much closer to understanding the neural substrates of thought. My purpose in this book is to explore recent literature regarding the participation of these structures in cognition. Specifically, I will emphasize language and memory both because these areas of cognition are the most frequently emphasized in the context of subcortical participation and because some agreement exists regarding the neuropsychological processes of language and memory. The book will be divided into two parts: language and memory. These subjects will be approached from a systems standpoint, that is, the assumption is made that subcortical structures, when they do play a role in cognition, do so as parts of complex brain systems.

It follows from this assumption that a knowledge of the neuroanatomy of the relevant subcortical structures is a prerequisite for understanding their role in cognition. In particular, understanding the way in which different subcortical nuclei and cortical areas are connected is the basis for understanding the flow of information from one structure to another and/or the regulatory or modulatory relationships between structures. The influence of one anatomic entity over another or the transfer of information from one anatomic entity to another is constrained by the way in which they are connected. Speculation regarding the role of a structure in language or memory must be done with an understanding of how it is connected to other structures participating in the same cognitive function if it is to be productive.

Thus, the first chapter for each part of this book will deal with the neuroanatomy of structures thought to be involved in language and memory, respectively. It is not the purpose of these chapters to give an exhaustive review of neuroanatomy. Rather, they will explore the systems of structures that may be involved in language and memory. Those readers with an intimate knowledge of neuroanatomy may find these chapters necessarily simplified due both to considerations of space and to the aim of this book to provide a survey for a broad variety of individuals who are interested in the participation of subcortical structures in cognition. Those readers who have a more limited background in neuroanatomy may want to supplement the information provided by perusing the relevant chapters of a good neuroanatomy text (e.g., Carpenter & Sutin, 1983; Nauta & Feirtag, 1986) or even by picking up a text discussing the neuroanatomy of one of these structures, such as the thalamus, in greater detail (e.g., Jones, 1985).

For more than 100 years, the neural substrates of language have been one of the most thoroughly studied functions from the standpoint of the the brain and cognition. The knowledge produced by over a century of study has provided an excellent backdrop against which to consider the participation of subcortical structures in language. For example, we have not only an idea of which cortical areas are involved in language, but also an idea of what these cortical areas contribute to language. Since subcortical structures do not participate in language or other cognitive functions in isolation from the cortex, this information regarding cortical functions will give us important hints regarding how subcortical structures supplement, modify, and/or regulate cortical contributions.

Thus, the first part of the book will concentrate on the participation (or nonparticipation) of various subcortical structures in language. The purpose of this part is not to arrive at definitive conclusions about the role of various subcortical structures in language; rather it is to explore the possibilities suggested by the currently available data. After discussing the neuroanatomy and the data concerning the thalamus and basal ganglia, I will devote some attention to theories regarding the participation of the thalamus and basal ganglia in language. In examining the latter issue, one must be cognizant of the role of theory at this early stage in the development of our knowledge. More specifically, the purpose of theory at such a time is primarily heuristic. In other words, current theories help to guide future research, which in turn will lead to more and more accurate models of brain–language processes.

Memory is also an extremely important function in cognition. Indeed, without memory there would be little meaningful cognition. For example, the ability of the human organism to acquire and use new language symbols and processes is necessary for the existence of language as a complex cognitive function. Further, there is an interface between language and memory that involves not only the acquisition of new symbols and procedures, but also the retrieval of already stored symbols for current usage. It is appropriate, therefore, to address issues of subcortical functions in memory, having language as a backdrop. A more complete understanding of brain processes in language and memory will lead to a greater appreciation for the overlapping and unique functions of these systems from a cognitive as well as an anatomical standpoint.

Thus, the second part of this book will be devoted to the role of subcortical structures in memory. Again, my focus will be upon exploring possibilities as opposed to reaching any definitive conclusions. I will address the thalamus, other diencephalic structures, the basal forebrain, and the basal ganglia regarding their possible role in memory; the connections between these structures are also addressed. I will then explore the relationship between current data regarding the participation of subcortical structures in memory and current neuropsychological assumptions regarding memory. I will discuss the extensive literature on memory in alcoholic Korsakoff's syndrome and Huntington's disease in some detail since these studies give us insight into what memory processes may be subserved by subcortical structures. Finally, I will examine memory theory in light of what the subcortical literature tells us about memory.

It is my belief that the addition of subcortical structures to neurocognitive models will provide for a degree of flexibility and complexity that does not exist in purely cortical models. However, we are only beginning to understand the potential roles of subcortical structures in cognitive functions. Do these structures serve to regulate and modulate cortical functions? Do they provide for the transfer (relay) of information from one structure to another? Or, do they perform more complicated information-processing functions? Do they integrate activities of various cortical structures? Are they involved in motivational functions? What does the literature tell us about their participation in language and memory? What does the way they are connected tell us about their operation in neurocognitive systems? These are some of the issues explored in this book.

1

SUBCORTICAL
STRUCTURES
IN LANGUAGE

1

Subcortical Neuroanatomy and Language

Discussing the evidence regarding subcortical structures and language without first addressing the relevant neuroanatomy would be like discussing the history of a country without knowing the facts of its geography. Just as geography determines many facets of history, neuroanatomy determines possibilities in the realm of cognition. For this reason, I shall begin with an exploration of those structures thought to be involved in language.

How information is processed and how actions are planned by a neural system depends upon what structures are available for these tasks and how these structures participate in processing and/or planning. Further, if we believe that a number of structures function together as a system in language analysis and production, how these structures are connected is also crucial. Since neuronal transmission of information occurs in one direction along axons, the direction of informational flow between structures limits the patterns of influence within the system. Cramon (1989) has made this point quite eloquently in his discussion of the memory system.

Thus, this chapter will focus on the neuroanatomy of those structures thought to be involved in language. It is not meant to be a comprehensive review of neuroanatomy; rather, it will discuss structures that have been implicated in language. Some emphasis will be placed upon how these structures are connected. Evidence regarding the participation of these structures in language will not be discussed in detail until later chapters of the book. The purpose of this chapter is simply to provide a foundation for discussing such evidence, to provide a road map of those structures that will be examined.

Much evidence exists to indicate that both the basal ganglia and the thalamus may be involved in language. In the basal ganglia, both the head of the caudate nucleus and the putamen have been studied (e.g., Alexander & LoVerme, 1980; Aram, Rose, Rekate, & Whitaker, 1983; Brunner, Kornhuber, Seemuller, Suger, & Wallesch, 1982; Damasio, Damasio, Rizzo, Varney, & Gersh, 1982; Demonet, 1987; Mazzocchi & Vignolo, 1979; Mehler, 1988; Naeser et al., 1982; Van Buren, 1963, 1966; Van Buren et al., 1966; Wallesch, 1985); the medial segment of the globus pallidus which receives a major portion of the efferent fibers from the caudate nucleus and putamen (Carpenter & Sutin, 1983), also seems like a likely area regarding language involvement (e.g., Svennilson et al., 1960; Wallesch, 1985). In the thalamus, both anterior and posterior regions have been implicated in language functions. The ventral lateral nucleus and pulvinar are frequently mentioned (Allen et al., 1966; Bell, 1968; Ciemans, 1970; Crosson et al., 1986; Gorelick, Hier, Benevento, Levitt, & Tan, 1984; Kameyama, 1976/1977; Ojemann, 1977; Puel et al., 1989; Selby, 1967; Van Buren, 1975; Van Buren & Borke, 1969; Wallesch & Papagno, 1988), but the anterior nucleus, the ventral anterior nucleus, the dorsal medial nucleus, and even the intralaminar nuclei have also received mention (e.g., Brown, 1977; Crosson, 1985; Graff-Radford, Damasio, Yamada, Eslinger, & Damasio, 1985; Schaltenbrand, 1965, 1975). I shall examine the basal ganglia first.

Before doing so, however, I need to say a word or two about how to approach reading this chapter. My goal was to provide enough detail regarding the neuroanatomy of the relevant subcortical structures that a moderately sophisticated reader could begin to conceptualize the relevant brain systems. I anticipate that many readers will have a significant degree of familiarity with neuroanatomy while others will have less experience with neuroanatomical concepts. The former group may see this chapter as somewhat oversimplified and may wish to refer to more extended texts such as Jones (1985) or Carpenter and Sutin (1983).

On the other hand, the latter group may find the detail in this chapter formidable. Such readers may wish to read the chapter for an overview as opposed to trying to absorb all the detail in an initial reading. For example, the minimum necessary detail regarding the basal ganglia includes knowledge of the caudate nucleus, putamen, both segments of the globus pallidus, and the connections of these structures with one another, the cortex, and the thalamus (see Table 1-1). Information regarding other connections, compartments within the striatum, and other connections of the nuclei is of lesser importance for the study of language and memory. The minimum necessary detail regarding the thalamus needed for understanding the rest of the book would be a familiarity with the major nuclei of the thalamus and their connections (see Table 1-2). Although a familiarity with the subdivisions of these nuclei would be helpful, it is not essential for further reading.

Indeed, after familiarizing oneself with the information of Chapter 1, it might thereafter be treated as a reference to which one can return if questions arise during perusal of the ensuing chapters. I hope that the detail of this chapter will not discourage readers from examining the following chapters. Rather, the interest generated by the other chapters of this book may help to determine how much of the anatomical detail the reader wishes to permanently absorb. Of course, the reader wishing a more in-depth familiarity with the various structures will need to consider the material presented in detail.

Potential Basal Ganglia Structures Involved in Language

Of the structures that different anatomists might include in the "basal ganglia," I shall focus upon the caudate nucleus, the putamen, and the globus pallidus because these are the structures that have been implicated in language. Collectively, these structures can be called the corpus striatum (Carpenter & Sutin, 1983). Figure 1-1 illustrates horizontal and coronal cuts through the left basal ganglia. At this level (horizontal cut), the head of the caudate nucleus, the putamen, and the globus pallidus are visible. Medially and toward the anterior portion of the caudate head lies the frontal horn of the lateral ventricle. Anterolateral to the caudate head is the frontal white matter, and posterolateral is the anterior limb and genu of the internal capsule.

The anterior limb of the internal capsule is the band of white matter that separates the head of the caudate nucleus from the putamen and the globus pallidus. Collectively, the putamen and the globus pallidus form a wedge-shaped area of gray matter sometimes called the lentiform nucleus. Lateral to the putamen are a thin band of white matter called the external capsule, a thin band of gray matter called the claustrum, and another thin band of white matter called the extreme capsule. Medial to the putamen lies the lateral segment of the globus pallidus, and more medially is the medial segment of the globus pallidus. The medial and lateral segments of the globus pallidus are separated from the thalamus by a band of white matter called the

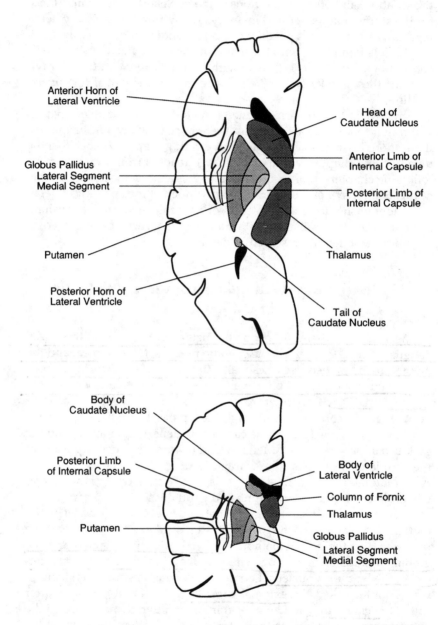

Figure 1-1. Sketch of horizontal and coronal cuts through the basal ganglia. (Drawings are composed to indicate relationships between structures but are not meant to be anatomically precise.)

posterior limb of the internal capsule, which rises over the lentiform nucleus from an inferior medial to a superior lateral position. Various white matter structures course beneath the lentiform nucleus.

The caudate nucleus (see Figure 1-2) is a long, arched nucleus that borders on the lateral ventricle for its entire length. The more bulky head of the caudate nucleus lies anterior to the thalamus and bulges into the frontal horn of the lateral ventricle, forming the posterolateral margin of the frontal horn. From there, the nucleus proceeds upward, arching gradually in the posterior direction. The body of the caudate nucleus forms a portion of the inferior lateral border of the lateral ventricle, becoming less prominent moving in a posterior direction. The superior portion of the caudate tail is lateral to the posterior-most portion of the thalamus and on the anterior wall of the trigone of the lateral ventricle. Inferiorly, as the trigone becomes the temporal horn, the caudate nucleus follows the ventricle anteriorly in the roof of the temporal horn. The caudate tail finally reaches the amygdaloid nucleus deep within the anterior portion of the temporal lobe (Carpenter & Sutin, 1983; Montemurro & Bruni, 1988; Netter, 1972).

Collectively, the caudate nucleus and the putamen are known as the neostriatum, or striatum for short. Their separation by the internal capsule is only partial. The head of the caudate nucleus and the putamen are joined inferiorly, and the caudate and putamen are connected by slender bridges of gray matter as the caudate turns

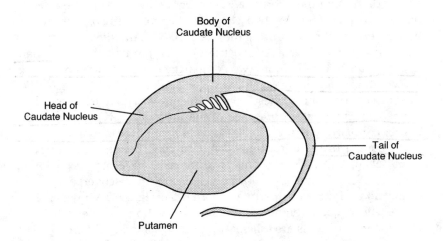

Figure 1-2. Sketch of a lateral view of the caudate nucleus and putamen. (Drawings are composed to indicate relationships between structures but are not meant to be anatomically precise.)

posteriorly (Carpenter & Sutin, 1983). Two structures that are related to the neostriatum are the nucleus accumbens and adjoining parts of the olfactory tubercle; they have connections that roughly parallel those of the caudate nucleus and the putamen, with their cortical input coming from limbic regions. Thus, the nucleus accumbens and adjoining parts of the olfactory tubercle, along with the inferior areas of the caudate and putamen, are sometimes referred to as the ventral striatum (Graybiel, 1984). The nucleus accumbens is inferior and somewhat medial to the more inferior portion of the caudate head and inferior to the inferior tip of the lateral ventricle's frontal horn (Haines, 1987).

To understand the potential role of these structures of the basal ganglia in language, it is necessary to know how they are connected to other structures that are also involved in language. The way in which language structures are connected will constrain the way in which they interact in language production and analysis. Eventually, knowledge that is still developing about the neurotransmitter systems and the histological characteristics of the relevant structures will also be necessary to give us a clearer picture of how the system operates. Below, I shall explore some of the relevant knowledge regarding the connections of the caudate nucleus, the putamen, and the globus pallidus.

The Caudate Nucleus and Putamen

Before discussing the afferent and efferent connections of the caudate nucleus, I must mention two characteristics of the neostriatum that have received attention during the late 1970s and the 1980s. First, it has been discovered that the neostriatum, in particular the caudate nucleus, can be divided into two compartments, sometimes called the "patch" and "matrix" compartments (e.g., Gerfen, 1985). One of the first discoveries about these compartments was that they could be defined by the relative presence of markers for acetylcholine in the matrix compartment and the relative absence of these markers in the patch compartment (Graybiel, 1984; Graybiel, Baughman, & Eckenstein, 1986). Other neurochemical differences have also been found (Gerfen, 1985; Graybiel, 1984). It has also been discovered that the connections of these compartments differ (Gerfen, 1985; Graybiel et al., 1986). The major afferent and efferent projections of the patch and matrix compartments are schematically represented in Figure 1-3. The functional significance of these compartments has been discussed, though it is not well understood.

A second characteristic of the striatum is that approximately 96% of the neuronal population consists of the spiny I-type neuron. Groves

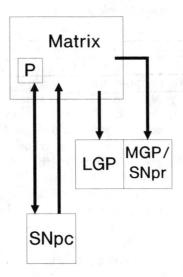

Figure 1-3. Schematic diagram of the connections of the patch (P) and matrix compartments of the striatum with the substantia nigra (SN) and the globus pallidus (GP). The patch compartment receives dopaminergic projections from pars compacta of the substantia nigra (SNpc) and projects back to pars compacta. The matrix compartment also receives dopaminergic input from pars compacta of the substantia nigra, but projects to pars reticulata of the substantia nigra (SNpr) and the medial and lateral pallidal segments (MGP and LGP, respectively).

(1983) is an excellent source for reviewing the characteristics of this striatal neuron in detail, but I will mention a few important properties here. First, spiny I neurons appear to project to targets outside the striatum and also to distribute collaterals to neighboring neurons within the striatum. These axon collaterals appear to terminate mainly within the space of the neuron's own dendritic fields (Preston, Bishop, & Kitai, 1980; Wilson & Groves, 1980). One of the main neurotransmitters of the neostriatal spiny I neuron is gamma-aminobutyric acid (GABA) (Wilson & Groves, 1980). Since GABA is thought generally to be an inhibitory neurotransmitter, these locally arborizing axon collaterals are assumed to have an inhibitory effect on neighboring cells (Groves, 1983). Thus, the firing of a spiny I cell may not only have external influences, but also may provide an inhibitory influence on neighboring neurons. The spiny II neuron is a second type of neostriatal neuron which is also suspected to project outside the striatum. Other potential neurotransmitters suggested for neostriatal efferents include substance P, angiotensin II, cholecystokinin, enkephalin, and dynorphin (Groves, 1983; Penney & Young, 1983, 1986).

Afferents of the Caudate Nucleus

There are several sources of afferents to the neostriatum (see Table 1-1); two of the main ones are the cortex and the substantia nigra. Projections from the cortex to the caudate nucleus are bilateral, though ipsilateral projections are more prominent. Projections from the cortex to the striatum are not collaterals from neurons projecting to the pyramidal motor system or the thalamus; a separate type of cell is probably involved which also has connections in local intracortical circuits. Cortico-striatal projections as a whole can be described as selective but not exclusive in terms of the relationship of specific cortical areas with specific striatal regions. For example, projections from the visual cortex to the striatum are small, while projections from other cortical areas can be quite substantial. Further, projections from

Table 1-1. Afferents and Efferents of the Basal Ganglia

Nucleus	Afferents	Efferents
Caudate nucleus	Cortex (primarily non–sensory-motor)	Globus pallidus, medial segment
	Substantia nigra, pars compacta	Globus pallidus, lateral segment
	Thalamic intralaminar nuclei	Substantia nigra, pars reticulata
		Substantia nigra, pars compacta
Putamen	Cortex (primarily sensory-motor)	Globus pallidus, medial segment
	Substantia nigra, pars compacta	Globus pallidus, lateral segment
	Thalamic intralaminar nuclei	Substantia nigra, pars reticulata
		Substantia nigra, pars compacta
Globus pallidus, medial segment	Caudate nucleus	Thalamic nuclei
	Putamen	Ventral anterior
	Nucleus accumbens	Ventral lateral
	Subthalamic nucleus	Dorsal medial
		Intralaminar
		Habenula
		Pedunculopontine nucleus
Globus pallidus, lateral segment	Caudate nucleus	Subthalamic nucleus
	Putamen	Substantia nigra
	Subthalamic nucleus	

the prefrontal cortex connect primarily with the caudate nucleus as opposed to the putamen, whereas fibers from the sensory-motor cortex project more heavily to the putamen. The premotor cortex projects to both the caudate nucleus and the putamen (Carpenter & Sutin, 1983).

At one time, it was felt that cortical projections to the caudate nucleus were organized primarily on an anterior-to-posterior basis with a particular region of the cortex projecting to that area of the striatum with which it is closest (Kemp & Powell, 1970). In other words, the prefrontal cortex projected to the head of the caudate nucleus, the parietal association cortex projected to the body of the caudate nucleus, and the temporal association cortex projected to the tail of the caudate nucleus. However, Yeterian and Van Hoesen (1978) showed that posterior areas of the cortex do indeed project to the head of the caudate nucleus, and anterior cortical areas do project to the body and tail of the caudate. In fact, their data suggested that cortical areas that are reciprocally connected project to partially overlapping areas within the caudate nucleus (see Figure 1-4[A]). Frequently, these areas of overlapping projections appear to be duplicated in multiple segments of the caudate nucleus.

The overlapping nature of projections to the striatum from reciprocally connected cortical areas has been questioned by Goldman-Rakic and Selemon (1986). These authors noted that Yeterian and Van Hoesen (1978) used separate preparations with a single labeling agent in their study and were not able, therefore, to compare projections from reciprocally connected cortical areas in a single preparation. Goldman-Rakic and Selemon's own data, in which a double labeling procedure was used, suggest that projections to the caudate nucleus from reciprocally connected cortical areas are adjacent as opposed to overlapping (see Figure 1-4[B]). Goldman-Rakic and Selemon suggested a medial to lateral organization of cortico-striatal projections in the caudate nucleus, with the posterior parietal cortex projecting dorsolaterally, the dorsolateral prefrontal cortex projecting centrally, and the orbitofrontal, superior temporal, and anterior cingulate cortices projecting ventromedially along the anterior to posterior extent of the nucleus.

The major neurotransmitter in all cortico-striatal pathways is thought to be glutamate (e.g., Penney & Young, 1986). Spencer (1976) showed that striatal cells are excited by cortical stimulation, and that this excitation can be suppressed in 90% of the striatal cells by application of a glutamate antagonist. Thus, glutamate is considered to be an excitatory neurotransmitter in cortico-striatal pathways.

Projections from the substantia nigra to the caudate nucleus are extremely important. Nigrostriatal projections come from a specific

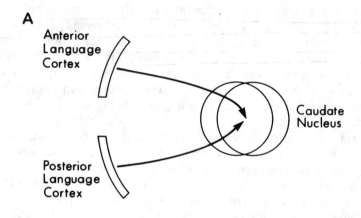

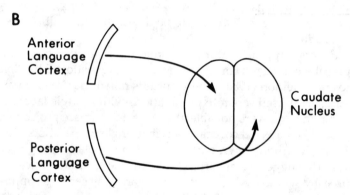

Figure 1-4. Schematic diagram of projections from reciprocally connected anterior and posterior cortex to the caudate nucleus. (A) Yeterian and Van Hoesen (1978) described projections as overlapping. (B) Goldman-Rakic and Selemon (1986) described projections as adjacent but not overlapping. From "Is the Striatum Involved in Language?" by B. Crosson, in press. In G. Vallar, C.-W. Wallesch, & S. Cappa (eds.), *Neuropsychological Disorders Associated with Subcortical Lesions,* New York: Oxford University Press. Reprinted by permission of Oxford University Press.

portion of the substantia nigra, pars compacta. These fibers provide dopamine input to both the patch and matrix compartments of the striatum (Penney & Young, 1986). Some controversy has existed regarding the influence of dopamine on striatal neurons (Cote & Crutcher, 1985). Some see it as excitatory (e.g., Kocsis, Sugimori, & Kitai, 1977), while others see it as inhibitory. However, a review of the evidence suggests that whether dopamine is excitatory or inhibitory may depend upon which neurons in the striatum and which striatal output one is investigating (for more detail, see Penney & Young, 1986). Pathology in the nigrostriatal neurons within pars compacta has been shown to be responsible for the symptoms of Parkinson's disease (Cote & Crutcher, 1985), which is most frequently treated using dopamine precursors or agonists (Bannister, 1985; Chusid, 1985).

One other source of caudate afferents should be mentioned. The intralaminar nuclei, lying deep within the internal medullary lamina of the thalamus, project to the striatum. The centre median nucleus projects to the putamen and the body of the caudate nucleus, the parafascicular nucleus projects to the putamen, and the smaller, more anterior intralaminar nuclei project to the caudate nucleus. It should be noted that the thalamic intralaminar nuclei receive afferents from the brain-stem reticular formation (Carpenter & Sutin, 1983). There is evidence that striatal spiny neurons show monosynaptic excitatory postsynaptic potentials during stimulation of the intralaminar nuclei (Kocsis et al., 1977).

Efferents of the Caudate Nucleus

Caudate efferents are shown in Table 1-1. The spiny I neuron of the striatum has been shown to project outside of the caudate nucleus and putamen (Kocsis et al., 1977; Preston et al., 1980; Somogyi & Smith, 1979; Wilson & Groves, 1980), and these projections are considered one of the main, if not the main, projection system from the caudate nucleus and putamen (e.g., Groves, 1983). As mentioned above, GABA is thought to be a major neurotransmitter in these projections. Traditionally, the main efferent target of the caudate nucleus has been considered to be the globus pallidus; however, caudate efferents reach other targets as well.

The two main targets for caudate neurons are the globus pallidus and the substantia nigra (Alexander, Delong, & Strick, 1986; Carpenter & Sutin, 1983). Yet, the story of striatal efferents is much more complex. First, striato-pallidal fibers reach both the lateral and medial segments of the globus pallidus (Carpenter & Sutin, 1983; Haines, 1987; Penney & Young, 1986). Fibers from the lateral pallidal segment project to the subthalamic nucleus, and the subthalamic nucleus, in turn, is assumed to project back to the lateral pallidum as well as to the medial pallidum (Penney & Young, 1986). Since lesions of the subthalamic nucleus are not generally felt to produce language deficits, the circuitry from the lateral pallidal segment to the subthalamic nucleus back to both pallidal segments is not of great interest in this discussion. But, fibers reaching the medial pallidal segment will be discussed in further detail below. Striato-pallidal fibers to both pallidal segments originate in the matrix compartment of the striatum (Penney & Young, 1986).

Striatofugal fibers also reach the substantia nigra, with neurons from the patch and matrix compartments reaching different targets. Fibers from the striatal matrix project to pars reticulata of the substantia nigra as well as to the globus pallidus (Gerfen, 1985; Graybiel et al., 1986; Penney & Young, 1986). Because of its projectional patterns, the pars reticulata is considered by many to be homologous with the globus pallidus (Alexander et al., 1986), that is, it projects to thalamic targets similar to those of the pallidum. Neurons within the patch compartment project to the pars compacta of the substantia nigra (Gerfen, 1985; Graybiel et al., 1986; Penney & Young, 1986), the structure that provides the dopaminergic afferents to the striatum.

To complicate the picture further, there is evidence of the presence of peptides within GABA-ergic spiny I neurons of the striatum. The peptide present may be substance P, enkephalin, neurotensin, or dynorphin. The dynorphin-containing neurons, and possibly the neurotensin-containing ones, appear to be located mainly in the patch compartment. Evidence regarding the substance P–containing neurons is more contradictory. The enkaphalin-containing neurons appear to project to the lateral globus pallidus, while the substance P–containing neurons project largely to the medial globus pallidus and the substantia nigra, pars reticulata. The dynorphin containing neurons project to the substantia nigra, pars reticulata, but the neurons containing neurotensin may project to pars compacta of the substantia nigra. The significance of these peptides is not currently known (e.g., see Penney & Young, 1986).

Afferents of the Putamen

Fibers projecting to the putamen are quite similar to those of the caudate nucleus (see Table 1-1). As noted above, cortical fibers show some preference for the caudate nucleus or the putamen based upon the area of the cortex from which they originate. Fibers from the somatosensory and motor cortices project more heavily to the putamen, causing many investigators to consider the putamen to be a motoric structure (Alexander et al., 1986; Carpenter & Sutin, 1983). Premotor fibers appear to project to both the caudate nucleus and the putamen, but fibers from the prefrontal cortex pass preferentially to the caudate nucleus. Dopaminergic innervation to the putamen comes from pars compacta of the substantia nigra. The parafascicular and centre median nuclei (thalamic intralaminar nuclei) project to the putamen (Carpenter & Sutin, 1983).

Efferents of the Putamen

The efferents of the putamen are similar to those of the caudate nucleus. The globus pallidus and pars reticulata of the substantia nigra are major targets, though the anterior portion of the putamen projects almost exclusively to the globus pallidus (Alexander et al., 1986; Carpenter & Sutin, 1983). As in the caudate nucleus, neurons from the matrix compartment are assumed to project to both pallidal segments and pars reticulata of the substantia nigra. Neurons from the patch compartment are assumed to project to the substantia nigra, pars compacta, from which the dopaminergic innervation of the striatum originates (Penney & Young, 1986).

The Globus Pallidus

As mentioned above, pars reticulata of the substantia nigra is often considered a homologous structure to the medial pallidal segment because of its similar connections (Alexander et al., 1986). There is some evidence that the globus pallidus may be involved in language (e.g., Brunner et al., 1982; Hermann et al., 1966; Svennilson et al., 1960), but there is no convincing evidence that pars reticulata of the substantia nigra plays a role in language. This being the case, the following discussion will focus on the lateral and medial pallidal segments.

Before discussing the specific connections of the globus pallidus, I must address one observation regarding the morphology of pallidal neurons. Yelnik, Percheron, and Francois (1984) studied the dendritic arborizations of Golgi-impregnated human and macaque brains. Neurons in the medial and lateral pallidal divisions were studied, and all neurons appeared to be of the same type. They had sparsely branched dendritic arborizations. These dendritic fields were disc shaped and parallel to the lateral border of the respective pallidal segment. Given this information, one could conclude that these disc-shaped dendritic fields are oriented perpendicularly to incoming striatal axons, and that they are probably traversed by a large number of striatal axons. This leaves pallidal neurons in a position to provide spatial and temporal summation of inhibitory inputs from different striatal areas. Percheron, Yelnik, and Francois (1984) further stated that this pattern suggests an integrative function for the globus pallidus.

Afferents of the Globus Pallidus

Unlike the striatum, the globus pallidus does not receive any projections from the cortex. Rather, the pallidum is a link between the striatum and other structures (see Table 1-1). Fibers from the putamen project medially into the globus pallidus and terminate in both the lateral and medial pallidal segments. Fibers from the caudate nucleus pass inferiorly and/or medially through the internal capsule to reach the pallidum. With the exception of the anterior putamen, both the putamen and the caudate nucleus also project to pars reticulata of the substantia nigra, considered to be a homologue of the globus pallidus (Alexander et al., 1986; Carpenter & Sutin, 1983). As mentioned above, the spiny I neuron appears to be the main source of the projections, and the primary neurotransmitter to both pallidal segments appears to be GABA (Carpenter & Sutin, 1983; Groves, 1983; Penney & Young, 1986). However, neuropeptides are also present in these neurons, with enkephalin-containing fibers projecting mainly to the lateral pallidum and the substance P–containing fibers projecting mainly to the medial pallidum (Penney & Young, 1986). Striato-pallidal fibers originate from the matrix compartment of the striatum (Graybiel et al., 1986; Penney & Young, 1986).

The other major source of input to the globus pallidus is the subthalamic nucleus. These fibers are distributed to both pallidal segments, though more heavily to the medial segment. Fibers from the subthalamic nucleus also reach pars reticulata of the substantia nigra, further indicating the homologous nature of pars reticulata to the medial pallidal segment (Carpenter & Sutin, 1983; Penney & Young, 1986).

Efferents of the Globus Pallidus

Projections from the medial pallidal segment (see Table 1-1) reach the thalamus, habenula, and the pedunculopontine nucleus. Fibers from the lateral pallidal segment project to the subthalamic nucleus and the substantia nigra. As noted above, fibers of the subthalamic nucleus project back to the medial and lateral pallidal segments (Carpenter & Sutin, 1983; Penney & Young, 1986). In the context of motor circuits, Penney and Young (1986) have speculated that this pallido-subtha-lamo-pallidal loop serves to suppress unwanted movements.

Pallido-thalamic projections appear to have GABA as their primary neurotransmitter and are assumed to have an inhibitory effect on thalamic targets (Penney & Young, 1986). Pallido-thalamic fibers from the medial pallidal segment either traverse the internal capsule and turn medially around the subthalamic nucleus or take a more ventral route inferior to the internal capsule and superior to the optic tract, then turn superiorly between the fornix and the subthalamic nucleus. These two efferent fiber systems from the pallidum merge in Forel's field H and ultimately enter the thalamic fasciculus (Carpenter

& Sutin, 1983). The thalamic targets for these pallidal efferents include the ventral anterior nucleus, the ventral lateral nucleus, the dorsal medial nucleus, and the centre median nucleus (one of the intralaminar nuclei) (Alexander et al., 1986; Carpenter & Sutin, 1983). Although cerebellar fibers also reach the ventral lateral nucleus, their projections are considered to be largely nonoverlapping with pallido-thalamic fibers in their terminal fields (Jones, 1985). Pallidal projections to the ventral anterior and ventral lateral thalamic nuclei are topographically organized with respect to their site of origin. For example, anterior parts of the medial pallidal segment project primarily to the principal part of the ventral anterior nucleus, and more posterior portions of the medial pallidal segment project to pars oralis of the ventral lateral nucleus (Carpenter & Sutin, 1983). This separation of fibers was emphasized by Alexander et al. (1986) as important in distinguishing different cortical-subcortical-cortical circuits and will be discussed further toward the end of this chapter.

As noted above, the medial pallidal nucleus also projects to the habenula, an epithalamic structure considered to be a part of the limbic system. The pedunculopontine nucleus, which receives projections from the medial pallidal segment, projects to pars compacta and receives projections from pars reticulata of the substantia nigra as well as receiving fibers from the cortex. The functions related to these connections of the pedunculopontine nucleus are not well understood. There appears to be some controversy regarding which segment of the substantia nigra projections from the lateral pallidum reach. As noted above, the lateral globus pallidus also projects to the subthalamic nucleus (Carpenter & Sutin, 1983).

Potential Thalamic Nuclei Involved in Language

The thalamus (see Figure 1-5) is an ovoidal gray mass deep within the cerebral hemispheres. Laterally, it is separated from the lenticular nucleus by the posterior limb of the internal capsule. The anterior-most tip of the thalamus borders on the posterior-most tip of the frontal horn of the lateral ventricle, in close proximity to the columns of the fornix anterior and medial to the thalamus. Anterior and somewhat lateral to the thalamus is the head of the caudate nucleus. The posterior-most tip of the thalamus borders on the trigone of the lateral ventricle, and portions of the hippocampal formation lie on the posterior medial margin of the thalamus. The medial portions of the right and left thalamus are separated from each other by the third ve.itricle, except where joined by the massa intermedia. The body of the lateral ventricle and some white matter tracts lie superior to the thalamus, and the hypothalamus and other white matter tracts lie inferior to the thalamus (Carpenter & Sutin, 1983).

The thalamus is divided into three nuclear groups by a band of fibers called the internal medullary lamina of the thalamus (see Figure 1-5). The three nuclear groups are known as the anterior, the medial, and the lateral nuclear groups. The anterior nuclear group consists of a large principal nucleus (anterior ventral) and accessory nuclei (anterior dorsal and anterior medial nuclei). Collectively, this nuclear group is sometimes referred to as the anterior nucleus. The medial thalamus contains the large medial or dorsal medial nucleus; some

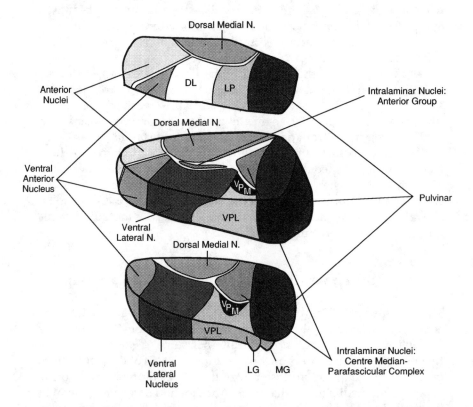

Figure 1-5. Sketch of the thalamus. (Full names of nuclei possibly involved in language are used, but abbreviations for other nuclei are used. DL = dorsal lateral; LG = lateral geniculate body; LP = lateral posterior; MG = medial geniculate; VPL = ventral posterior lateral; VPM = ventral posterior medial. Drawings are composed to indicate relationships between structures but are not meant to be anatomically precise.)

midline nuclei also border on the third ventricle and in the massa intermedia. The greatest number of subdivisions lie in the highly differentiated lateral nuclear group, which can be divided into a ventral tier of nuclei, the dorsal nuclei, and the large posterior pulvinar. A group of nuclei within the internal medullary lamina of the thalamus are known as the intralaminar nuclei. The intralaminar nuclei include the centre median and parafascicular nuclei as well as smaller, more anterior nuclei.

The ventral lateral nucleus has been one of the most frequently mentioned nuclei with respect to language. Since this thalamic structure was the target of surgical lesions for Parkinson's disease or related disorders, we possess data about language dysfunction after surgically created lesions (e.g., Allen et al., 1966; Bell, 1968; Selby, 1967) or electrical stimulation of the nucleus as a result of implantation of electrodes for these operations (e.g., Ojemann, 1975, 1977; Ojemann, Blick, & Ward, 1971; Ojemann & Ward, 1971). The ventral lateral thalamus also is occasionally mentioned in studies of aphasia after vascular lesion of the thalamus (e.g., Gorelick et al., 1984). The other frequently mentioned nucleus is the pulvinar. The functions of this thalamic nucleus have been studied by means of electrical stimulation during operative procedures (e.g., Ojemann, 1977; Ojemann et al., 1968), and though less frequently than the ventral lateral thalamus, there is some negative data after surgical ablation (e.g., Brown, 1975, 1979). A few cases of retrograde degeneration of the pulvinar after cortical aphasias are known (e.g., Van Buren, 1975; Van Buren & Borke, 1969), and the dominant pulvinar sometimes has been implicated in aphasia after vascular lesion (e.g., Ciemans, 1970; Crosson et al., 1986; Puel et al., 1989).

Other nuclei are mentioned less commonly. The ventral anterior nucleus has been mentioned in stimulation work regarding language (Schaltenbrand, 1965, 1975), in some studies of aphasia after vascular lesion (Gorelick et al., 1984; Graff-Radford et al., 1985) and in some theoretical works (Crosson, 1985; Crosson & Hughes, 1987; Crosson, Novack, & Trenerry, 1988; Wallesch & Papagno, 1988). The anterior nucleus is mentioned in some studies of vascular lesion (Graff-Radford et al., 1985) and in stimulation research (Schaltenbrand, 1965, 1975). The dorsal medial nucleus has been mentioned mainly in a theoretical context (e.g., Brown, 1975, 1979), but dorsal medial lesions rarely produce significant aphasia (e.g., Choi, Sudarsky, Schachter, Biber, & Burke, 1983; Cramon, Hebel, & Schuri, 1985; McEntee, Biber, Perl, & Benson, 1976; Speedie & Heilman, 1983). The intralaminar nuclei have been mentioned in a few vascular lesion studies (e.g., Mori, Yamadori,

& Mitani, 1986), and have been assigned a more indirect role in theoretical works (e.g., Crosson, 1985). The following discussion of anatomy and pathways of thalamic nuclei will be limited to those nuclei for which there has been at least some evidence of language involvement.

The Ventral Lateral Nucleus

The ventral lateral nucleus (see Figure 1-5) lies in the middle of the ventral tier of the lateral nuclear group. At its anterior extent, it is bordered by the ventral anterior nucleus. According to Jones (1985), the ventral anterior nucleus and the ventral lateral nucleus inter-digitate at their interface. In his view, one difference between the ventral anterior and the ventral lateral nuclei at this point is that the ventral lateral nucleus receives fibers from the cerebellum but the ventral anterior nucleus does not. Jones also maintains that the ventral lateral nucleus receives pallidal fibers but the ventral anterior does not, though this view is not universally accepted. At its posterior extent, the ventral lateral nucleus is adjacent to the ventral posterior lateral and ventral posterior medial nuclei. The ventral lateral nucleus can be divided into three main parts: pars oralis, pars caudalis, and pars medialis. "Area X" on the anterior medial border of the ventral lateral nucleus is usually considered a part of the nucleus (Carpenter & Sutin, 1983).

Afferents of the Ventral Lateral Nucleus

The connections of the ventral lateral nucleus are outlined in Table 1-2. There have been some discrepancies regarding input to the ventral lateral thalamus, primarily regarding the overlap versus the lack of overlap between cerebellar, pallidal, and nigral input. For example, Carpenter and Sutin (1983) state that all divisions of the ventral lateral nucleus have been described as receiving contralateral cerebellar input, with some suggestion that cerebellar input to pars oralis may be sparse. Based partly on work by Asanuma, Thach, and Jones (1983a, 1983b, 1983c), Jones (1985) has maintained that fibers from the cerebellum project only to pars caudalis and to a portion of area X.

Carpenter and Sutin (1983) wrote that fibers from the medial pallidal segment project to pars oralis and the lateral portion of pars medialis. The most prolific connections to pars oralis originate in the posterior part of the medial pallidal segment. Pars medialis of the ventral lateral nucleus receives input from pars reticulata of the substantia nigra, considered to be a homologue of the globus pallidus

Table 1-2. Afferents and Efferents of Thalamic Nuclei[a] That Are Candidates for Involvement in Language

Nucleus	Afferents	Efferents
Ventral lateral	Globus pallidus, medial segment Substantia nigra, pars reticulata Cerebellum Motor cortex Premotor cortex Spinothalamic tract Vestibular nucleus	Motor cortex Premotor Cortex Supplementary motor area
Pulvinar	Occipital cortex Primary visual cortex Superior temporal lobe Inferior parietal lobe Frontal cortex Superior colliculus Pretectal area	Occipital cortex Primary visual cortex Superior temporal lobe Inferior parietal lobe Frontal cortex
Ventral anterior	Globus pallidus, medial segment Substantia nigra, pars reticulata Thalamic intralaminar nuclei Premotor cortex Frontal cortex Parietal cortex	Premotor cortex Frontal cortex Parietal cortex Thalamic intralaminar nuclei Dorsal medial thalamus
Dorsal medial	Amygdala Olfactory tubercle Substantia innominata Globus pallidus, medial segment Substantia nigra, pars reticulata Thalamic intralaminar nuclei Ventral anterior thalamus Prefrontal cortex	Prefrontal cortex (broad distribution)
Anterior nuclei	Mammillary bodies Parahippocampal gyrus Cingulate gyrus Retrosplenial cortex	Retrosplenial cortex Cingulate gyrus Parahippocampal gyrus
Intralaminar nuclei	Brainstem reticular formation Globus pallidus, medial segment	Putamen Caudate nucleus Ventral anterior thalamus

(cont.)

Table 1-2 *(cont.)*

Nucleus	Afferents	Efferents
Intralaminar nuclei *(cont.)*	Prerolandic cortex Perirolandic cortex Cerebellum Spino-thalamic tract Pretectal area	Cortex (broad distribution)

ªSince the connections of different subdivisions of thalamic nuclei are relevant to function, and since connections of some nuclei are controversial, this table can be used only as a rough guide. Readers should refer to the text and/or the cited literature for more detail.

(Alexander et al., 1986). But Jones (1985) argues that projections from the globus pallidus terminate exclusively in pars oralis and projections from pars reticulata of the substantia nigra terminate exclusively in pars medialis. Thus, Jones (1985) sees cerebello-thalamic, pallido-thalamic, and nigro-thalamic projection fields as maintaining distinct boundaries within the ventral lateral nucleus, while Carpenter and Sutin (1983) allow for some overlap of these projection systems.

Cortical projections from the motor and premotor cortex (areas 4 and 6, respectively) reach the ventral lateral nucleus. Projections from the motor cortex reach the three major divisions, though projections from the motor cortex to pars caudalis are not as prolific as those from the premotor cortex. The premotor cortex also projects to area X (Carpenter & Sutin, 1983). Jones (1985) also mentions inputs to pars caudalis of the ventral lateral nucleus from the spino-thalamic tract and the vestibular nucleus.

Efferents of the Ventral Lateral Nucleus

As with many thalamic nuclei, thalamo-cortical connections are reciprocal with cortico-thalamic connections. Thus, the most prominent target of ventral lateral efferents is the motor cortex. These projections are topographically arranged. There is some evidence that ventral lateral projections make monosynaptic contact with corticospinal tract neurons and exert a strong influence on motor cortex output. Efferents from the ventral lateral nucleus may also reach the premotor cortex (Carpenter & Sutin, 1983). Again, there is some controversy regarding the termination of fibers from various parts of the ventral lateral nucleus in the cortex, in particular regarding whether the portion receiving cerebellar input (pars caudalis) and the portions receiving pallidal and nigral inputs (pars oralis and pars medialis, respectively) project to separate or overlapping cortical areas. Jones (1985) states that pars caudalis projects primarily to the motor cortex (area 4), while pars oralis projects to the premotor cortex (area 6). Thus, according to Jones, the cerebellar and pallidal systems maintain separate projection fields even at the level of the second order thalamo-cortical fibers. The premotor projections of pars oralis are reputed by Jones to include the supplementary motor area in the medial cortex. Jones speculates based on this anatomy that the globus pallidus (along with the supplementary motor area) plays a role in planning movement stratagems.

The Pulvinar

The pulvinar (see Figure 1-5) is the large nuclear mass forming most of the posterior part of the thalamus. Superiorly, the anterior portion of the pulvinar borders on the lateral posterior nucleus, and the remaining portions of the anterior border of the pulvinar are with the ventral posterior lateral and ventral posterior medial nuclei. The anterior portion of the medial border of the pulvinar is on the posterior portion of the internal medullary lamina. The medial and lateral geniculate nuclei are located on the anterior inferior margin of the pulvinar. The pulvinar is divided into four segments: pars oralis, pars inferior, pars medialis, and pars lateralis. The names are for the most part descriptive of location, with pars oralis lying in the anterior segment of the nucleus. Many neuroanatomists include the lateral posterior nucleus as a closely related structure to the pulvinar, referring to the pulvinar-lateral posterior complex (Jones, 1985).

Afferents of the Pulvinar

The pulvinar has prolific connections with numerous cortical areas. Pars inferior and portions of pars lateralis receive input from the occipital cortex, including the primary visual reception area (Carpenter & Sutin, 1983; Jones, 1985). Both the superior temporal lobe and the inferior parietal lobe project to both pars lateralis and pars medialis of the pulvinar. There is some evidence that more anterior portions of the superior temporal lobe project to pars medialis while more posterior portions of the superior temporal lobe project to pars lateralis (Trojanowski & Jacobson, 1975). In monkeys, portions of the inferior parietal lobule project to pars medialis, pars lateralis, and pars oralis, and these parietal projections are thought to originate from distinct cortical areas (Asanuma, Andersen, & Cowan, 1985). Projections from the medial pulvinar to the frontal cortex (lateral prefrontal and lateral orbital) (Asanuma et al., 1985; Bos & Benevento, 1975; Trojanowski & Jacobson, 1974) are assumed to be reciprocated (Carpenter & Sutin, 1983). Noncortical input to the pulvinar includes the superior colliculus, the pretectal area (which contains visually related nuclei), and possibly the optic tract (Jones, 1985).

Efferents of the Pulvinar

The arrangement of efferent fibers of the pulvinar are essentially reciprocal to the cortical inputs noted above. Thus, pars medialis, pars lateralis, and pars oralis each project to different portions of the inferior parietal lobe (Asanuma et al., 1985; Jones, 1985). Pars oralis and pars lateralis also project to different portions of the superior parietal lobe (Jones, 1985). Pars medialis projects to the anterior portion of the superior temporal gyrus, while pars lateralis is the main projection to the posterior temporal gyrus (Trojanowski & Jacobson, 1975). The lateral and inferior pulvinar project to the occipital cortex, including the primary visual cortex (Jones, 1985). As noted above, there is evidence for projections from the medial pulvinar to the dorsal lateral prefrontal cortex and to the lateral orbital cortex (Asanuma et al., 1985; Bos & Benevento, 1975; Trojanowski & Jacobson, 1974). Although Jones (1985) is skeptical regarding such projections, Asanuma and colleagues (1985) present convincing data that neurons of pars medialis projecting to the dorsal lateral prefrontal cortex are comingled with neurons projecting to the inferior parietal lobule, though these are not the same neurons.

The Ventral Anterior Nucleus

The ventral anterior nucleus lies at the extreme anterior portion of the ventral tier of the lateral nuclear group. Medial to the ventral anterior nucleus and separated from it by the internal medullary lamina is the anterior nuclear group. Posteriorly, the nucleus becomes restricted to the more medial portion of the ventral tier. In general, the posterior border of the nucleus is formed by pars oralis of the ventral lateral nucleus. This nucleus has two divisions: pars magnocellularis, occupying the posteromedial portion of the nucleus, and pars principalis, occupying the anterolateral portion (Carpenter & Sutin, 1983; Jones, 1985). Apparently, the connections of the ventral anterior nucleus are not entirely certain; one problem is difficulty delimiting the nucleus in some species (Jones, 1985).

Afferents of the Ventral Anterior Nucleus

One must keep the above caveat in mind when considering the afferents of the ventral anterior nucleus. According to Carpenter and Sutin (1983), pars principalis of the ventral anterior nucleus receives afferents from the medial segment of the globus pallidus, primarily the anterior portion of the medial pallidal segment. These fibers traverse the internal capsule or the area just beneath the internal capsule and enter the ventral anterior nucleus from the thalamic fasciculus. Pars magnocellularis, in contrast, receives fibers from pars reticulata of the substantia nigra. These fibers progress medially and anteriorly from the substantia nigra, then turn superiorly paralleling the mammillothalamic tract. Some neuroanatomists report cerebellar projections to pars principalis, but Jones (1985) maintains that these cerebellar fibers reach anterior segments of the ventral lateral nucleus which interdigitate with the ventral anterior nucleus. Indeed, Jones appears to believe that the nigral and pallidal projections described above may also belong to the ventral lateral nucleus. For the purposes of this book, I shall assume that fibers from the anterior portion of the medial pallidal segment and from pars reticulata of the substantia nigra do reach the ventral anterior nucleus; this assumption has been made in other important works (e.g., Alexander et al., 1986).

There is evidence that the intralaminar nuclei, particularly the centre median nucleus, project to the ventral anterior nucleus (Nauta & Whitlock, 1954), but this evidence is difficult to evaluate because of the retrograde degeneration technique used and the numerous fibers passing through the ventral anterior nucleus, possibly including some thalamo-cortical fibers from the intralaminar nuclei (Jones, 1985). There is also evidence that the ventral anterior nucleus modulates the cortical effects of activity in the intralaminar nuclei (Carpenter & Sutin, 1983), but this evidence is difficult to evaluate for the same reasons.

Concerning cortical afferents to the ventral anterior nucleus, Jones (1985) emphasized connections of the anterior parietal lobe with the ventral anterior nucleus. But others consider pars principalis to receive input from the premotor cortex, and pars magnocellularis to receive fibers from the cortex just anterior to the premotor cortex (Carpenter & Sutin, 1983). In a study primarily concerned with the connections of pars medialis of the pulvinar, Asanuma et al. (1985) found the inferior parietal cortex to project to pars magnocellularis of the ventral anterior nucleus. The motor cortex does not project to the ventral anterior nucleus (Carpenter & Sutin, 1983). Again, for the purposes of this work, I shall assume the frontal connections to be established in keeping with other works (Alexander et al., 1986).

Efferents of the Ventral Anterior Nucleus

Traditionally, the ventral anterior is considered to project to frontal cortex anterior to the motor cortex; Carpenter and Sutin (1983) interpreted data existing as of 1983 to indicate that frontal projections of the ventral anterior nucleus were widespread. Again, Jones (1985) is skeptical regarding this point; however, Asanuma et al. (1985) did indicate some projections to the dorsal lateral prefrontal cortex from the magnocellular division of the ventral anterior nucleus. If one were to assume reciprocity, this would support the assumption of projections from the frontal cortex to the ventral anterior nucleus. Inferior parietal connections are also reciprocal (Asanuma et al., 1985; Jones, 1985).

There is some evidence of intrathalamic projections from the ventral anterior nucleus. Carpenter and Sutin (1983) consider two such pathways to be established. The first is a projection from pars magnocellulis of the ventral anterior nucleus to pars principalis of the ventral anterior nucleus. This projection is not reciprocated by pars principalis. The second pathway is projections from portions of pars principalis of the ventral anterior nucleus to the intralaminar nuclei and the dorsal medial nucleus.

The Dorsal Medial Nucleus

The dorsal medial thalamus (see Figure 1-5) occupies most of the space medial to the internal medullary lamina in the thalamus. It can be divided into three divisions. Pars magnocellularis lies in the anterior superior medial portion of the nucleus. Pars parvicellularlis, the largest division, occupying 50% or more of the dorsal medial nucleus, lies posteriorly, superiorly, and laterally. Pars paralaminaris, the smallest division of the dorsal medial nucleus, lies adjacent to the internal medullary lamina (Carpenter & Sutin, 1983).

Afferents of the Dorsal Medial Nucleus

Pars magnocellularis of the dorsal medial nucleus receives heavy inputs from the olfactory and limbic systems. These inputs include the amygdala, the pyriform cortex, and the olfactory tubercle. This division also receives input from the temporal neocortex and the substantia innominata (Carpenter & Sutin, 1983). Another input to pars magnocellularis emphasized by Alexander and colleagues (1986) is from the anterior lateral portion of the internal pallidal segment. Pars paralaminaris receives fibers from pars reticulata of the substantia nigra. The dorsal medial nucleus is thought to receive input from the centre median and other thalamic intralaminar nuclei and from members of the lateral thalamic nuclei (Carpenter & Sutin, 1983).

The most prolific source of cortical input to the dorsal medial nucleus is the prefrontal cortex. Pars magnocellularis receives fibers from the posterior orbitofrontal cortex. Pars parvicellularis appears to receive input from all divisions of the frontal cortex (orbital, dorsal lateral, mesial) anterior to the premotor cortex. Pars paralaminaris has input from the frontal eye field (area 8) and possibly from the premotor cortex (Carpenter & Sutin, 1983).

Efferents of the Dorsal Medial Nucleus

The prolific inputs from the prefrontal cortex to the dorsal medial nucleus are reciprocated. Indeed, some investigators have suggested that the prefrontal cortical regions should be defined as the cortical projection fields of the dorsal medial thalamus (e.g., Fuster, 1980; Leonard, 1969; Rose & Woolsey, 1948). But Reep (1984) has objected to such a characterization of the prefrontal cortex because it tends to obscure the "structural and functional heterogeneity present in these cortical areas" (p. 12). At any rate, the connections of pars magnocellularis with the posterior orbitofrontal cortex; the connections of pars parvicellularis with the orbital, dorsal lateral, and mesial divisions of the prefrontal cortex; and the connections of pars paralaminaris with the frontal eye fields and possibly the premotor cortex are all thought to be bidirectional.

The Anterior Nuclei

The anterior thalamic nuclei lie lateral and anterior to the dorsal medial nucleus and medial to the ventral anterior nucleus. The anterior nuclei are separated from the ventral anterior and dorsal medial nuclei by the internal medullary lamina. As mentioned above, the anterior ventral nucleus is the largest of the anterior nuclei. Two smaller nuclei, the anterior dorsal and the anterior medial nuclei, are also a part of this nuclear complex (Carpenter & Sutin, 1983).

Afferents of the Anterior Nuclei

There are two very prominent projections into the anterior nuclei: the mammillothalamic tract and the fornix. The latter is the major fiber bundle from the hippocampal formation and projects to both the anterior nuclei and the mammillary bodies which, in turn, project back to the anterior nuclei. Fibers from the medial mammillary nucleus project to the ipsilateral anterior ventral and anterior medial nuclei, but the lateral mammillary nucleus projects bilaterally to the anterior dorsal nucleus but not to other subdivisions of the anterior nuclei. The pathway of the mammillothalamic tract is of some interest: as it courses superiorly toward the anterior nuclei, it passes through the medial ventral anterior nucleus (Carpenter & Sutin, 1983; Jones, 1985).

Fibers of the fornix project bilaterally to the anterior ventral and anterior medial nuclei. Later studies indicate that these projections originate from the more mesial portions of the parahippocampal gyrus (subiculum, presubiculum, parasubiculum) as opposed to originating from the hippocampus proper (i.e., the portion of the hippocampal formation between the subiculum and dentate gyrus) (Jones, 1985). One should note that the entorhinal cortex projects to both the hippocampus proper and to the subiculum (Carpenter & Sutin, 1983). Other sources of cortical input to the anterior nuclei include the anterior cingulate area, other portions of the cingulate gyrus, and the superior and inferior retrosplenial cortex (Jones, 1985).

Efferents of the Anterior Nuclei

The cortical projections of the anterior nuclei largely reflect the heavy relationship to the limbic system, as do the cortico-thalamic projections. A principal target of the anterior ventral nucleus is the superior retrosplenial cortex, but there are also projections to the inferior retrosplenial cortex, the anterior cingulate area, other parts of the cingulate gyrus, and the presubiculum. A major target of the anterior medial nucleus is the inferior retrosplenial cortex, but there are also projections to anterior cingulate area, other parts of the cingulate gyrus, the superior retrosplenial area, the presubiculum, and the parasubiculum. The major projection of the anterior dorsal nucleus appears to be to the inferior retrosplenial cortex, but this nucleus also projects to the presubiculum. Thus, there is a great deal of overlap between the cortical projections of the three anterior nuclei (Jones, 1985). Projections from the anterior nuclei to the cingulate cortex are thought primarily to traverse the anterior limb of the internal capsule (Carpenter & Sutin, 1983), though there are probably other routes (Jones, 1985). There has been some conjecture that projections from anterior nuclei to the cingulate and retrosplenial cortices may be, at least in part, cholinergic, but Jones (1985) concludes that further study on the matter is needed. The habenula and mammillary bodies may be subcortical projection areas for the anterior nuclei (Carpenter & Sutin, 1983).

The Intralaminar Nuclei

The intralaminar nuclei are a group of related nuclei that lie more or less within the internal medullary lamina. The intralaminar nuclei can be divided into two groups: one that lies more anteriorly and superiorly and the other that lies more posteriorly and inferiorly with respect to the other. The more anterior group includes the paracentral, central lateral, and central medial nuclei (Carpenter & Sutin, 1983). The rhomboid nucleus is sometimes included in this group (Jones, 1985). The more posterior and inferior group includes the centre median and the parafascicular nuclei.

Afferents of the Intralaminar Nuclei

The intralaminar nuclei receive both cortical and subcortical afferents. One important source of subcortical afferents is the brain-stem reticular formation. These fibers originate in the reticular formation of the medulla, pons, and midbrain, and terminate in the centre median–parafascicular complex as well as in the paracentral and central lateral nuclei. These fibers are thought to be primarily unilateral and may be responsible for the role of the intralaminar nuclei in arousal (Carpenter & Sutin, 1983; Jones, 1985). The centre median nucleus receives heavy input from the medial pallidal segment; these projections may be collaterals of input to the ventral lateral nucleus (Jones, 1985). If so, the projections probably rely on GABA as a neurotransmitter. The centre median nucleus may also receive fibers from pars reticulata of the substantia nigra, the superior colliculus, and the vestibular nuclei (Carpenter & Sutin, 1983). Spinothalamic fibers reach the central lateral and other nuclei in the more anterior intralaminar nuclei. The pretectal region may also contribute afferents to the intralaminar nuclei. The central lateral nucleus and adjacent portions of the parafascicular nucleus are targets of cerebellar afferents (Jones, 1985).

The cerebral cortex sends fibers to the intralaminar nuclei; some of these may be branches of axons which also terminate in the striatum (Jones, 1985). These data would suggest glutamate as a candidate for the neurotransmitter in these connections. Most of the cortical afferents originate from the prerolandic or perirolandic cortex. The posterior prefrontal cortex and mesial limbic cortex target the paracentral and central medial nuclei; the premotor area projects to the central lateral and parafascicular nuclei; and the motor cortex targets the centre median nucleus and/or the adjacent parts of the central lateral nucleus. The somatosensory cortex and anterior parietal lobe send fibers to the posterior part of the central lateral nucleus. There are probably negligible or no projections to the intralaminar nuclei from the lateral temporal or occipital cortices (Carpenter & Sutin, 1983; Jones, 1985).

Efferents of the Intralaminar Nuclei

The major projection of the intralaminar nuclei is to the striatum. The projections are relatively widespread, though some nuclei project preferentially to one area of the striatum more than to other areas. Older retrograde degeneration studies indicated that the anterior and posterior parts of the centre median nucleus project to the anterior and posterior parts of the putamen, respectively. Anterior portions of the head of the caudate nucleus receive more projections from the central medial nucleus, and the central lateral and paracentral nuclei project to the posterior parts of the caudate head (Jones, 1985).

Carpenter and Sutin (1983) mention the ventral anterior thalamus as receiving fibers from the intralaminar nuclei. Jones (1985) discussed evidence of such connections in the context of the cortical "recruiting response" which can be elicited by stimulation of the intralaminar nuclei, and at a shorter latency from the ventral anterior nucleus. Small lesions in the ventral anterior nucleus can abolish the recruiting response to intralaminar stimulation. Jones appears to favor the hypothesis that thalamo-cortical fibers from the intralaminar nuclei pass through the ventral anterior nucleus without synapsing and are responsible for the stimulation and ablation effects on the recruiting response noted from the ventral anterior nucleus. Jones states that there is no direct evidence for a projection from the intralaminar nuclei to the ventral anterior nucleus. The Golgi impregnation study of Scheibel and Scheibel (1966) was suggestive of terminals from the ipsilateral and contralateral intralaminar nuclei, though later studies have apparently not confirmed this fact (Jones, 1985).

Although the major projection of the intralaminar nuclei is to the striatum, there are less prolific but more diffuse projections to the cerebral cortex. These fibers seem most concentrated in the medial and dorsolateral frontal cortex, but there appear to be a few fibers to almost every cortical area (Jones, 1985). The sparse and diffuse nature of the projections led Carpenter and Sutin (1983) to conclude that the heavier projections to the intralaminar nuclei from the more anterior cortex were not reciprocated.

Cortico-Subcortical Loops Potentially Involved in Language

Recent theory regarding neural substrates of behavior and cognition have turned decidedly toward the consideration of complex neural systems. Although Luria's works (e.g., 1973, 1980) stand as exceptional examples of a "functional systems" approach to neuropsychology, his emphasis was mainly on the interaction of cortical components in the generation of cognition. More recently, Alexander et al. (1986) have emphasized cortico-striato-pallido-thalamo-cortical loops that may play roles in movement, visual-motor behavior, emotion, and cognition. As far back as 1942, Bucy conjectured the importance of such a loop in movement disorders. Paillard (1982) discussed a loop involved in praxis. More recent theoretical treatises regarding the importance of the cortico-striato-pallido-thalamo-cortical loop in movement have been accomplished by Penney and Young (1983, 1986). These loops have also been implicated in psychiatric disturbance (Early, Posner, Reiman, & Raichle, 1989a, 1989b; Swerdlow & Koob, 1987). The cortico-striato-pallido-thalamo-cortical loops have also been regarded by some investigators and theoreticians as important in language (e.g., Brunner et al., 1982; Buckingham & Hollien, 1978; Crosson, 1985; Crosson & Hughes, 1987; Crosson et al., 1988; Wallesch & Papagno, 1988).

Actually, the work of Penney and Young (1983, 1986) mentioned multiple cortico-subcortical loops as relevant to movement. Among these loops are a cortico-striato-pallido-thalamo-cortical loop, a cortico-thalamo-cortical loop, a striato-pallido-nigro-striatal loop, and a pallido-subthalamo-pallidal "loop." The former two concepts are relevant for language. Discussion of the possible function of these loops in language will be reserved for the later chapter on theory. The discussion that follows will focus on the neuroanatomy of these loops, and to a lesser extent, on the neurochemistry of the loops.

Cortico-Thalamo-Cortical Loops

The idea of cortico-thalamo-cortical loops has been derived from the fact that many cortico-thalamic connections are reciprocated by thalamo-cortical projections (e.g., see Carpenter & Sutin, 1983, or Jones, 1985). To Penney and Young (1983), the cortico-thalamo-cortical loop serves a specific purpose. These authors have noted that cells in the ventral lateral nucleus that project to the cortex receive collaterals from corticospinal tract neurons, which are responsible for movement. They further cite evidence that the cortico-thalamic neurotransmitter is glutamate, which is known to be an excitatory transmitter. The thalamo-cortical neurotransmitter is not known in this case, but it is thought to be excitatory. According to Penney and Young's (1983) model, the function of the cortico-thalamo-cortical circuit is a positive feedback loop. That is, the corticofugal fibers excite thalamic neurons, which in turn reexcite the same cortical neurons, which in turn continue to excite the thalamic neurons. The result is to maintain the activity of both cells once one cell becomes active.

This concept of maintenance of behavior may be relevant to language and the tonic activity of the language cortex. Yet, there may be another aspect to cortico-thalamo-cortical loops relevant to language. Two of the thalamic nuclei sometimes implicated in language, the ventral anterior nucleus and the pulvinar, have projections not only to posterior areas associated with language, but also to anterior areas that may play a role in language (Asanuma et al., 1985). It should be noted that the anterior projections may be less prolific in these cases. The reader will recall that reciprocally connected cortical regions project to overlapping and/or adjacent areas of the striatum (Goldman-Rakic & Selemon, 1986; Yeterian & Van Hoesen, 1978). Although this pattern has not been noted in the thalamus, the above mentioned data cause one to wonder if this type of principle may not apply to certain thalamic nuclei as well. More importantly, these anatomic data raise the possibility that cortico-thalamo-cortical transmission may occur in an anterior cortex-to-thalamus-to-posterior cortex or in a posterior cortex-to-thalamus-to-anterior cortex fashion, though this hypothesis must be considered conjectural.

Cortico-Striato-Pallido-Thalamo-Cortical Loops

As noted above, cortico-striato-pallido-thalamo-cortical loops have received much attention lately regarding movement, cognition, and psychopathology. They are specifically mentioned in works discussing subcortical language functions. These loops have been most clearly outlined by Alexander et al. (1986). These reviewers noted five cortico-striato-pallido-thalamo-cortical loops: a motor loop, an oculo-motor loop, a dorsolateral prefrontal loop, a lateral orbitofrontal loop, and an anterior cingulate loop. However, they stated that other loops may well be discovered in the future. The point was also made that these circuits maintain their anatomical integrity at all levels without a large degree of overlap between them. For example, the lateral dorsomedial portion of the internal pallidal segment and the anterior lateral portion of substantia nigra, pars reticulata, are involved in the dorsolateral prefrontal loop while the ventral lateral portion of the

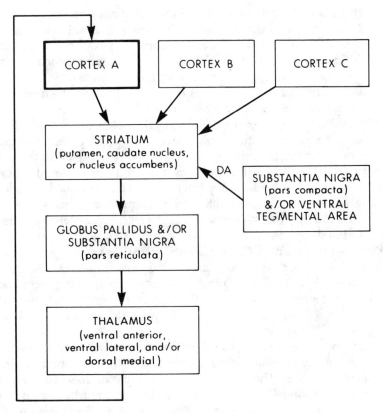

Figure 1-6. Basic structure of cortico-striato-pallido-thalamo-cortical loops. Cortex A represents the prerolandic portion of the cortex specific to a particular loop, while Cortex B and Cortex C represent postrolandic areas also projecting into the loop. Note that the loop is only partially closed since only the prerolandic cortical area receives thalamic projections.

internal pallidal segment and the posterior lateral portion of pars reticulata of the substantia nigra are involved in the motor circuit.

The basic structure of these loops is indicated in Figure 1-6. Multiple areas of the cerebral cortex project into the striatal component of the loop. The cortical components projecting into the striatal part of the circuit always include a prerolandic area to which the loop eventually projects back. The striatal component then projects to two structures: a specific portion of the medial segment of the globus pallidus and a specific part of pars reticulata of the substantia nigra. The pallidal and nigral components in turn project into one or two thalamic areas. The loop is completed when the thalamic component(s) projects back to the prerolandic region that originally projected into the striatal component of the same loop. Reflecting on the above review of anatomy, it should be noted that the cortico-striatal, striato-pallidal, and pallido-thalamic portions of these loops are unidirectional, but the thalamo-cortical connections are usually reciprocated.

A great deal of speculation has occurred regarding the function of these loops, but one ostensible function of these circuits would be for postrolandic cortex to participate in regulation of the activity of the prerolandic segment of the circuit. Alexander and his colleagues (1986) noted one further property of these cortico-striato-pallido-thalamo-cortical loops: the cortical regions projecting into the loop are functionally related and usually interconnected. Presumably, the loop through the striatum, pallidum, and thalamus performs a different function than the cortico-cortical connections. This concept appears to be validated by the fact that the cortico-cortical connections are reciprocal (Yeterian & Van Hoesen, 1978), whereas postrolandic components project to prerolandic components through the loop, but the reverse is not true. In other words, the pre- and postrolandic components influence each other through cortico-cortical connections, but only the postrolandic component can influence the prerolandic component through the loop.

The putative neurotransmitters for these cortico-striato-pallido-thalamo-cortical loops are also of interest since their nature can help to define the function. The most integrated discussion has been done by Penney and Young (1983, 1986) in their discussion of the motor loop. The cortico-striatal neurotransmitter is considered to be glutamate, and glutamate has an excitatory influence on striatal neurons. These facts seem fairly clearly established (Koscis et al., 1977; Preston et al., 1980; Spencer, 1976).

The primary striato-pallidal and striato-nigral neurotransmitter is thought to be GABA (Penney & Young, 1983), but, in addition to GABA, there are different neuropeptides present in these projections. These neuropeptides appear to reside in the GABA-ergic neurons. Substance P and dynorphin appear to be contained in striatal projections to the medial pallidal segment. Penney and Young (1986) note that these neuropeptides might function as modifiers of GABA's effects, as trophic factors, or as primary neurotransmitters. GABA is assumed to have an inhibitory effect on its pallidal targets. Finally, it should be noted that the projections to the medial pallidal segment and to pars reticulata of the substantia nigra originate from the matrix compartment of the striatum (Penney & Young, 1986).

The pallido-thalamic and nigro-thalamic components of the loop are assumed to use GABA as a neurotransmitter. As with the striato-pallidal component, GABA is thought to have an inhibitory influence on its thalamic component. The thalamo-cortical transmitter is unknown, but it is thought to be excitatory, as noted above (Penney & Young, 1983, 1986).

Conclusion

This concludes my discussion of neuroanatomy for the language system. At this time, the reader should be reminded that much of the evidence for participation of subcortical structures in language comes from naturally occurring vascular lesions. In considering such data, it is extremely important to remember that both the gray matter structures and the pathways between them must be considered. Interruption of the input from one structure to another may have the same effect as a lesion of the structure from which the fibers originated. A further complication is that a distance of a few millimeters may make a dramatic difference as to whether fibers directed to the important portion of a nucleus are damaged versus the target portion of the nucleus itself is damaged. Crosson (1989) noted that in the case of inhibitory projections, the effects of these two types of lesions may be entirely the opposite. Damaging an inhibitory input may lead to disinhibition of the target structure (i.e., increased output or other activity characteristic of decreased inhibition) (see Steriade & Deschenes, 1984) at times when the inhibitory input would normally be active. On the other hand, damage to a target structure itself will lead to elimination of or decrease in output.

Finally, one must consider that in the cortico-striato-pallido-thalamo-cortical loops, many of the interconnecting pathways run very close to the gray structures. In many instances of vascular lesion, both gray structures and multiple pathways are involved. In such instances, we must look at the damaged structure or pathway that is furthest downstream in the loop to assess the relationships between behavior and anatomy.

2

The Basal Ganglia and Subcortical White Matter in Language

The role of the basal ganglia in language is a problematic area. Indeed, some investigators (e.g., Alexander, Naeser, & Palumbo, 1987) have questioned whether the basal ganglia have any definite role in linguistic processes. One problem in studies of patients with vascular lesions of the basal ganglia is that basal ganglia structures are seldom damaged without injury to other structures. Of critical importance in this respect are the white matter pathways surrounding the basal ganglia. There is reason to believe that some of these pathways are involved in language processes.

Other types of research concerning the basal ganglia and language are equally troublesome. For example, large enough samples of patients with degenerative diseases affecting the basal ganglia (e.g., Parkinson's and Huntington's diseases) are available for studying language processes. However, it is uncertain if one can attribute the subtle language changes seen in these cases to basal ganglia pathology because atrophic changes in the anterior cortex are also common as these disorders progress. Further, it has been argued that language changes associated with these disorders are secondary to changes in more basic cognitive processes necessary to support language. Surgical lesion and stimulation cases would offer another source of data, but such studies involving the basal ganglia are not nearly as plentiful as those for the thalamus. Finally, study of cerebral blood flow and metabolism with SPECT or PET techniques (e.g., Baron et al., 1986;

Metter et al., 1983, 1984, 1986, 1987, 1988, 1989; Wallesch et al., 1985) may eventually provide evidence in this area, but the number and diversity of studies is still limited at this time. Thus, the most definitive statement that currently can be made is that the topic of basal ganglia involvement in language is hotly debated.

The purpose of this chapter is to explore in greater detail both the evidence regarding the involvement of the basal ganglia and surrounding white matter in language and the problems with this evidence. Various viewpoints will be briefly explored and critiqued. In the process of exploring these issues, I will also cover some foundation areas, the most important of which is a discussion of relevant language phenomena. This discussion will be rather brief; the reader wishing more comprehensive discussion of language phenomena as they relate to the brain should read a more basic text concerned with language disorders (e.g., Goodglass & Kaplan, 1983). Next, the discussion will turn to neurosurgical lesion and stimulation data regarding the basal ganglia. I will then review vascular lesion studies of the basal ganglia and subcortical white matter. This topic necessitates some discussion of the blood supply for the basal ganglia and surrounding white matter. The next topic concerns evidence from childhood language disorders, cerebral blood flow and metabolism data, and degenerative disorders affecting the basal ganglia. Finally, I will offer a few tentative conclusions.

Language Phenomena Relevant to Subcortical Aphasia

Language disorders can be described in many ways. For example, a complete evaluation of language disorders involves exploration of both spoken and written language functions. Unfortunately, most studies of language after subcortical lesions have focused primarily upon spoken language. Written language phenomena are typically excluded, examined in only the most cursory way, or ignored in the interpretation of data. Four dimensions have been explored most commonly in studies of subcortical language phenomena: fluency of spoken language, auditory-verbal comprehension, semantic versus phonemic substitutions, and repetition.

The definition of fluency most commonly used is that of Goodglass and Kaplan (1983). Basically, this dimension of language functioning involves the flow of language maintained by patients with *aphasia,* that is, language disturbance after brain injury. A patient's degree of fluency is observed in his/her conversational or narrative language. Operationally, Goodglass and Kaplan have described fluency as involving the intonational contours of language, articulatory agility, the number of words spoken before a pause, and the variety of grammatical forms present. If patients are unimpaired in these areas, their speech will flow in a relatively normal fashion. Patients who are severely impaired in these areas will show speech that is monotonic, demonstrates groping for sounds, is marked by pauses after every one or two words, and shows simplified grammar consisting primarily of nouns or nouns and verbs. In short, the flow of language is impaired, and is referred to as *nonfluent*.

Alexander (1989) distinguishes between *nonfluent language* and *nonfluent speech*. To understand this distinction, one must first understand the distinction between language and speech. Language consists of linguistic processes involving semantics (meaning), phonology (sound), and grammar (structure). The ultimate goal of language is to communicate through the use of symbols. Speech is the motor act through which language is realized. It involves movement of the lips, tongue, soft palate, larynx, and other structures. For Alexander, intonational contours and articulatory agility involve speech fluency, and variety of grammatical forms and number of words before a pause involve language fluency. Alexander made this distinction in discussing language after nonthalamic subcortical lesion; it will be discussed at length later in the chapter.

Unfortunately, some investigators have confused tasks involving "word fluency" with the fluent versus nonfluent language and speech discussed above. Word-fluency tasks involve the generation of as many words as one can that are in a certain semantic category (e.g., animals) or that begin with a given letter of the alphabet. These tasks are thought to reflect frontal lobe functioning, especially of the dominant frontal lobe. However, patients with impaired "word fluency" may show normal fluency in conversational language. In other words, there is no simple one-to-one correspondence between performance in "word fluency" and conversational fluency. The use of the term *fluency* to describe the former type of task is unfortunate because sometimes, reviewing the literature, one has difficulty distinguishing whether an investigator is talking about "word fluency" or describing the flow of conversational language. Such confusion can invalidate comparisons between studies on this dimension. Use of the term *fluency* should be reserved to refer to the flow of language and speech as described above; this usage will dictate my use of the terms *fluent* and *nonfluent* in this text. Hereafter I will refer to the ability to generate words of a certain type as "word-list generation."

"Comprehension," of course, refers to the ability to understand the linguistic communication of another person. In clinical examinations, comprehension is frequently measured by the ability to perform spoken commands. In many cases, a distinction is made between whether a patient can perform simple or both simple and complex commands. Presumably, simple commands involve one or two steps with a limited number of elements, whereas a complex commmand might involve more than two steps and/or have multiple elements (*Steps* refers to actions; *elements* refers both to actions and to distinctions that might be made between potential objects of the action). For example, "Tap each shoulder twice with two fingers, keeping your eyes closed" (Goodglass & Kaplan, 1983) has two actions (tap, keep eyes closed) and five elements (tap/each shoulder/twice/with two fingers/keeping your eyes closed). This command would be considered complex. "Make a fist," a command consisting of one action and one element, would be considered a simple command. One problem with this method of examining comprehension is that patients' ability to comprehend language can be confused with their ability to plan and execute movement if the examination is not carefully conducted. Memory and attention can also be involved in complex commands.

At one time, few distinctions were made between types of comprehension deficits. But during the 1980s it was noted that patients with Broca's aphasia had difficulty understanding certain types of syntax (e.g., Blumsteim, Goodglass, Stetlender, & Biber, 1983). This group of patients frequently had been considered to have minimal comprehension deficits. It can be inferred from other studies (e.g., McCarthy & Warrington, 1984; Ojemann, 1983) that the ability to process the phonological and semantic aspects of language also may be to some degree separable.

The semantic aspects of language are those processes that deal with meaning. One simple way to address semantics in aphasic language production is to examine the type of substitutions (paraphasias) a patient makes in spoken language. Substitutions of one sound for another (called literal or phonemic paraphasia) deal more with the phonological and/or motor-programming aspects of language. Some authors (e.g., Robin & Schienberg, 1990) also believe that neologisms (a word in which less than 50% of the sounds are from the target word and which carries no meaning in the respective language) are signs of a breakdown in phonological production. But when a patients' paraphasias are primarily substitution of one word for the correct word (semantic or verbal paraphasia), the disturbance may be semantic in nature.

Repetition is another important function studied during investigations of subcortical aphasia. Repetition can be done at the level of the single word, the phrase, or the sentence. Some types of aphasias are classified on the basis of how repetition compares to other aspects of language. For example, conduction aphasia is defined by repetition being disproportionately worse than other language functions. The transcortical aphasias (e.g., transcortical sensory and transcortical motor aphasia) show relatively preserved repetition in the face of impairment of other language functions. Transcortical motor aphasia demonstrates relatively intact repetition and comprehension with nonfluent output; transcortical sensory aphasia shows relatively spared repetition with fluent but paraphasic output and impaired comprehension. Some investigators (e.g., McCarthy & Warrington, 1984) believe that the relatively spared repetition in the transcortical aphasias is due to sparing of a phonological route to language production while other (semantic) mechanisms are damaged. Thus, some investigators see examination of repetition performance as one way to evaluate the intactness of phonological language-production mechanisms.

Thus, the fluency dimension relates to language production, and the comprehension dimension relates to language decoding. The study of semantics could relate either to language production or to language decoding, though the semantic phenomena most often cited in the subcortical aphasia literature relate to the production side of the equation. Changes in repetition frequently have been interpreted as related to phonological decoding and/or production. The exclusion of other phenomena from the preceeding discussion does not mean that these other processes are not valid or important; it simply reflects the fact that the four phenomena that I have discussed are the most frequently explored phenomena in the literature on subcortical aphasia.

Studies of Basal Ganglia Language Functions in Stereotactic Surgery Cases

During the 1940s and 1950s it was discovered that lesions in the ventral lateral thalamus and globus pallidus would relieve some of the symptoms of Parkinson's disease (Gillingham, Watson, Donaldson, & Naughton, 1960). An originally serendipitous discovery led to stereotaxic neurosurgical operations to help control Parkinson's disease. Because the operations involved the globus pallidus alone in the initial stages of the technique and evolved into thalamectomies that created lesions in specific portions of the ventral lateral thalamus, just a few studies exist that investigate the behavioral effects of operative lesion on the globus pallidus. Moreover, most studies that report the effects of pallidal lesions on language do not separate those cases in which only pallidal lesions were made from those cases in which thalamic lesions were made (Allen et al., 1966; Cooper, 1958; Gillingham et al., 1960). In these cases, language dysfunction after pallidectomy and/or thalamectomy occurred primarily after lesions in the left hemisphere with the percentage of cases showing aphasia after left hemisphere lesion reaching a figure as high as 16% (Allen et al., 1966). In general, the language dysfunction was reported to remit rapidly.

Only Svennilson et al. (1960) reported separate results for 81 pallidectomies. Aphasia occurred in 24% of patients with dominant-hemisphere pallidectomies and dilated ventricles and 7.5% of patients with dominant-hemisphere lesions without dilated ventricles. Language symptoms were not extensively described but included word-finding difficulty and paraphasia. One patient described their language symptoms as reflecting a "lack of coordination between thought and speech." (Separate studies of thalamectomies were much more common and will be discussed in the next chapter.)

These stereotaxic operations also gave investigators an opportunity to electrically stimulate some structures of the basal ganglia and note the results on language. Stimulation was sometimes used to ensure proper location of the electrode before ablation. Hermann et al. (1966) reported the interruption of ongoing language with stimulation of the globus pallidus. Unfortunately, the authors did not specify whether there were any differences between dominant- and nondominant-hemisphere stimulation in these cases. In fact, the frequency of this phenomenon in general was not mentioned.

Van Buren and colleagues (Van Buren, 1963, 1966; Van Buren et al., 1966) noted an interesting linguistic phenomenon related to stimulation of the head of the caudate nucleus. These authors found that a number of "psychic" phenomena appeared during or after stimulation in the vicinity of the caudate head (Van Buren, 1963). These psychic phenomena often included language output consisting of short sentences or phrases that were irrelevant to the experimental situation. A careful reading indicates that language onset most often occurred at stimulation offset. A reevaluation of the data (Van Buren, 1966) showed that irrelevant language and other psychic phenomena were associated with stimulation within the caudate head, while stimulation of the white matter lateral and/or anterior to the caudate head produced only arrest of ongoing speech with no "psychic" phenomena.

Spontaneous, irrelevant language was associated with stimulation in and around the left caudate head in 4 of 14 patients. Only 1 of 11 right-handed patients demonstrated spontaneous language in association with stimulation of the right caudate head. One of three left-handed patients showed language during stimulation of both the right and the left caudate head (Van Buren et al., 1966). Since the caudate head has not been the target of operations, it has only rarely been stimulated in other studies. From a scientific viewpoint, it is unfortunate that there have not been attempts to replicate Van Buren's findings in terms of stimulation of the dominant caudate head. Such findings in an isolated study would be of questionable interest; however, Schaltenbrand (1965, 1975) has reported remarkably similar findings with respect to language when stimulating in and around the dominant ventral anterior thalamus. Since the caudate head is connected to the ventral anterior thalamus through the globus pallidus, Schaltenbrand's findings can be considered as related to those of Van Buren.

Thus, data developed on the basal ganglia and language during stereotaxic surgery are limited. More extensive data regarding the thalamus developed from stereotaxic studies will be discussed in the next chapter. The development of aphasia after lesion of the dominant pallidum (Svennilson et al., 1960) is of interest because this stereotaxic lesion study is probably the one place in the literature where the pallidum has lesions in the absence of lesions to surrounding structures. Thus, it suggests that the dominant globus pallidus may be involved in language. Of course, it can be argued that the striatal dysfunction from the Parkinson's disease of these patients means that their brain was not functioning normally to begin with. The other finding of interest is the production of spontaneous language at the offset of stimulation of the dominant caudate head.

Vascular and Other Naturally Occurring Lesions of the Basal Ganglia and Surrounding White Matter

Blood Supply

Before I discuss language functions after vascular lesion to the basal ganglia, the reader needs to understand the blood supply of the basal ganglia and surrounding structures. The pattern of blood supply to these structures, of course, will determine patterns of lesion during infarction in the area since infarction is caused by occlusion of the

Table 2-1. Blood Supply of the Basal Ganglia and Internal Capsule[a]

Artery	Structures supplied
Medial striate artery	Head of caudate nucleus (anterior, medial part) Anterior limb of internal capsule
Lateral striate arteries	Lateral globus pallidus (lateral part) Head of caudate nucleus (posterior, lateral part) Body of caudate nucleus Putamen Anterior limb of internal capsule Posterior limb of internal capsule (superior part)
Anterior choroidal artery	Tail of caudate nucleus Putamen (posterior most part) Lateral globus pallidus (medial part) Medial globus pallidus (lateral part) Posterior limb of internal capsule (inferior part) Retrolenticular internal capsule
Branches of posterior communicating artery	Medial globus pallidus (medial part)
Branches of internal carotid artery	Genu of internal capsule

[a]According to Carpenter & Sutin (1983)

blood supply. The internal capsule, in particular, shares blood supply with the basal ganglia. Intracerebral hematomas from a hemorrhage, however, do not necessarily respect the boundaries of arterial supply. Our ability to interpret the results of a hematoma as isolated to the immediate area that it occupies is also limited because normally pressure effects from the hematoma extend beyond its boundary (e.g., Graff-Radford et al., 1985; McFarling, Rothi, & Heilman, 1982).

Table 2-1 lists the parts of the basal ganglia and internal capsule supplied by the various arteries. According to Carpenter and Sutin (1983), the anterior, medial caudate head is supplied by the medial striate artery, and the caudate tail and posterior extreme of the putamen receive blood supply from the anterior choroidal artery. The remainder and bulk of the putamen, the posterior lateral portions of the caudate head, body of the caudate nucleus, and lateral portion of the lateral pallidal segment are supplied by the lateral striate arteries. The medial portion of the lateral pallidal segment and the lateral portion of the medial pallidal segment receive blood supply from the anterior choroidal artery, while the most medial portion of the medial pallidal segment is nourished by branches of the posterior communicating artery.

A large portion of the anterior and posterior limbs of the internal capsule are supplied by the lateral striate arteries. However, the medial striate artery supplies the anterior-most portion of the anterior limb, and the anterior choroidal artery nourishes the inferior-most portion of the posterior limb and the retrolenticular portion of the internal capsule. The genu of the internal capsule receives arterial branches directly from the internal carotid artery.

Thus, infarction in the territory of the medial striate artery might affect the anterior, medial caudate head and anterior-most anterior limb of the internal capsule. An infarct in the lateral striate arteries might damage a large portion of the internal capsule, portions of the head and the body of the caudate nucleus, and large portions of the putamen. Ischemic damage in the territory of the anterior choroidal artery might affect both the medial and lateral pallidal segments, the posterior limb and retrolenticular portion of the internal capsule, and possibly even parts of the thalamus.

The following discussion will cover language dysfunction after vascular lesion of the basal ganglia and/or the surrounding white matter. There are many ways of approaching such a discussion, of which I shall use two. The first is to compile lesions that include the various structures of the corpus striatum and/or parts of the internal capsule and to look at the symptoms associated with these various structures. This approach has some flaws, which will be discussed below. Moreover, treatment of the periventricular white matter, which also accompanies such lesions, has been quite variable and does not allow for extensive inclusion in this discussion. However, the role of the periventricular white matter in language symptoms after deep vascular lesions will play a prominent role in the second approach to reviewing the literature. This second approach will be to discuss studies that have emphasized somewhat different ways of analyzing the anatomy and/or somewhat different ways of analyzing language symptoms. Some of these investigations have yielded definite hypotheses regarding the origins of subcortical language symptoms.

Deficits in written language will be handled under a separate subsection, because studies treating this topic have been very inconsistent. The issues of frequency and persistence of language dysfunction are critical because a lack of persistence or a small incidence of language dysfunction after lesion to the basal ganglia and/or surrounding white matter would call into question the participation of these structures in language. These issues will also be addressed. Studies of cerebral blood flow and metabolism will be included under a separate section, since this type of study includes unique methodological considerations.

Compilation by Structure

In order to gain some insight into how different subcortical structures excluding the thalamus are involved in language, I compiled the results of several studies to examine what symptoms were associated with what structures. The symptoms addressed were those discussed above: fluent versus nonfluent language, auditory comprehension, repetition, and semantic versus phonemic paraphasias. If I noted that a structure was involved in a particular lesion, the case was tabulated with other cases that included that structure. For example, if a lesion included the head of the caudate nucleus, the anterior limb of the internal capsule, and the putamen, I tabulated the symptoms associated with this lesion under all three structures. Thus, a case might be tabulated under multiple structures if each of the structures was included in the lesion. Because hemorrhage and infarction are different processes that might have different effects on involved structures, I tabulated these two entities separately. Due to the varying frequencies for which the different language symptoms were described, total numbers of patients classified will vary from symptom to symptom. Data from children were not included in the tabulation because of indications that lesions of certain cortical areas produce different types of aphasia in childhood than in adulthood (e.g., Blumstein, 1981). Cases were tabulated from the following studies: Alexander and LoVerme (1980); Alexander, Naeser, and Palumbo (1987); Basso, Sala, and Farabola (1987); Bladin and Berkovic (1984); Brunner et al. (1982); Cappa, Cavallotti, Guidotti, Papagno, and Vignolo (1983); Damasio et al. (1982); Fisher (1979); Fromm, Holland, Swindell, and Reinmuth (1985); Hayashi, Ulatowska, and Sasanuma (1985); Knopman, Selnes, Niccum, and Rubens (1984); Lieberman, Ellenberg, and Restum (1986); Mazzocchi and Vignolo (1979); Metter et al. (1983); Murdoch, Chenery, and Kennedy (1989); Naeser et al. (1982); Ramsberger and Hillman (1985); Robin and Schienberg (1990); Tanridag and Kirshner (1985); Wallesch (1985); Yamadori, Ohiro, Seriu, and Ogura (1984).

Table 2-2 shows the compiled data for fluent versus nonfluent language. It can be seen that lesion to some structures favors nonfluent versus fluent output: head of the caudate nucleus (62% vs. 38%), globus pallidus (71% vs. 29%), anterior limb of internal capsule (66% vs. 34%), and genu of internal capsule (100% vs. zero%). Other structures seem to be evenly split between nonfluent and fluent aphasias when lesioned: putamen (44% vs. 56%), posterior limb of internal capsule (53% vs. 47%). However, an interesting phenomenon is observed if one considers hemorrhage and infarction separately. For example, in the putamen, 14 hemorrhagic cases fell into the fluent category of aphasia

Table 2-2. Frequency of Fluent versus Nonfluent Aphasia When Vascular Lesion Includes Various Subcortical Structures

Structure	Form of aphasia					
	Fluent			Nonfluent		
	H	I	%	H	I	%
Putamen	14	20	44	2	42	56
Head of caudate nucleus	5	8	38	1	20	62
Globus pallidus	4	4	29	0	21[a]	71
Anterior limb of internal capsule	4	12	34	3	28	66
Genu of internal capsule	0	0	0	0	9	100
Posterior limb of internal capsule	4	6	53	0	9	47

[a]Includes one case of pallidal lesion secondary to anoxia.
H = hemorrhagic lesion; I = infarction

while only two fell into the nonfluent category. In fact, if we were to remove the hemorrhagic cases entirely from Table 2-2, leaving only cases of ischemic lesions, every structure would show substantially more nonfluent than fluent aphasias. Perhaps the most impressive finding in Table 2-2 is that hemorrhagic lesions overwhelmingly produce fluent aphasias, while infarctions tend less strongly to produce nonfluent aphasias. Although the reasons for this finding are unclear, it strongly suggests that hemorrhage and infarction should be treated as separate entities.

Table 2-3 shows how lesions of different structures affect auditory comprehension. Functioning in auditory comprehension has been divided into three categories: intact, mildly to moderately impaired, and severely impaired. The reader will note that most cases of nonthalamic subcortical lesion demonstrate some impairment of comprehension, with relatively few cases being unaffected in this function. For the putamen, hemorrhagic cases seem somewhat less impaired than infarction cases, but this does not hold true for other structures.

Table 2-4 displays how lesions of different structures affect repetition. The reader can see that more patients have unimpaired repetition than unimpaired auditory comprehension, with the possible exceptions of patients with lesions in the globus pallidus and/or posterior limb of the internal capsule. Nonetheless, impairment of repetition is also a common occurrence with all structures noted in Table 2-4. For repetition, there are few consistent differences for hemorrhage and infarction.

Table 2-3. Impairment of Comprehension When Vascular Lesion Includes Various Subcortical Structures

Structure	Level of impairment								
	Intact			Mild-Moderate			Severe		
	H	I	%	H	I	%	H	I	%
Putamen	1	4	8	13	17	49	7	19	43
Head of caudate nucleus	0	3	9	1	10	32	6	14	59
Globus pallidus	0	2	11	2	3	28	2	9	61
Anterior limb of internal capsule	0	1	2	5	14	41	7	19	57
Genu of internal capsule	0	1	13	0	5	63	0	5	25
Posterior limb of internal capsule	0	0	0	1	6	41	2	8	59

H = hemorrhage; I = infarction

Table 2-4. Impairment of Repetition When Vascular Lesion Includes Various Subcortical Structures

Structure	Level of impairment								
	Intact			Mild-Moderate			Severe		
	H	I	%	H	I	%	H	I	%
Putamen	3	13	34	10	6	34	6	9	32
Head of caudate nucleus	3	9	44	1	4	19	1	9	37
Globus pallidus	0	2	15	1	1	15	4	5	69
Anterior limb of internal capsule	2	11	38	4	3	21	3	11	41
Genu of internal capsule	0	1	20	0	1	20	0	3	60
Posterior limb of internal capsule	0	0	0	2	1	33	2	4	67

H = hemorrhage; I = infarction

Table 2-5 displays cases that were noted to have a predominance of either semantic or phonemic paraphasias. There were only enough cases for the putamen and the globus pallidus to be displayed. The reader should note that in both structures hemorrhagic cases that show a predominance of one type of paraphasia tend to produce a predominance of semantic over phonemic paraphasias, while infarctions tend to favor phonemic over semantic paraphasias. This finding reinforces the idea that hemorrhage and infarction should be treated as separate entities. Perhaps some advance in the area of subcortical aphasias might be made if one could determine why there are differences in the affects of hemorrhage and infarction.

Although the findings with respect to hemorrhage and fluent versus nonfluent language seem robust, other findings in the above discussion must be considered within the context of the difficulties with this type of compilation. Alexander (1989) has pointed out some of the inconsistencies of the previous literature, which include the examination of patients at variable times postonset. The later the examination is conducted, the more likely the symptoms will have changed due to spontaneous recovery and/or compensation. Further problems exist with the way in which various investigators have defined fluent versus nonfluent language. There also has been inconsistency in the type of measures used between studies. These inconsistencies in definition and measures make it difficult to make comparisons between studies, and I had to use my own judgment to decipher several patient descriptions and equate them to the categories used.

One further problem with this type of analysis involves anatomical and functional considerations. If one believes that the cortico-striato-pallido-thalamo-cortical loops discussed in Chapter 1 are the important structures for language, then one might gain some insight by looking at the structure farthest "downstream" in the loop as the structure that determines patterns of cognitive deficit. Such an

Table 2-5. Predominance of Phonemic versus Semantic Paraphasias When Vascular Lesion Includes Different Subcortical Structures

Structure	Paraphasias					
	Phonemic			Semantic		
	H	I	%	H	I	%
Putamen	0	7	37	8	4	63
Globus pallidus	0	1	17	4	1	83

H = hemorrhage; I = infarction

approach assumes that the prerolandic cortex to which the loop projects is the end point of the loop and what is "downstream" can be determined from this reference point. Thus, the last link in the chain of influences that is damaged will determine the symptom pattern. In this context, it would make sense to focus on the anterior limb of the internal capsule since this pathway leads from the thalamus to the cortex and is the final pathway in the loop before reaching the prerolandic component of the loop. A glance at Tables 2-2 through 2-4 is somewhat disappointing in this respect, since the effects of lesions in the anterior limb of the internal capsule lead to mixed effects on language with respect to fluent versus nonfluent output, auditory comprehension, and repetition.

These mixed results for the anterior limb of the internal capsule simply demonstrate the problems with this approach. In the first place, we are not only uncertain about which portion of the anterior limb of the internal capsule might carry fibers important for language, but in most cases discussed in the literature we are also uncertain as to which portion of the anterior limb has been injured. A further problem with this approach is that a difference of a few millimeters might well make a significant difference in what symptoms are seen. For example, Figure 2-1 shows a hypothetical area L in the ventral anterior thalamus related to language and inhibitory fibers traversing other portions of the ventral anterior thalamus to reach L. Lesion X within the ventral anterior thalamus would interrupt the inhibitory input to L, decrease the inhibitory input to L at times when the input to L from the pallidum would normally be active, and lead to increased output from L at these times. On the other hand, a lesion Y within L itself would interrupt the source of output from L, thereby reducing output at times when L would normally be active. Again, the problem is that we do not know what areas in what structures might be relevant to language, and we therefore have a difficult time assessing whether inputs to or outputs from language-related areas are being interrupted. We are perhaps closer to this type of analysis in memory (e.g., Cramon et al., 1985). Nonetheless, limitations in both anatomical knowledge and imaging techniques will limit our ability to address such issues.

Studies Emphasizing Unique Anatomical and/or Language Analysis

Thus, studies that simply tabulate lesions in different structures and try to correlate them with patterns of language dysfunction are flawed by a number of difficulties. Advancing knowledge regarding the role of the basal ganglia and/or surrounding pathways in language requires

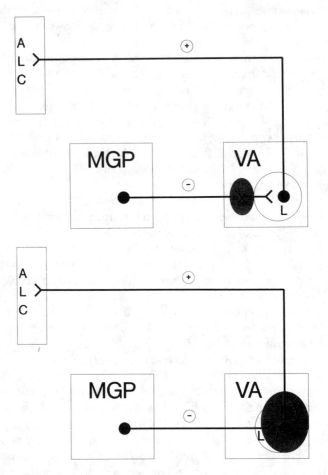

Figure 2-1. Two depictions of a hypothetical area L within the ventral anterior thalamus. A lesion X involving the inhibitory pallidal input to area L would have the opposite impact of a lesion Y to area L itself under circumstances in which the inhibitory pallidal input would normally be active.

researchers to use ingenuity to design unique ways of addressing this problem. Fortunately, examples of such ingenuity do exist. In general, such studies involve devising unique ways of examining either the anatomical aspects of the question, or the language aspects of the question, or both.

Some of the best studies in this vein have come from the Boston group, Naeser, Alexander, and their colleagues. A seminal study in this series was Naeser et al. (1982). There are two important aspects to this study. First, the authors noted that capsular/putaminal lesions showed different syndromes depending upon which of the surrounding white matter pathways were involved. Patients with capsular/putaminal lesions that extended into the anterior, superior white matter showed grammatical but slow, dysarthric output with relatively intact comprehension. Patients with capsular/putaminal lesions that extended into the posterior subcortical white matter, including the auditory radiations in the temporal isthmus, showed fluent, paraphasic output with significant auditory comprehension problems. Patients with capsular/putaminal lesions extending both anteriorly and posteriorly were globally aphasic. Cappa et al. (1983) had similar findings.

The second important finding in Naeser and colleagues' (1982) study was that patients with capsular/putaminal lesions extending in the anterior, superior direction showed some characteristics of nonfluent aphasia but not others. In particular, their speech was slow and showed impaired articulatory agility, but it was not agrammatic. Discussion of the different aspects of nonfluency has been an important facet of their later papers.

Another strong paper in this series was that of Alexander, Naeser, and Palumbo (1987). In this paper, the authors used phrase length and variety of grammatical forms as measures of fluency versus nonfluency in language production. Articulatory agility was assumed to be a measure of dysarthria. The investigators examined 16 cases of aphasia with primarily subcortical lesions, one case with cortical and subcortical lesion, and two cases of insular and limited subcortical involvement. The authors noted that lesions limited primarily to the putamen or caudate nucleus tended to cause no language disturbance or only mild word-finding deficits, though cases involving the posterior putamen were associated with hypophonia. Additional extension into the anterior limb of the internal capsule or limited superior extension into the periventricular white matter resulted in no language disturbances and only mild disturbances in prosody. Involvement of the anterior, superior periventricular white matter yielded limited language output with hesitation and slow initiation, considered to represent a mild form of transcortical motor aphasia. More extensive lesions to the deep frontal white matter were noted to produce a more classical transcortical motor aphasia (i.e., nonfluent output with relatively spared repetition and comprehension). It was suggested that such lesions interrupt fibers from the supplementary motor area to Broca's area. These fibers were seen as important in conveying the drive to speak from the limbic cortex (via the supplementary motor area) to the lateral language cortex.

Lesions that disrupted both the posteromedial anterior limb of the internal capsule and the genu of the internal capsule and/or the superior periventricular white matter are seen as responsible for dysarthria because of interruption of descending output of Broca's area and the inferior motor cortex. When damage to both the anterior periventricular white matter and to the superior periventricular white matter occurs, output is hesitant and slow. Patients show the capacity for longer utterances and the use of grammatical structures, but language is frequently limited to the use of short phrases with simple grammatical constructions. The authors define this output as fluent, focusing on the patients' capacity rather than their more typical output. More consistent impairment in phrase length and grammatical form is seen with extension of lesions in the periventricular white matter past the frontal horn of the lateral ventrical, possibly including portions of the genu of the corpus callosum.

Finally, lesions of the putamen with posterior extension across the temporal isthmus lead to fluent aphasia with neologistic output and impaired comprehension. The authors speculated that the neologistic language and impaired comprehension could be related to interruption of thalamo-cortical fibers to the temporal lobe. The degree to which extension across the posterior periventricular white matter is important is not clear. Auditory association pathways between the temporal association cortices are found in this area. According to these investigators, lesion to the posterior putamen itself might be responsible for the hypophonia sometimes seen in these cases. Thus, Alexander et al. (1987) concluded that lesion to the caudate nucleus and putamen might be responsible for speech dysfunction, but that language dysfunction is caused primarily by lesion of specific white matter pathways.

This study is important for two reasons. First, it focuses attention on the issue of which symptoms of nonfluent aphasia might be more related to language and which symptoms might be more related to speech. As noted above, impairment of phrase length and agrammatism are seen as indicators of language dysfunction, while articulatory agility is seen as related to speech. Thus, these authors might see a case as fluent with respect to language that other authors might classify as nonfluent because of articulatory agility or prosody problems. Another way in which these authors might classify a patient as fluent that other authors would classify as nonfluent is that they regard the patient's potential as opposed to their more common response as the criterion for classification. In spite of this somewhat unusual approach to classification of fluent versus nonfluent output, all five hemorrhagic patients were fluent. Five of 12 patients with ischemic lesions were seen as nonfluent, while seven were classified as fluent.

The second important facet of this paper is that it focuses attention on the role of subcortical white matter pathways in language. However, the reader should realize that Alexander and colleagues' view that white matter lesions are responsible for language dysfunction in nonthalamic subcortical lesions is not shared by everyone. For example, Wallesch et al. (1983) showed that postacute patients with left-basal-ganglia lesions demonstrated significantly worse performance on language tasks than patients with right-basal-ganglia lesions. Patients with left-hemisphere lesions primarily involving the subcortical white matter did not differ from patients with similar lesions in the right hemisphere. The implication is that it is the basal ganglia and not necessarily the white matter that is important in language. Further, Basso, Sala, and Farabola (1987) did not note a particularly high incidence of aphasia in their ten patients with lesions primarily confined to the white matter. Five were nonaphasic, three were minimally aphasic, one had anarthria, and only one had a reasonably severe nonfluent aphasia. Likewise, Cappa and Vallar (1989) state that there is no reason to believe that the basal ganglia are uninvolved in language.

Further, it must be remembered that Alexander and colleagues' cases with lesions confined to the caudate nucleus or the putamen were among the smaller lesions described in the literature. There is evidence that small lesions, whether cortical or subcortical, do not cause severe and lasting aphasia (Brunner et al., 1982; Ludlow et al., 1986). In particular, Brunner et al. found that lesions of Broca's area did not cause severe or lasting aphasia unless associated with an extension of the lesion into the basal ganglia. Similarly, posterior cortical and posterior plus anterior cortical lesions caused more severe and lasting aphasia when lesions extended into the basal ganglia. Finally, with respect to Alexander and colleagues' (1987) claim that the basal ganglia are not involved in language, it must be noted that the white matter regions they investigated not only carry cortico-cortical connections but also contain thalamo-cortical, cortico-thalamic, striato-pallidal, pallido-thalamic, and cortico-striatal pathways.

In some respects, this latter issue is addressed in the 1989 study by Naeser, Palumbo, Helm-Estabrooks, Stiassny-Eder, and Albert. This study compared patients with no speech output or speech output limited to stereotypies to patients with Broca's aphasia, that is, nonfluent speech and language with better preservation of auditory comprehension. The authors found two structures consistently damaged in the group with more severe output problems that were not damaged in the patients with Broca's aphasia: the medial subcallosal fasciculus and the portion of the periventricular white matter carrying sensory information of the mouth, lips, and tongue to the cortex and carrying messages away from the mouth, lips, and tongue area of the motor cortex. Both areas must be damaged to produce lack of output or output limited to stereotypies. It is obvious that the latter pathways are important for the execution of speech. The medial subcallosal fasciculus is known to contain fibers coursing from the supplementary motor area and anterior cingulate gyrus to the caudate nucleus. The authors see this pathway as important in connecting the limbic system with the speech and language system, providing the "motivation" for speaking. It would seem that this latter function would be important in both language and speech.

Finally, Alexander (1989) has discussed further advances in the work of the Boston group. In this paper, both speech and language are considered to have nonfluent characteristics, and the nonfluent characteristics of speech and the nonfluent characteristics of language can be separated from one another. Impaired articulatory agility, disturbed melodic line, and hypophonia are considered to be the essence of nonfluent speech. Decreased phrase length and agrammatism comprise nonfluent language. Thirteen patients with nonthalamic subcortical lesions were examined. Variability in time postonset, which had provided a confound in previous studies, was controlled by performing behavioral assessments at 2 to 3 weeks postonset. Some patients were examined again at 6 to 10 weeks postonset. Problems with pressure effects in the hemorrhagic lesions in early stages was controlled by including cases of ischemic lesions only. Using the above criteria, 12 of 13 patients had fluent language at the first evaluation, though truncation of utterances or elision were frequent. Speech fluency, in contrast, was impaired in all subjects. In addition, nine cases had delays in initiation of all utterances. The dissociation between speech and language fluency occurred whether or not there was involvement of the caudate nucleus or putamen. Repetition and oral reading were unimpaired in all but two cases. Comprehension was functionally normal, but some impairments were found in testing of more complex material. All patients showed word-retrieval deficits and produced semantic paraphasias, but phonemic paraphasias were relatively uncommon. Thus, the author concluded that nonfluent speech is relatively common in subcortical aphasia, but nonfluent language is relatively rare. It must be noted that patients do have problems in speech and language initiation that are hard to separate, and lexical deficits are probable. Some of the cases in the literature previously classified as generally nonfluent could potentially be reclassified as having fluent language according to Alexander's criteria. The distinction drawn between nonfluent speech and nonfluent language is potentially a very important one and deserves further exploration.

Mehler (1988) presented an interesting paper that explored different aspects of subcortical aphasias. He found three partially dissociable symptoms that he believed to be associated with caudate nucleus pathology: intrusions (abrupt, nonrelevant, semantically incorrect phrases), fluctuating nonfluency, and pervasive perseverations. The author suggested that these partially dissociable symptoms were the product of disruption of temporo-caudate, striato-pallidal, and fronto-caudate pathways, respectively.

A final study of interest is the one in which Albert, Bachman, Morgan, and Helm-Estabrooks (1988) found decreased latencies and improved naming in a case of transcortical motor aphasia when they administered bromocriptine, a dopamine agonist. Although the authors submitted that the action of this drug was at the level of the cortex, it is also clear that the lesion in their patient included parts of the caudate nucleus and putamen. Such a lesion could interrupt the dopamine supply from the substantia nigra, pars compacta to the striatum, and the dopamine agonist may have been active in the striatum where the dopamine supply was limited by the lesion.

In summary: Alexander, Naeser, and their colleagues have suggested that nonfluent speech commonly occurs after nonthalamic subcortical lesions, but that nonfluent language is relatively rare. Delayed initiation of speech and language is also frequent, and may be due to the interruption of fibers between the supplementary motor/anterior cingulate areas and Broca's area in some cases. No language output or language confined to stereotypes happens only when both the medial subcallosal fasciculus and the periventricular white matter are injured together. The research of the Boston group has served to focus attention on the subcortical white matter as important in language. Mehler (1988) has suggested that partially dissociated symptoms after nonthalamic subcortical lesion may be due to the differential interruption of anterior and posterior cortical input to the striatum or striatal output to the globus pallidus. There are some preliminary indications that dopamine agonists may improve language functions to some degree in some types of aphasia (Albert et al., 1988).

Written Language after Lesion of the Basal Ganglia and/or Subcortical White Matter

Evaluation of written language functions after lesion of the basal ganglia and/or subcortical white matter has been infrequent, though somewhat less so than after thalamic lesion. Cappa et al. (1983) mentioned agraphia in five of five nonthalamic subcortical aphasias, though descriptions of error types were not given. Alexia was mentioned in two of these five patients. Kertesz (1989) studied agraphia in 15 patients with dominant-hemisphere subcortical lesions and 12 patients with dominant-hemisphere cortical lesions. Significant agraphia was present in all 15 patients with subcortical lesion: severe in 5, prominent in 5, and mild in 5. Severity of limb apraxia and aphasia did not correlate with agraphia, but verbal apraxia was related to agraphia. Better preservation of reading was usually present. The anterior limb of the internal capsule and the neostriatum were the most commonly involved structures. All 15 cases also showed naming deficits. Agraphia was more variable in the cortical cases. The author notes that cortico-striato-pallido-thalamo-cortical loops may help to modulate cortical functions related to writing.

In spite of a nonfluent aphasia, Fisher (1979) noted no writing deficit in his case of lesion in the posterior limb of the internal capsule and putamen. Tanridag and Kirshner (1985) reported three cases of dominant subcortical lesion in which writing was disproportionately impaired in comparison to other language functions, including oral reading and reading comprehension. Lesions involved the putamen, subcortical white matter, and/or the posterior limb of the internal capsule. In eight patients with minimal aphasia and nine with fluent aphasia, Basso et al. (1987) reported written language to be more sensitive to subcortical lesions than spoken language. Writing was generally nonfluent in the patients with fluent spoken output, that is, they were able to produce only isolated letters to a few words. These authors reported no spontaneous written language in four patients with nonfluent aphasia. Dysgraphia was the most striking symptom in three other patients. The authors noted that a frequent dissociation between relatively preserved oral production and poorly preserved writing. Lieberman et al. (1986) described written as well as spoken language deficits in three patients with lesions of the interior capsule, head of the caudate nucleus, globus pallidus, and/or subcortical white matter. Writing was severely impaired in all cases, nonfluent in two patients, and fluent in one patient. Reading comprehension was moderately-to-severely impaired in all cases.

Hayashi et al. (1985) described a patient who made frequent semantic substitutions or made no response during oral reading tasks. Reading comprehension was good for high-frequency concrete nouns, but more impaired for complex material. For both oral reading and reading comprehension, the patient read better in kanji (Japanese writing using ideograms) than in kana (Japanese writing characterized by correspondence between script and syllables). The hemorrhagic lesion was in the dominant putamen, anterior limb of the internal capsule, and subcortical white matter.

A few tentative conclusions may be drawn from this literature. First, writing may be impaired after nonthalamic subcortical lesions of the dominant hemisphere. In fact, writing may be disproportionately impaired compared to other language functions. Second, in some cases writing appears to be nonfluent while spoken language is fluent. Third, reading may also be impaired in lesions of the basal ganglia and surrounding white matter, but, at least in some cases, it is less severely or less frequently impaired than writing.

Incidence and Persistence of Aphasia after Lesions of the Dominant Basal Ganglia and Subcortical White Matter

Incidence and persistence of aphasia after subcortical lesion are important issues because the probability that structures and pathways participate in language must be judged, to some extent, from the context of incidence and persistence. If aphasia occurs only infrequently after lesion of a subcortical structure, it might be argued that such a structure is not normally involved in language. Conversely, if aphasia is usually seen after lesion to a specific structure or pathway, then the phenomenon demands explanation. If the structure is not directly involved in language, then why does aphasia occur? The issue of persistence is more complicated. A good recovery of language function after an initial aphasia does not necessarily mean that the involved structure does not participate in language. For example, such a recovery might mean that there are alternative ways of performing the linguistic activity in which the structure was participating. Nonetheless, a lack of persistence of aphasia symptoms after lesion of a structure could mean the structure does not participate in language. Therefore, if the structure is thought to be involved in language, then a lack of persistence of aphasia after lesion to the structure will eventually require explanation.

Incidence of aphasia after nonthalamic subcortical lesion varies from study to study. In addition to the obvious issues of location and type of lesion, other relevant variables may affect the percentage of cases that demonstrate aphasia. Examples of variables affecting incidence include the following: the nature of referrals of patients into a center or study, the sensitivity of a clinical examination versus a standardized test of aphasia, and the sensitivity of an aphasia instrument to subtle language dysfunction.

In lesions of the internal capsule, Fisher (1979) found one of six patients (17%) demonstrated aphasia. In this patient, the lesion extended into the caudate nucleus and putamen. In ten patients with infarcts of the dominant (left) caudate head, Caplan et al. (1990) found two cases (20%) with language abnormalities. One case, which involved extension into the anterior limb of the internal capsule and anterior putamen, exhibited "stuttering" and omission of consonants. The second case, which involved extension into the anterior limb of the internal capsule, exhibited stammering and word-finding difficulty. Caplan et al. did not perform extensive language testing on their sample. Cappa et al. (1983) found six patients with strictly subcortical lesions of the dominant hemisphere who were admitted to their service in an 8-month period. Lesions included infarcts and hemorrhages and were confined to the basal ganglia, centrum semiovale, internal capsule, and external capsule. The six patients were given an aphasia evaluation between 15 and 44 days postonset, and two of six (33%) were noted to have aphasia.

Other studies have shown a higher incidence of aphasia. Hier, Davis, Richardson, and Mohr (1977) noted that five of seven patients (71%) with dominant-hemisphere putaminal hemorrhage who were conscious initially presented with aphasia. Bladin and Berkovic (1984) noted that five of six patients (83%) with dominant-hemisphere subcortical infarction had aphasia. Lesions included the head of the caudate nucleus, putamen, and anterior limb of the internal capsule.

Basso et al. (1987) reviewed the files of 1500 patients examined at their aphasia unit over an 8½-year period. Thirty-seven patients were found who were right-handed, had a single left-hemisphere lesion sparing the convexity, had no cortical atrophy, and had a CT scan and neuropsychological evaluation between 15 and 60 days postonset. Lesions were extrathalamic or extended beyond the thalamus in 36 of 37 cases. Of these 36 patients, 29 had infarcts and 7 had hemorrhages. The insula was involved in nine cases. There was no aphasia in 8 of these 36 cases (22%) with extrathalamic lesions. Another eight patients (22%) had borderline language deficits. Three (8%) were primarily anarthric, and a significant degree of aphasia was noted in the remaining 17 patients (47%). It should be noted that this group cannot be considered a random sample because it consisted of patients referred to an aphasia unit. Thus, the authors noted that the degree of neuropsychological disorders might be overestimated.

Data are also variable with regard to persistence of language symptoms. Scott and Miller (1985) noted on cases of putaminal hemorrhage in which symptoms remitted rapidly; two of four dominant-hemisphere lesions had aphasia. Brunner et al. (1982), on the other hand, reported significant language deficits in patients with left-hemisphere subcortical lesions at 6 months postonset. In their cases of aphasia with lesions of the dominant caudate head, putamen, and anterior limb of the internal capsule, Bladin and Berkovic (1984) reported that comprehension recovered more completely than fluency. Wallesch (1985) noted improvement in all seven cases of nonthalamic subcortical aphasia he reported, but all patients had some residual symptoms at 3–8 months postonset. Robin and Schienberg (1990) were able to conduct extended followups on six of ten patients with aphasia secondary to lesion of the basal ganglia and surrounding white matter. In one patient, symptoms cleared by 8 weeks postonset, and in another symptoms cleared by 40 weeks postonset. The other four patients had persistent symptoms of varying degrees anywhere from 16 to 56 weeks postonset.

Also of interest are the cases of combined cortical and subcortical lesions with aphasia. For example, Mazzocchi and Vignolo (1979) reported that in 11 of 16 cases with chronic Broca's aphasia with cortical lesions, the basal ganglia and/or internal capsule were involved. But the basal ganglia were involved in only two of five cases of chronic Wernicke's aphasia, and in zero of three cases of chronic conduction aphasia. Brunner et al. (1982) reported that lesions of Broca's area alone did not cause lasting or severe aphasia. However, when a lesion of Broca's area extended through the subcortical white matter into the basal ganglia, aphasia was more severe and long lasting. Aphasias with posterior and posterior plus anterior cortical lesions were more severe and long lasting if they extended into the basal ganglia. At 6 months postonset, Knopman et al. (1984) reported fluent output with predominantly phonemic paraphasia. Of course, the implications of Naeser and colleagues' (1989) paper is that the medial subcallosal fasciculus and periventricular white matter are involved in patients with no output or only stereotypies on a chronic basis.

To summarize: Aphasia with small lesions of the dominant internal capsule may be relatively rare (Fisher, 1979). With larger, dominant-hemisphere lesions of the basal ganglia and subcortical white matter, aphasia has varied between 33% (Cappa et al., 1983) and 83% (Bladin & Berkovic, 1984). A safe bet is that the rate is somewhere between these two figures and may be lower at longer times postonset. Regarding persistence of deficits, patients often make a significant degree of recovery (e.g., Wallesch, 1985), though evidence of language dysfunction frequently does persist. In some cases, residual deficits may be significant. Aphasias where cortical lesions are present are made more severe and persistent by lesion of the subcortical white matter and basal ganglia (Brunner et al., 1982; Mazzocchi & Vignolo, 1979).

Studies of Cerebral Blood Flow and Metabolism and the Basal Ganglia

The relatively recent development of positron emission tomography (PET) and single photon emission computerized tomography (SPECT) have offered investigators the opportunity to look at cerebral blood flow and/or cerebral metabolism in normal subjects and in patients with brain lesions. These scans provide images of the functional integrity of the brain, as opposed to computerized tomography (CT) or magnetic resonance (MR) scans that yield images of the structural integrity of the brain. A look at regional changes in brain functions for patients with aphasia, for example, could provide insights into the way the brain's language system operates. Because of the interconnection of language-system components, it is quite likely that structural damage to one part of the system will affect activity in other undamaged parts of the system to which it is directly or indirectly connected. There are, of course, also complications in the interpretation of PET and SPECT data; these will be addressed at the end of this section.

Metter and his colleagues have performed a series of PET studies on patients with aphasia. In their investigations, this group has studied regional metabolism of glucose while subjects were in a resting state in a quiet room with eyes and ears unoccluded. (^{18}F)-fluorodeoxyglucose was used to measure glucose metabolism. Regions of interest were specified a priori, and left-hemisphere metabolism for each region of interest usually was compared to right-hemisphere metabolism for the homologous region using a ratio of left < right. Because individual rates of glucose metabolism are highly variable, this method provided a measure that was comparable between subjects.

Metter et al. (1983) found mild depression of cortical glucose metabolism in patients with subcortical aphasia. Patients with cortical aphasias showed depression of glucose metabolism in the caudate nucleus as well as in the thalamus. Metter et al. (1984) examined correlations between language measures and glucose metabolism in various regions of interest for 11 aphasic patients. Level of glucose metabolism in the dominant caudate head was correlated with three of nine language measures: a reading comprehension and a writing measure from the Boston Diagnostic Aphasia Examination (Goodglass & Kaplan, 1983), and a speaking measure from the Porch Index of Communicative Ability (Porch, 1971). Some correlations were also seen with dominant thalamic glucose metabolism (see Chapter 3).

Metter et al. (1986) found that patients with left midputaminal hemorrhages and aphasia demonstrated diffuse left < right cortical glucose metabolism asymmetries. These asymmetries were most prominent in the temporal or temporoparietal regions but extended to a lesser degree to the frontal regions as well. Patients with aphasia and left posterior putaminal damage with lesion extending into the temporal, temporoparietal, and/or insular cortex demonstrated left < right temporoparietal metabolic asymmetries, but frontal metabolism was symmetric. One patient with aphasia and an old hemorrhage in the posterior lenticular nuclei and posterior limb of the internal capsule demonstrated left < right metabolic asymmetry in the temporoparietal cortex.

Metter et al. (1987) found greater relative metabolic decreases in the left hemisphere in the caudate head, thalamus, and cortical areas for aphasic patients demonstrating cerebellar metabolic asymmetries than for aphasic patients without cerebellar metabolic asymmetries. However, it should be noted that some patients had lesions extending into the caudate nucleus. These data would imply some relationship of cerebellar functioning to subcortical and cortical structures.

In another study of regional glucose metabolism, Metter et al. (1988) used path analysis and found damage to subcortical structures, including the anterior and posterior limbs of the internal capsule, the head of the caudate nucleus, the lenticular nuclei, the thalamus, and the insula, was correlated with frontal glucose metabolism that was in turn related to fluency. Damage to subcortical structures also had a direct effect on fluency. Of the subcortical structures examined, the anterior limb of the internal capsule seemed to have the greatest influence on frontal metabolism, but the posterior limb of the internal capsule seemed to have the greatest direct affect on fluency.

Metter et al. (1989) compared cortical and subcortical damage and glucose metabolism in patients with Broca's, Wernicke's, or conduction aphasia. Patients with Broca's aphasia had significantly greater metabolic asymmetries in the head of the caudate nucleus and thalamus than did patients with Wernicke's or conduction aphasia. However, patients with Broca's aphasia also demonstrated greater structural changes in most subcortical structures than patients with Wernicke's or conduction aphasia. Patients with Broca's and Wernicke's aphasia demonstrated greater metabolic asymmetry in the caudate head than controls.

Olsen, Bruhn, and Oberg (1986) studied regional cerebral blood flow in eight cases of aphasia due to infarction or hemorrhage of the dominant lentiform nuclei. All patients showed good-to-excellent recovery. Decreased cerebral blood flow was found in the cortex overlying the deep lesions, with flow sufficient for tissue viability but not sufficient for normal tissue function. The authors stated that the decreased cortical blood flow was invariably in the territory of the occluded artery. They suggested that language symptoms were due to the decreased cortical blood flow, which was related to arterial occlusion and not functional relationships between the lentiform nuclei and the cortex. It should be noted that this is not the common interpretation of subcortical aphasia.

Demonet et al. (1989) studied regional cerebral blood flow in cortical and subcortical aphasias using SPECT. In this study, blood flow for various regions of interest was indexed to the average within-hemisphere blood flow. This choice of measures renders comparisons between hemispheres difficult. Mean left-hemisphere cerebral blood flow was related to severity of aphasia in the cortical, but not the subcortical, aphasias. Impaired repetition in the subcortical cases (representing phonological disturbance) was associated with lower cerebral blood flow in the perisylvian region than for subcortical cases with lesser impairment in repetition. The cases with greatest impairment of repetition had lenticulo-capsular lesions. The relationship between subcortical lesions and perisylvian cortex may represent participation in common systems (Alexander et al., 1986) or commonality of supply from major arteries. In subcortical cases, patients without major impairment of comprehension demonstrated higher cerebral blood flow to the right temporoparietal region.

Alexander (1989) described four cases of nonthalamic subcortical aphasia which he considered protypical. That is, the patients had impaired speech fluency with normal language fluency, word-finding difficulties with semantic paraphasias, moderate-to-severe initiation problems on initial evaluation, and impaired auditory-verbal comprehension only at more complex levels. Infarcts were located in the putamen, caudate nucleus, internal capsule, periventricular white matter, and/or subcortical white matter. Blood flow and oxygen metabolism were measured in a resting state using PET technology. Regions of interest were defined and left/right metabolic ratios were calculated. Left-hemisphere regions showing the greatest relative decline included the frontal operculum, the lower motor cortex, the posterior parietal region, and the thalamus. These results are consistent with the findings of Metter et al. (1988) that subcortical structures influence fluency through frontal lobe structures as well as independently; however, Alexander's findings contradict the findings of Metter et al. (1986) which indicated that dominant putaminal lesions causing aphasia were most frequently associated with temporoparietal, but not frontal, hypometabolism.

A few studies of cerebral blood-flow changes in normals performing language tasks have appeared in the literature. Wallesch, Henriksen, Kornhuber, and Paulson (1985) used SPECT to compare language-production tasks (oral and silent story retelling) to nonlanguage oral-motor tasks (oral movements, counting, saying vowel-consonant syllables). In general, increases in cerebral blood flow bilaterally in the head of the caudate nucleus and unilaterally in the left pallidal/thalamic region were observed in the language production as compared to the oral-motor tasks. In a PET study, Petersen, Fox, Posner, Mintun, and Raichle (1988, 1989) were unable to detect any changes in subcortical blood flow during semantic word-production tasks.

To summarize: Decreased glucose metabolism in the region of the dominant caudate head, as well as in the dominant thalamus, has often been associated with aphasia. Some care must be exercised in interpreting these changes in glucose metabolism. Previous studies (Mata et al., 1980; Schwartz et al., 1979) have indicated that glucose metabolism changes in neural structures are the result of synaptic activity (i.e., the level of input to a structure) rather than the result of the firing rate of the involved neurons (i.e., the level of output of a structure). These findings seemed to be confirmed in a study of experimental chorea (Mitchell, Jackson, Sambrook, & Crossman, 1989). Implications for cerebral glucose-metabolism studies in aphasic patients exist. For example, decreased glucose-metabolism changes in the caudate head would represent decreased synaptic activity in this area. This decreased synaptic activity might be due to destructive lesion of the caudate nucleus which, of course, includes the synapses, or due to decreased synaptic activity secondary to reduced input to the caudate nucleus. Keeping these implications in mind, reduction in glucose metabolism in the dominant caudate head and thalamus was greater for Broca's than for Wernicke's or conduction aphasia. But lesions of the caudate nucleus, thalamus, and other subcortical structures were also more common in Broca's aphasia. Although not unequivocal, certain aspects of subcortical aphasias appear to be associated with decreased metabolism in prerolandic cortex. The question has been raised as to whether cortical changes in blood flow after subcortical lesion may be due simply to circulatory dysfunction, as opposed to being a product of the functional relationship between cortical and subcortical structures. SPECT and PET studies of language production in normals do not yet provide unequivocal evidence regarding the participation of the basal ganglia in language.

Childhood Language Disorders and the Basal Ganglia

Both because of the different implications of lesion location in childhood aphasia, and because of the implications of developmental language disturbance, it is worth discussing childhood language disorders separately. Two cases of childhood aphasia after lesion to subcortical structures can be found. Ferro, Martins, Pinto, and Castro-Caldas (1982) described a case of aphasia in a 6-year-old, left-handed girl with a right-hemisphere infarction of the putamen, globus pallidus, internal capsule, and insula. After a few hours of muteness, she demonstrated decreased spontaneous speech with nonfluent output and intact comprehension. After two weeks, only some articulation errors in spontaneous speech and repetition persisted. Aram, Rose, Rekate, and Whitaker (1983) described a 7-year-old, right-handed girl with a hemorrhagic infarction of the left putamen, head of the caudate nucleus, anterior limb of the internal capsule, and subcortical white matter. Like the case of Ferro et al., this girl was initially mute, but unlike the Ferro et al. case, she had moderate impairment of comprehension. At 40 days postonset, the patient showed nonfluent output, semantic paraphasia, and moderately impaired repetition, but intact comprehension. After 6 1/2 months, she demonstrated normal language. Aram et al. noted dysarthria but normal language in an 11-year-old, right-handed girl with an infarction of the left posterior medial putamen, posterior globus pallidus, posterior limb of the internal capsule, and body of the caudate nucleus.

There is also a description of a developmental language disorder in the literature that may have some implications for the role of the basal ganglia in language. Fisher, Kerbeshian, and Burd (1986) noted a syndrome involving pervasive developmental disorder, a tic disorder, and a characteristic pattern of speech and language impairment. Patients with this syndrome demonstrated prosodic deficiencies, mumbling, motor and/or vocal tics, repetitive stereotyped utterances, and severe developmental delays in language output and comprehension. When the authors' four patients were treated with haloperidol (a dopamine antagonist) for the tics, all four demonstrated rapid and dramatic improvement in language output, and three of four patients demonstrated rapid and dramatic improvement in language comprehension. When one patient had to be discontinued from haloperidol treatment, the language gains were lost. It is unlikely that language could have developed so rapidly after the administration of haloperidol. Rather, it is likely that some language skills had been developed in spite of the tic disorder but were unable to be used by patients until treatment for tics was initiated. If the haloperidol was acting at the level of the striatum, the implication is that a disturbance in the nigrostriatal dopamine system prevented the use of language, although some language development occurred and was latent until treatment of tics with the dopamine antagonist. One might speculate, then, that an excess level of dopamine activity within the striatum inhibited the use of the language that had developed. It should be noted, however, that the dopamine antagonist could have been active at other levels of the nervous system, including the limbic system or the cortex.

In summary: Both cases of subcortical aphasia in children have reported initially nonfluent language with eventual recovery. Given the propensity for nonfluency in childhood aphasia, even with posterior temporal lesions (Blumstein, 1981), and given the small number of cases, the importance of the nonfluent symptoms is hard to judge. The developmental disorders described by Fisher et al. (1986) suggest that the basal ganglia may be involved in the ability of people to use language, with some acquisition occurring in spite of a lack of ability to use it. This suggestion comes from the fact that some language development seemed to occur in Fisher and colleagues' patients in spite of their inability to use language prior to pharmacologic treatment. However, it should be remembered that the effects of their dopamine antagonist on language may have been operative at other levels of the nervous system than the basal ganglia.

Language and Degenerative Diseases of the Basal Ganglia

Although many problems arise in looking at language in degenerative diseases affecting the basal ganglia, some insights might be gained by exploring this topic. For the most part, degenerative diseases affecting the striatum, such as Parkinson's and Huntington's diseases, have not been thought to produce language dysfunction. This is in contrast to Alzheimer's disease, a form of dementia extensively affecting the cerebral cortex, where language dysfunction resembling transcortical sensory aphasia has been reported (e.g., Cummings, Benson, Hill, & Reed, 1985), and language dysfunction is particularly common in the more severe stages of the disorder (Faber-Langendoen et al., 1988). Actually, language dysfunction resembling the more classical forms of aphasia have not been widely reported to accompany either Parkinson's or Huntington's disease, but some studies have found more subtle dysfunctions in the language system in these disorders.

Studies comparing language abilities of patients with Parkinson's disease to neurologically normal controls have produced mixed results. The inconsistency of results is partly due to the fact that some studies have used instruments on which most of the normal subjects have received the highest score possible. This type of performance is called a "ceiling effect" for the normal subjects because their performance has reached the top level possible (ceiling) on the test. The implication is that tests on which subjects show ceiling effects do not measure the full range of the ability; when a majority of subjects demonstrate such a performance, it is uncertain what level of difficulty the test measures, so the ability of the test to detect subtle deficits is in question.

For example, studies using naming tests on which normals clearly demonstrate ceiling effects fail to show differences between normals and patients with Parkinson's disease (Bayles & Tomoeda, 1983; Cummings, Darkins, Mendez, Hill, & Benson, 1988; Pillon, Dubois, Lhermitte, & Agid, 1986; Pirozzolo, Hansch, Mortimer, Webster, & Kuskowski, 1982). On the other hand, studies utilizing naming tests which do not show ceiling effects in normals have found subnormal naming for Parkinson's disease (Globus, Mildworf, & Melamed, 1985; Matison, Mayeux, Rosen, & Fahn, 1982). From a methodological standpoint, it should be noted that these latter two studies excluded patients with a diagnosable dementia; therefore, the inclusion of patients with Alzheimer's disease cannot be the reason differences between the Parkinson's disease and normal groups were found.

Occasionally, other differences between Parkinson's disease patients and neurologically normal controls have been found. For example, below normal repetition (Matison et al., 1982) and below-normal auditory comprehension (Globus et al., 1985) have also been described. Globus et al., however, did not find that Parkinson's disease patients diverged from normal controls in verbal expression. But Cummings et al. (1988) did find decreased phrase length, decreased grammatical complexity, decreased melodic line in oral expression, and writing difficulties in addition to motor speech difficulties in 35 idiopathic Parkinson's patients without dementia, in spite of the fact that normals performed "nearly perfectly" on the test battery. Illes (1989) did not find changes in syntax during discourse for Parkinson's disease patients; however, her Parkinson's group did show longer-than-normal hesitations in discourse that were judged to be linguistic in nature as opposed to purely motoric.

Word-list-production tests, which require a subject to give as many words as possible in a certain category within a given time limit, do not usually demonstrate ceiling effects in a normal population. Results of word-list-production tasks in patients with Parkinson's disease have been mixed: patients performed below normal controls on five of ten word-list-production measures from five studies that were reviewed (Globus et al., 1985; Lees & Smith, 1983; Matison et al., 1982; Pillon et al., 1986; Taylor et al., 1986).

Studies with asymmetric Parkinson's disease affecting the right side of the body are of some interest because one would expect such patients to have greater dysfunction in the dominant striatum than the nondominant striatum. Some studies have found that patients with right asymmetric Parkinson's disease perform below patients with left asymmetric symptoms on naming (Spicer, Roberts, & LeWitt, 1988) or word-list generation (Spicer et al., 1988; Taylor et al., 1986). Yet, other studies have found no differences between right asymmetric Parkinson's patients and normals on naming (Direnfeld et al., 1984) or word-list generation (Starkstein, Leiguarda, Gershanik, & Berthier, 1987). The lack of consistency between studies may be due to the fact that significant asymmetry is frequently seen during the initial stages of Parkinson's disease, and cognitive symptoms may be less severe at this point.

Finally, some studies have compared the performance of Parkinson's disease patients to the performance of Alzheimer's disease patients on language tasks. These comparisons are important because it has been assumed that Alzheimer's disease patients show definite language dysfunction, while such an assumption has been questioned with Parkinson's disease. In spite of this assumption, results of these studies have been equivocal. Some studies have failed to show differences between the two types of patients on naming (Bayles & Tomoeda, 1983; Direnfeld et al., 1984; Pillon et al., 1986) or on word-list generation (Pillon et al., 1986) in spite of the fact that the Alzheimer's patients did show worse performance than controls for some tasks. In one study (Bayles & Tomoeda, 1983) the lack of differences between Parkinson's and Alzheimer's patients may be due to the use of less-than-severely demented Alzheimer's disease patients, who are less likely to show aphasic symptoms (Faber-Langendoen et al., 1988). Finally, Cummings et al. (1988) demonstrated differences between these two types of patients on 12 of 32 tasks in spite of ceiling effects for normals.

Studies of language phenomena have been less plentiful for patients with Huntington's disease. A lack of differences between Huntington's patients and neurologically normal controls has been found both for a naming task with ceiling effects for controls (Bayles & Tomoeda, 1983) and a naming task without a ceiling effect (Butters, Sax, Montgomery, & Tarlow, 1978). On the other hand, Kennedy, Fisher, Shoulson, and Caine (1981) found Huntington's disease subjects to show below-normal performance in naming and auditory comprehension. Smith, Butters, White, Lyon, and Granholm (1988) demonstrated that both mildly and moderately impaired Huntington's patients scored below normal controls in a naming task without ceiling effects. The latter authors hypothesized that the degree of association between words in the lexico-semantic system was weakened for Huntington's disease.

In comparison to naming tasks, performance in word-list-generation tasks has been consistently below normal in patients with Huntington's disease (Butters, Granholm, Salmon, Grant, & Wolfe, 1987; Butters et al., 1978; Butters, Wolfe, Granholm, & Martone, 1986; Kennedy et al., 1981). In addition to the interpretation describing weakening of associations between words, Butters and his colleagues have also seen word-list-generation deficits to represent problems in retrieval of information from long-term verbal-memory stores in these patients.

Some changes in spoken discourse of Huntington's disease patients have been found. In fact, Gordon and Illes (1987) reported reduction in the number of words produced in discourse tasks, diminished syntactic complexity, reduction of melodic line, increased paraphasic errors, increased word-finding difficulty, and increases in unfilled pauses for Huntington's disease patients versus controls at risk for the disease. The authors hypothesized that the types of language symptoms found depend upon the area of the caudate head that degenerates and the cortical connections of the area. They believed that a progression of symptoms begins with the anterior medial caudate head and progresses to the posterior caudate head. Because the anterior medial caudate head is connected to the dorsolateral frontal cortex, symptoms like transcortical motor aphasia develop first, gradually progressing to the more prolific paraphasia seen in Wernicke's aphasia. Actually, other studies have not found quite so obvious language deficits in Huntington's disease.

Wallesch and Fehrenbach (1988) noted a decrease in subordinate clauses and syntactic complexity, greater difficulty in naming, and a decrease in auditory verbal comprehension in late versus early Huntington's disease. When compared to controls with Friedreich's ataxia, the Huntington's disease patients in Wallesch and Fehrenbach's study demonstrated greater difficulty with naming and decreased auditory-verbal comprehension. Similar to the findings of Wallesch and Fehrenbach (1988), Podoll, Caspary, Lange, and Notch (1988) also found simplified syntactic structure without agrammatism, auditory-comprehension deficits correlating with the general level of dementia, loss of initiative in conversation, and visually related naming errors. The changes in syntactic complexity in Huntington's disease patients found in both studies are similar to changes found by Cummings et al. (1988) for Parkinson's disease patients. Illes (1989), however, found reduced syntactic complexity in discourse for Huntington's, but not Parkinson's, disease patients. Huntington's disease patients also showed longer-than-normal pauses and greater-than-normal self-corrections during discourse in this study.

Changes in syntactic complexity in Huntington's disease also bear some similarity to the two frontal lesion patients discussed by Nadeau (1988) whose lesions included but were not limited to the inferior frontal gyrus. For the most part, language difficulties were only minimally evident; however, the patients' spontaneous language gave the impression of decreased syntactic complexity, and impairment in the use of more complex syntactic structures was confirmed on formal testing.

To summarize: patients with Parkinson's disease showed below-normal performance on naming in at least two instances when the instruments used did not produce ceiling effects in normals, but their performance on word-list-generation tasks was variable from one study and one task to the next. Huntington's disease patients have shown variable performance in naming tasks, but they have shown consistently below-normal performance on word-list generation. Both Parkinson's and Huntington's disease patients have shown decreased use of complex syntactic structures that bears some similarities to frontal patients, but these changes in syntax have been more consistently found for Huntington's than Parkinson's disease patients. It would be tempting to surmise that the cortico-striato-pallido-thalamo-cortical loops are impaired in these degenerative diseases affecting the striatum, and that this impairment is responsible for the subtle language problems that resemble those of frontal patients. This hypothesis is particularly appealing when one remembers that the partial closing of these subcortical loops is to the prerolandic cortical component. However, there is one prominent problem with this interpretation: patients with Parkinson's disease, and particularly those with Huntington's disease, can show frontal atrophy at later stages in the disease, which indicates direct involvement of the frontal lobes. Of course, this may not be a question of either the frontal involvement or the basal ganglia involvement causing the subtle language difficulties since the frontal and striatal changes may well be directly related in the disease process. In other words, degeneration in these diseases may involve a system including both the striatum and the frontal cortex, and changes in language may reflect the involvement of the whole system, as opposed to either structure in isolation.

Conclusions

Data concerning the basal ganglia and various subcortical white matter structures in language can be a bit confusing, especially if one views the different types of data in isolation from one another. Considering any one source of data alone, one would have to draw the conclusion that involvement of the basal ganglia in language functions is an open question and that this question may not be resolved in the context of our current technology, our current understanding of the relationship between vascular lesion processes and cognition, and our current understanding of disease processes. But if one integrates information across several sources of data, some tentative conclusions can be derived.

One such conclusion is that subcortical white matter pathways are without question involved in language. This proposition must be true because these pathways are the means by which the various components of the language system communicate with one another. Without such communication, the coordinated output of spoken language in conversation would be impossible. Naeser, Alexander, and colleagues (Alexander, 1989; Alexander et al., 1987; Naeser et al., 1982, 1989) have made some preliminary efforts at better mapping the white matter pathways of importance in the language system. The pathways implicated in language include the medial subcallosal fasciculus which carries fibers from the mesial frontal cortex (supplementary motor area and anterior cingulate) to the caudate nucleus and may be involved in the initiation of language and speech. Other subcortical white matter pathways connect one cortical area with another, such as the connections between the supplementary motor area and Broca's area, or the connections between posterior and anterior language areas which are contained in the arcuate fasciculus. It must be remembered that subcortical white matter pathways also carry cortico-thalamic connections, thalamo-cortical connections, other cortico-striatal connections including pathways between the posterior language cortex and the head of the caudate nucleus, striato-pallidal connections, and pallido-thalamic connections. All these fiber tracts could have implications for language.

If Van Buren's (Van Buren, 1963, 1966; Van Buren et al., 1966) data indicating that irrelevant language is elicited at the offset of electrical stimulation of the caudate head are viewed in isolation, the importance of his observations is questionable. The phenomenon was seen only in a few patients and not replicated because few other studies of caudate stimulation exist. However, Schaltenbrand (1965, 1975) also described compulsory language during stimulation of the ventral anterior thalamus (see Chapter 3). Given the connections between the caudate head and the ventral anterior thalamus through the globus pallidus, these strikingly similar findings can be considered a replication of sorts and suggest that the head of the caudate nucleus and the ventral anterior thalamus are linked in language. This is consistent with the suggestion of Alexander et al. (1986) that cortico-striato-pallido-thalamo-cortical loops other than those already known will be found. Whether this loop might play a role in formulating the content of language, or might play a role in regulating language function without participating in formulation, is the question of interest. Naeser et al. (1989) and Alexander (1989) indicate that cortico-striatal connections might be important for language initiation, but they reject the idea that the corpus striatum is involved in the formulation of language. Of course, it is also possible that the phenomena reported by Van Buren and Schaltenbrand have other explanations. Theoretical implications will be further reviewed in Chapter 4.

Vascular lesion data are quite variable in most respects. Alexander et al. (1987) suggest that most of the variability can be accounted for by what white matter pathways are injured. One consistency in the data is that hemorrhagic lesion in the lentiform nuclei and head of the caudate nucleus almost invariably lead to fluent output in cases where aphasia is present. Future investigation of this phenomenon might reveal a reason for this pattern. Further, Alexander's (1989) division of nonfluent output into speech aspects and language aspects is an advance that may yield further clarity to the investigation of nonthalamic subcortical aphasias. His finding of generally fluent language (with the possible exception of initiation) in the presence of nonfluent speech will require careful replication.

Of course, there are many complications in interpreting vascular lesion data. The difficulty in determining which of the lesioned structures in aphasia may be important in language has already been discussed. A further complication is the variable time postonset in many studies, though the studies of Alexander (1989), Basso et al. (1987) and others have controlled this problem to some degree. But, in the end, the problems with time postonset may not be entirely resolvable. Acute phenomena may bring involvement of structures surrounding the lesioned structures and demand postponement of cognitive evaluation for at least a few days. Yet, the system may already be compensating for disruption by this time, obscuring the actual relationship between the lesioned structure and language.

It is also useful to look at the results of language studies in patients with degenerative diseases affecting the striatum in combination with recent vascular lesion data. Like Alexander's (1989) vascular lesion patients, patients with Parkinson's and Huntington's diseases show dysarthria but generally fluent language. However, Parkinson's and Huntington's patients do show subtle changes in that they use simplified syntax (Cummings et al., 1988; Podoll et al., 1988; Wallesch & Fehrenbach, 1988). Alexander (1989) did not explore this aspect in his subcortical patients. Several good paradigms for exploring syntax and morphology were used by Nadeau (1988) who found that patients with frontal lesions including Broca's area also had difficulties in the use of complex syntax. Future studies must explore the use of complex syntax in nonthalamic subcortical aphasias. The absence of syntactic deficits in nonthalamic subcortical aphasias would suggest that the deficit in Parkinson's and Huntington's patients is due to direct involvement of the frontal lobes. However, the presence of such deficits in the vascular-lesion, subcortical-aphasia population would emphasize the importance of the cortico-striato-pallido-thalamo-cortical loops in complex syntax.

PET studies of patients do appear to implicate the head of the caudate nucleus in some sort of language function (Metter et al., 1983, 1984, 1989), though the nature of the function is unclear. It also appears that lesions that include the basal ganglia will affect frontal metabolism and blood flow (Alexander, 1989; Metter et al., 1988). One interpretation of these data are that they support the participation of cortico-striato-pallido-thalamo-cortical loops in language, since these loops partially close by thalamic projections to the prerolandic cortex. PET and SPECT studies of neurologically normal subjects are too few to draw firm conclusions, though one wonders if the basal ganglia may be involved in narrative but not single-word production when the results of Wallesch et al. (1985) are compared to those of Petersen et al. (1988, 1989).

There are also too few studies in the area of childhood language disorders to draw firm conclusions about the participation of the basal ganglia in childhood language. It should be noted, however, that if these structures do play a regulatory role in language, the implications of this role may vary with the stage of development of the system. A definitive contribution to this literature would be welcome.

One conclusion that can be drawn about the role of the basal ganglia in language is that their role in formulation of language content may be limited. They may be involved in regulatory processes such as initiation. Such regulatory processes may have some bearing upon syntactic operations. From the standpoint of lesion studies, the role of subcortical white matter structures and the basal ganglia are almost inextricably intertwined since subcortical lesions typically involve both. At this time, it would appear that small lesions limited to one structure of the basal ganglia do not cause severe or lasting aphasia. But, one must remember that lesions confined to a single cortical structure also do not tend to cause severe or lasting aphasia (e.g., Brunner et al., 1982), and small lesions in the subcortical white matter do not tend to cause severe or lasting aphasias either (e.g., Basso et al.,

1987; Wallesch et al., 1983). One pertinent question to be addressed is whether the nervous system compensates easily for small lesions in the cortex, white matter, or basal ganglia, or whether some other process explains these phenomena.

3

The Thalamus in Language

Frequently, consideration of the effects of thalamic lesions can be simpler than trying to separate the effects of vascular basal ganglia lesions from the concomitant damage to surrounding white matter pathways. Moreover, studies of surgical lesion and electrical stimulation studies concerning the thalamus are more plentiful. The current controversy regarding the role of the dominant thalamus in language concerns not whether at least some thalamic nuclei play a direct or indirect role in language, but rather what nuclei within the thalamus are involved. The two major candidates are the pulvinar and a group of nuclei in the more anterior portion of the thalamus that includes the anterior nucleus, the ventral anterior nucleus, and the ventral lateral nucleus. Evidence that the pulvinar is involved in language derives from postmortems after hemorrhagic lesions, electrical stimulation studies, and retrograde degeneration studies. Surgical lesion studies and investigations of series of thalamic infarction cases, however, call the participation of the dominant pulvinar into question. Regarding the more anterior portions of the thalamus, surgical lesion studies, electrical stimulation data, and investigations of thalamic infarction series provide support for the involvement of these nuclei. But the comparative frequency of anomia with pulvinar versus ventral lateral stimulation calls into question the importance of the latter.

In this chapter I will explore the evidence for the involvement of the dominant thalamus in language. In addition to addressing what thalamic nuclei might be involved in language, the current chapter will also discuss the most common symptom cluster after dominant thalamic lesion and begin to explore what the role of the dominant thalamus in language might be. I will start by exploring the results of surgical lesion studies, move on to discuss electrical stimulation studies, and subsequently address vascular lesion studies. Cerebral blood flow and metabolism research as it applies to study of the role of the thalamus in language will also be covered. I will set forth a few conclusions about the meaning of this research at the end of the chapter.

Studies of Surgical Lesions of the Thalamus

As noted in Chapter 2, a serendipitous discovery revealed that interruption of the connections between the globus pallidus and the ventral lateral thalamus could mitigate symptoms of Parkinson's disease. Given the position of these nuclei in cortico-striato-pallido-thalamo-cortical loops, and given the involvement of the striatum in Parkinson's disease because of depletion of the nigrostriatal dopamine supply, this result is not surprising. This discovery eventually led to stereotactic surgeries, especially during the 1950s and 1960s, for the relief of motor symptoms of Parkinson's disease. With the increasing effectiveness of pharmacological control for Parkinson's disease, this type of neurosurgical procedure is not widely practiced today, though it is still performed in a few locations.

Although initial surgeries focused on the globus pallidus as well as the thalamus, in most locations, the standard protocol evolved into creating limited lesions in the posterior portion of the ventral lateral nucleus (e.g., Cooper et al., 1968). Many studies attempted to assess cognitive changes after these neurosurgical procedures: one frequent finding was aphasia that did not exist prior to the surgery. As I shall discuss below, such aphasic symptoms remitted rather rapidly in most cases. Many earlier texts that mention the phenomenon of thalamic aphasia rely upon these descriptions of thalamectomy as their source of information, leading them to the erroneous conclusion that thalamic aphasia inevitably remits within a few days or weeks.

Crosson (1984) reviewed the literature regarding aphasia after thalamectomy. Given the rarity of these surgeries today, no significant data has accumulated since this review. The conclusions of Crosson's 1984 review will be briefly summarized below; the reader interested in greater detail is referred to the original text. Important issues with respect to aphasia after thalamectomy include incidence of aphasia, relative incidence for left- versus right-sided lesions, target of lesion within the thalamus, and persistence of aphasia. Since ventral lateral lesions were much more common than lesions of the pulvinar, studies that deal with aphasia or language symptoms after ventral lateral lesions are much more common.

With respect to the relative incidence for left- versus right-sided lesions in the ventral lateral thalamus, the cumulative results of studies in the literature are not entirely unequivocal. Two studies (Cooper et al., 1968; Waltz et al., 1966) reported no difference between the incidence of aphasia and/or dysarthria for left- versus right-hemisphere lesion. The Waltz et al. study clearly suffered from a lack of separation of aphasia and dysarthria. (The former represents an actual impairment of language while the latter is due to paralysis or weakness of the muscles needed for articulation.) Another study (Gillingham et al., 1960) reported aphasia only in patients who received bilateral thalamectomies. However, a clear majority of studies indicate a greater incidence of aphasia after left unilateral ventral lateral thalamic as opposed to right ventral lateral thalamic lesions (Allen et al., 1966; Asso et al., 1969; Bell, 1968; Cooper, 1958; Darley, Brown, & Swenson, 1975; Samra et al., 1969; Selby, 1967). Other studies have taken the approach of studying specific language functions after ventral lateral thalamectomy. These studies have shown decreases in naming, word fluency, and comprehension to be greater after left-hemisphere operations (Ojemann, 1975; Riklan et al., 1969; Vilkki & Laitinen, 1974, 1976).

The actual percentages for incidence of aphasia vary considerably, depending upon how the researcher breaks down the data. In studies where the incidence cannot be retrieved from the manuscript by side of lesion, the figure varies from 3% (Gillingham et al., 1960) or 7% (Cooper, 1958) to approximately 13% (Waltz et al., 1966). However, if one considers those studies broken down by side of lesion, the incidence of aphasia after left ventral lateral thalamectomy varies from 16% (Allen et al., 1966) to approximately 42% (Selby, 1967), with the median for seven studies being 25% (Allen et al., 1966; Bell, 1968; Cooper et al., 1968; Darley et al., 1975; Riklan et al., 1969; Samra et al., 1969; Selby, 1967). The incidence of aphasia after right ventral lateral operations (excluding patients who are left-handed and show aphasia) varies from zero% (Allen et al., 1966; Bell, 1968; Riklan et al., 1969; Samra et al., 1969) to as high as 25% (Cooper et al., 1968). The reader should note that four of these six studies showed a figure of zero% (Darley et al., 1975, is the sixth study). Figures for aphasia after bilateral ventral lateral thalamectomies range from 7% (Allen et al., 1966) to 50% (Samra et al., 1969). The median for six studies is 24% (Allen et al., 1966; Asso et al., 1969; Bell, 1968; Darley et al., 1975; Riklan et al., 1969; Samra et al., 1969), which is consistent with the incidence of aphasia after unilateral left ventral lateral thalamectomy. The consistency between the figures for left and bilateral ventral lateral operations indicates that the addition of a right-hemisphere lesion does not increase the likelihood of aphasia, though some investigators would not agree (e.g., Gillingham et al., 1960). If one simply looks at an increase in naming difficulty from preoperative levels, Ojemann (1975) found such an increase in seven of ten patients.

The persistence of symptoms after ventral lateral thalamectomies varies. Some investigations give the impression that changes in language disappear almost entirely after a few weeks (Cooper, 1958; Riklan et al., 1969; Waltz et al., 1966). Others note the persistence of aphasia in a few cases (Samra et al., 1969; Selby, 1967). The finding of persistent aphasia after ventral lateral thalamic ablation is rare, but Bell (1968) did report persistent symptoms for 4–48 months in 40% of those patients who experienced postoperative aphasia.

Only two studies explored changes in language after pulvinar lesion. Brown, Riklan, Waltz, Jackson, & Cooper (1971) found that only 1 of 11 patients showed postoperative changes in language, and that patient had an aphasia preoperatively. Vilkki and Laitinen (1976) indicated that patients with left pulvinar lesions did not show the same language changes as patients with left ventral lateral lesions.

Thus, studies reporting language changes after thalamectomy exhibit some variability. The possible reasons for this variability are numerous. Operative protocols in different locations are one potential source of variability. In ventral lateral thalamectomies, the posterior portion of the nucleus was usually the target. Perhaps the proximity of the lesion to the more anterior portions of the ventral lateral nucleus or even to the neighboring nucleus, ventral anterior, had some effects on the incidence or permanence of aphasia. Since lesions were electrolytic, cryogenic, or chemically induced, the type of lesion created could also have some differing effects on surrounding tissues. The method of observation may have had an effect on the incidence of aphasia reported. Most studies were conducted before the advent of standardized aphasia testing, so unstandardized clinical observations and examinations were used. The abilities of different clinical techniques and different clinicians to observe language deficit could vary considerably. When Ojemann (1975) used a standard naming test on a pre- and postoperative basis in a small sample, he did note changes in naming ability in 70% of the patients with left ventral lateral lesions. A further possible source of variance is the way in which speech and language symptoms were separated: Some studies did not separate language (cognitive) and speech (motor) symptoms.

If one considers thalamectomy studies in isolation, one might conclude that the dominant ventral lateral thalamus might be involved in language. However, in reaching such a conclusion, one would have to account for the fact that aphasia after ventral lateral thalamectomy usually remits within a few days. Crosson (1984) concluded that the effects of ventral lateral lesion might arise from temporary disturbance of tissue in areas surrounding but not included in the lesion. Based upon the examination of thalamectomy data, one might conclude that the pulvinar is not involved in language. On the other hand, examination of electrical stimulation data leads us to a different conclusion.

Studies of Electrical Stimulation of the Thalamus

During the course of therapeutic thalamectomies for movement disorder, pain, or other problems, neurosurgeons would implant electrodes and perform electrical stimulation to help verify localization for ablation (Ojemann, 1983; Selby, 1967). This protocol also enabled some investigators to study the effects of electrical stimulation of the thalamus on language. As with the thalamectomy data discussed above, only a few new studies have been published since Crosson's (1984) review of the literature. Stimulation studies will be briefly reviewed below. The reader wishing more detail is referred to Crosson (1984) or the original studies.

Most of the more carefully controlled studies in this area have been performed by Ojemann and his colleagues (Ojemann, 1975, 1977; Ojemann & Fedio, 1968; Ojemann, Fedio, & Van Buren, 1968; Ojemann & Ward, 1971). It is worth noting their technique because it has some specific advantages over many other stimulation studies. Their task required subjects to say "This is a...," then to name the object shown to them on a slide. Naming errors were only considered to have been made when the patient was able to say the phrase "This is a..." without being able to correctly name the object on the slide.

The biggest advantage of this technique is that it allows for separation of errors in naming (i.e., errors of language) from inability to speak at all. This distinction is important because an inability to speak at all may be caused by an inability to move or initiate movement in the muscles involved in speech. Such an interruption of motoric function does not necessarily imply impairment of the formulation or comprehension of language. On the other hand, failure to correctly name an object when the capability of speaking has not been affected can be considered an error in language.

Ojemann and his colleagues studied language during stimulation of both the pulvinar and ventral lateral thalamus. Ojemann et al. (1968) demonstrated naming errors in five of eight patients with left pulvinar stimulation. One left-handed patient showed anomia with right pulvinar stimulation; no other patients demonstrated anomia with right pulvinar stimulation. Errors included omission of the object name, substitution of the name of another object, and perseveration-- errors also made with thalamic aphasia. Errors in naming photographs from memory (as opposed to naming the object while looking at its photograph) (Ojemann, 1977; Ojemann & Fedio, 1968) can also be elicited by stimulating the dominant pulvinar either during presentation of the stimulus or during recall of the object name. Although the authors consider these results as reflecting verbal-memory abilities, it seems more likely that they represent difficulties in object naming, whether the patient is naming from the actual stimulus or from his/her memory of it.

Ojemann and Ward (1971) found that 4 of 13 patients with left ventral lateral stimulation showed anomia; 2 others showed perseveration. Perseveration and anomia could not be elicited with right ventral lateral stimulation. Similarly, Ojemann (1975) reported anomia or perseveration from 7 of 17 patients with left ventral lateral stimulation. Errors in naming photographs from recall increased from baseline levels when left ventral lateral stimulation was performed during recall but decreased from baseline levels when stimulation was performed during presentation of the pictures (Ojemann, 1975; Ojemann, Blick, & Ward, 1971). Again, one must exercise caution in interpreting the results as reflecting verbal memory functions because the task can be interpreted as requiring naming of objects under slightly different conditions than the original naming studies (i.e., naming the object from a visual memory as opposed to recalling the word after having seen the picture).

Rates of anomia during ventral lateral versus pulvinar stimulation are most easily compared by reading Ojemann (1977). Nine of 21 cases (43%) stimulated in the dominant ventral lateral thalamus showed anomia, while 15 of 18 cases (83%) stimulated in the dominant pulvinar demonstrated this phenomenon. There were no cases of anomia after stimulation of the nondominant ventral lateral nucleus or pulvinar. Thus, it should be noted that there is a greater density of naming errors with stimulation of the dominant pulvinar than with stimulation of the dominant ventral lateral thalamus.

Schaltenbrand (1965, 1975) reported a rather different phenomenon with stimulation of nuclei in the more anterior portions of the thalamus (ventral anterior; ventral lateral, pars oralis; anterior ventral). Schaltenbrand described compulsory language that could not be inhibited even if the patient was asked to do so. In such instances, the patients uttered phrases or short sentences that had little relevance to the experimental situation. Sometimes, repeated stimulation would elicit the same verbalization; at other times, repeated stimulation would elicit different verbalizations. This phenomenon was primarily noted in the dominant thalamus; it was shown in 6 of 12 patients with dominant thalamic stimulation, but only 2 of 14 with nondominant thalamic stimulation. In the later work (1975), Schaltenbrand noted that compulsory language was elicited from about one-quarter of his patients, more commonly with stimulation of the dominant thalamus. Although this phenomenon was not universal, it is quite important. Schaltenbrand (1965, p. 839) noted that stimulation of the cortex never leads to the production of words or sentences. Penfield and Roberts (1959) or Ojemann (1983) can be consulted to confirm the lack of elicitation of language with cortical stimulation. It is of interest that Schaltenbrand (1975) speculated that the role of the thalamus in language might be the "releasing and silencing of preformed patterns" (including phonemes, words, half sentences, and whole sentences).

Actually, as discussed in the previous chapter, there is one other place in the nervous system from which language can be evoked with electrical stimulation: the dominant caudate head (Van Buren, 1963, 1966; Van Buren et al., 1966). When one compares the language evoked from caudate and thalamic stimulation, the similarities are striking. In both instances, patients utter words, phrases, or short sentences that are irrelevant to the experimental context. However, one important difference should be noted: language tends to be elicited at the offset of stimulation in the caudate head, but from Schaltenbrand's descriptions, language is apparently elicited during the electrical stimulation in the rostral nuclei of the thalamus. I will discuss the probable relationship between these striatal and thalamic phenomena in the next chapter.

Two studies have appeared in the generally available literature since 1984. Both examined the effects of dominant thalamic stimulation on dichotic listening for words. Ojemann (1985) stimulated the dominant ventral lateral nucleus (9 cases) and the nondominant ventral lateral nucleus (5 cases) during a dichotic listening task. The task involved the simultaneous presentation of different words to the left and right ears. The words differed with respect to only one speech sound. Under normal circumstances, subjects will report correctly a greater number of words from the right ear than the left ear. This "right-ear effect" has been interpreted as a sign of left-hemisphere dominance for language. Ojemann found that his subjects who were stimulated in the left ventral lateral thalamus during dichotic listening showed improved performance for dichotic words in both ears (i.e., subjects demonstrated the same degree of right-ear effect as during the unstimulated trials). For patients stimulated in the right ventral lateral thalamus during dichotic listening, no significant change over the unstimulated condition was observed. The author accounted for increased performance during left thalamic stimulation by hypothesizing an alerting response for language specific to the left ventral lateral thalamus.

Bhatnager et al. (1989) gave a dichotic listening task to one patient both before and after therapeutic thalamic stimulation for chronic pain. The electrode for this stimulation was implanted in the left centre median nucleus, and the period of stimulation was 20 minutes. Surprisingly, the patient demonstrated an improvement in left-ear response when the consonant-vowel-consonant words were presented simultaneously or with minimal lag in the presentation between the words. Because SPECT images indicated increased blood flow to the thalamus bilaterally after the stimulation period, the authors hypothesized the increased left-ear performance to be due to improved transmission of linguistic information from the right to the left hemisphere. Right-ear performance did not improve, according to the authors, because it was at near-maximum performance before stimulation. The authors accounted for the bilateral effects on SPECT by assuming that stimulation near the junction of the midbrain and thalamus allowed for spread of the stimulation effects from the left hemisphere to the right hemisphere through the midbrain reticular formation.

In summary: Anomia has been produced after both dominant ventral lateral and dominant pulvinar stimulation. The percentage of patients showing anomia is higher in pulvinar than ventral lateral stimulation. Anomia is not shown when the nondominant ventral lateral nucleus and nondominant pulvinar are stimulated, indicating lateralization of language function at the level of the thalamus (Ojemann, 1977). Spontaneous, irrelevant language has been reported from stimulation of the more anterior portions of the dominant thalamus, and very occasionally from the more anterior portions of the nondominant thalamus (Schaltenbrand, 1965, 1975). More recently, improvement in dichotic listening has been shown with stimulation of the dominant ventral lateral nucleus and the dominant intralaminar nuclei, but not with stimulation of the nondominant ventral lateral nucleus (Bhatnager et al., 1989; Ojemann, 1985). One hypothesis regarding the ventral lateral nucleus suggests that it is involved in an alerting response specific to language.

Some cautions must be applied when interpreting subcortical electrical stimulation data. Ojemann (1976) noted that the most likely explanation for anomia during thalamic stimulation was that the electrical stimulation introduces a signal into the system that cannot be interpreted by the system and interferes with the processing of other signals. Thus, such stimulation acts somewhat like a temporary lesion of the stimulated area. Crosson (1984) noted several possible explanations: (1) electrical stimulation could have excited some process contradictory to language; (2) stimulation could have excited mechanisms that inhibit certain language functions; (3) electrical stimulation could have "overloaded" language mechanisms, temporarily making them refractory to further neural responses; (4) stimulation could have spread locally beyond the target structure into surrounding structures; or (5) stimulation could have been conducted along neural pathways to distant structures that may be more directly involved in language. Ojemann (1976) did note controls used in his studies to prevent the local spread of stimulation. He and his colleagues stimulated below levels that would elicit motor responses (ruling out spread to the internal capsule) and below levels that would elicit somatosensory sensations (ruling out spread from the nuclei stimulated to adjacent sensory nuclei). I will discuss the potential meaning of these stimulation data more fully in the next chapter.

Studies of Vascular Lesion in the Thalamus

Blood Supply

Studies of vascular lesion of the thalamus are not quite so problematic as studies of the basal ganglia. Although lesions of other structures can accompany thalamic vascular lesions, the fact that the thalamus is primarily supplied by the terminal portions of four or five small arteries or arterial groups means that some vascular lesions can be confined to this structure. In their discussion of thalamic infarction, Graff-Radford et al. (1985) and Bogousslavsky, Regli, and Uske (1988) discussed thalamic circulation. It should be noted that Bogousslavski et al. did not include the anterior choroidal artery as supplying the thalamus, noting this as a controversial matter. Graff-Radford et al. did not include the posterior choroidal arteries.

Table 3-1 notes the nuclei in the territory of each of the five arteries or arterial groups described in one or both of the studies mentioned above (Bogousslavsky et al., 1988; Graff-Radford et al., 1985). It can be seen that the posterior lateral portions of the thalamus are supplied by the geniculothalamic arteries, themselves derived from the posterior cerebral artery. Anterior lateral portions of the thalamus are supplied by the tuberothalamic artery, also known as the polar artery. The tuberothalamic artery is usually derived from the posterior communi-

Table 3-1. Arterial Territories of the Thalamus[a]

Artery	Thalamic Nuclei Supplied
Tuberothalamic (polar) artery	Ventral anterior nucleus Ventral lateral nucleus (partial) Dorsal medial nucleus (partial) Anterior nuclei (partial)
Thalamic paramedian (interpeduncular profundus) artery	Intralaminar nuclei Dorsal medial nucleus (partial) [Zona incerta] [Red nucleus]
Geniculothalamic arteries	Ventral posterior lateral nucleus Ventral posterior medial nucleus Medial geniculate body Pulvinar (partial) Centre median nucleus (partial)
Anterior choroidal artery	Pulvinar (partial) Ventral lateral (partial) [Globus pallidus] [Posterior limb of internal capsule]
Posterior choroidal arteries	Lateral geniculate body Anterior nuclei Dorsal medial nucleus (partial) Pulvinar (partial)

[a]Because of individual variations, the territories described in this table cannot be considered invariate. For example, Castaigne et al. (1981) described variations of the thalamic paramedian artery. References used for this table include: Archer, Ilinsky, Goldfader, & Smith (1981), Bogousslavsky, Regli, & Uske (1988), Castaigne et al. (1981), Gorelick, Hier, Benevento, Levitt, & Tan (1984), Graff-Radford, Damasio, Yamada, Eslinger, & Damasio (1985), and Percheron (1973).

cating artery. The thalamic paramedian artery, also known as the interpenduncular profundus artery, supplies portions of the medial thalamus. The thalamic paramedian artery also supplies the red nucleus at the level of the midbrain and the zona incerta. This artery is derived from the posterior cerebral artery. The posterior choroidal arteries, derived from the posterior cerebral artery, supply the region of the lateral geniculate body. Finally, the anterior choroidal artery supplies portions of the lateral thalamus, as well as portions of the basal ganglia and internal capsule. The anterior choroidal artery is derived directly from the internal carotid artery in many cases, but from the middle cerebral artery or the posterior communicating artery in some cases (Carpenter & Sutin, 1983). Thus, it can be seen that there is some overlap in circulation between the thalamus and other structures, but not nearly so much as in the basal ganglia.

Table 3-2. Criteria of Cambier et al. (1982)[a] and Crosson (1984) for Thalamic Aphasia

Cambier et al. (1982)	Crosson (1984)
Paraphasia in naming (primarily semantic)	Frequent paraphasia (primarily semantic)
Incoherence in narrative discourse	Jargon
Absence of significant comprehension deficits	Less severe deficits in auditory comprehension
Normal repetition	Intact or minimally impaired repetition
Reduced vocal volume (increasing across the course of a verbalization)	
Aspontaneity in oral expression	
Pauses in oral expression	
Word-finding deficit (with frequent perseveration)	

[a]Cited by Demonet (1987).

Before discussing data concerning language and vascular lesion of the thalamus, I must pay some attention to the way in which thalamic aphasia has been defined. In his 1984 review concerning the role of the thalamus in language, Crosson noted three questions with respect to the issue of "thalamic" aphasia. First, is there a unique cluster of symptoms after thalamic lesion that defines a syndrome that differs from other types of aphasia? Second, if a pattern of language deficits exists, is it directly attributable to thalamic language functions, or can some other explanation account for the phenomena? Third, does aphasia after thalamic lesion last long enough to justify consideration of the thalamus as mediating important language functions?

Varying answers have been given to the syndrome question. Table 3-2 compares the symptoms of thalamic aphasia according to Crosson (1984) and Cambier, Elghozi, and Graveleau (see Demonet, 1987). Crosson's definition included four criteria: (1) fluent output with frequent paraphasia, primarily semantic (i.e., the substitution of one word for another), is present; (2) sometimes paraphasia is so severe that it deteriorates into jargon; (3) auditory comprehension is less severely impaired than language output; (4) repetition is minimally impaired. Cambier and colleagues' definition is a bit more restrictive, requiring the absence of significant comprehension deficits and normal repetition. Cambier et al. added further characteristics, including reduced vocal volume, aspontaneity in oral expression, pauses in oral expression, and word-finding deficit with frequent perseveration.

Demonet (Demonet et al., 1989) and Puel (Puel et al., 1984, 1986) have termed this syndrome "dissident aphasia." Demonet and colleagues (1989) noted that the syndrome occurs in cases of dominant subcortical lesion other than thalamic lesion and that not all symptoms occur in all cases. They noted as primary symptoms reduced spontaneous speech, verbal paraphasias and perseverations, absence of severe comprehension disorders, and normal word repetition. Thus, there are similarities between authors in the way thalamic aphasia is defined, with the main differences being which symptoms should be included and the degree to which different symptoms are shown.

The following discussion will deal with the questions of syndrome, cause, and persistence of aphasia after vascular thalamic lesion. Since these questions might be answered differently depending upon whether patients have hemorrhage or infarction, these two entities will be covered in different sections. It should be further noted that the problems with interpreting infarction versus hemorrhage data also vary, further justifying the need to consider these categories of lesion separately.

Aphasia after Dominant Thalamic Hemorrhage

Crosson's (1984) review contained 37 cases of aphasia after thalamic hemorrhage from 18 different studies (Alexander & LoVerme, 1980; Bugiani, Conforto, & Sacco, 1969; Cappa & Vignolo, 1979; Chesson, 1983; Ciemans, 1970; Crosson, Parker, Warren, LaBreche, & Tully, 1983; Fazio, Sacco, & Bugiani, 1973; Glosser, Kaplan, & LoVerme, 1982; Horenstein, Chung, & Brenner, 1978; Jenkyn, Alberti, & Peters, 1981; Kirshner & Kistler, 1982; Maiuri, Signorelli, Colella, & Gangemi, 1983; Metter et al., 1983; Mohr, Watters, & Duncan, 1975; Penfield & Roberts, 1959; Reynolds, Harris, Ojemann, & Turner, 1978; Reynolds, Turner, Harris, Ojemann, & Davis, 1979; Wahoske, Johnson, & Rubens, 1976). All but two cases had their hemorrhage in the left thalamus. In the two cases with right thalamic lesion, the right hemisphere was assumed to be the language-dominant hemisphere. In general, cases of thalamic hemorrhage with aphasia have not been published widely since the 1984 review, because the number of previous reports has made such cases less interesting, and because difficulties in the interpretation of behavioral symptoms after hemorrhage exist (see discussion below). Nonetheless, Demonet (1987) did have a large series of aphasia cases after subcortical lesion. This series included 12 cases of thalamic lesion, who were examined in the acute phase (one month or less postonset), of which 11 were hemorrhagic.

The first issue I will address for these cases of aphasia after dominant thalamic hemorrhage is how well they fit criteria established for the syndrome of thalamic aphasia, such as those of Cambier et al. (1982) or Crosson (1984). In considering this issue, let us turn first to the cases reviewed by Crosson (1984). Twenty-three of the 37 thalamic hemorrhage cases he reviewed provided enough data to assess all four of his criteria for thalamic aphasia. Ten of these 23 cases met all four criteria for thalamic aphasia. An additional 12 met all but one of the four criteria for thalamic aphasia; in all 12 cases paraphasia, but not jargon, was mentioned. It is probable that many of these 12 cases had a milder form of the syndrome. Only one case (Glosser et al., 1982) did not meet at least three of the four criteria; in this case, the mass effect was felt to extend from the thalamus as far as the lateral putamen and external capsule acutely, and a late CT scan showed a lesion in the region of the external capsule and lateral putamen. Thus, in the case that did not meet the 1984 definition of thalamic aphasia, the acute effects extended from the thalamus into other structures.

In his dissertation, Demonet (1987) provided enough information to assess his 12 cases of thalamic aphasia with evaluations between 1 week and 1 month postonset by both Crosson's (1984) and Cambier and colleagues' (1982) criteria for thalamic aphasia. If all criteria had to be met, 9 of the 12 cases of thalamic aphasia met Crosson's criteria, but only 2 of 12 cases met all of Cambier and colleagues' criteria. In the latter instance, the reasons that cases did not fit Cambier and colleagues' criteria included absence of a reduction in spontaneous language (2), absence of hypophonia (4), and the presence of some comprehension deficit (6).

A case reported in 1983 by Papagno and Guidotti was not picked up by the 1984 review. The patient showed a lack of fluent speech, minimally impaired repetition, some impairment of comprehension, and a predominance of neologisms. Thus, this case cannot be said to match the four ciriteria for thalamic aphasia. One other case of thalamic hemorrhage with aphasia reported since 1984 is worth mentioning. Robin and Schienberg (1990) reported a case of dominant thalamic hemorrhage with aphasia including fluent output, a predominance of neologisms and phonemic paraphasias, mildly impaired auditory comprehension, and severely impaired repetition. Thus, this case, too, did not meet or approximate the 1984 criteria for thalamic aphasia. In this regard, it should be noted that the lesion was reported to extend from the anterior and medial thalamus into the anterior limb of the internal capsule; this unusual extension into the anterior limb of the internal capsule could account for the impaired repetition.

When one considers the criteria of Cambier et al. (1982) and Crosson (1984), the bulk of the evidence does suggest certain conclusions. First, in cases of aphasia after dominant thalamic hemorrhage, hypophonia, reduced spontaneity, total absence of comprehension deficit, and jargon may be found, but they are not essential components of the aphasia syndrome. Second, paraphasia (primarily semantic), comprehension less impaired than output, and relatively intact repetition can be considered as part of the syndrome. In many cases, the aphasia may be mild, but in some cases the aphasia may be severe enough that output deteriorates to jargon.

The next issue I will address is intrathalamic localization. In most cases of thalamic hemorrhage, precise statements about localization cannot be made due to possible pressure effects; however, some trends can be found in cases where postmortems were performed. In some cases, hemorrhage was reported to include virtually the entire dominant thalamus (Bugiani et al., 1969; Ciemans, 1970; Fazio et al., 1973; Mohr et al., 1975). In one case of thalamic aphasia (Mohr et al., 1975), hemorrhage involved more anterior portions of the dominant thalamus and surrounding structures. However, Kameyama (1976/77) notes aphasia showed up in only two of 42 cases of thalamic (ventral posterior lateral) lesion, and in both cases the lesion was hemorrhagic and extended into the pulvinar. Both Ciemans (1970) and Mohr et al. (1975) reported cases of aphasia in which lesions were confined to the dominant pulvinar and surrounding nuclei. Finally, the case of Crosson et al. (1983, 1986) had a lesion in the dorsal nucleus that extended into the anterior superior pulvinar. This lesion (actually a hemorrhagic infarction) extended from lateral to medial in a horizontal plane in this part of the pulvinar.

In one post-1984 study, Kawahara et al. (1986) reported aphasia in 6 of 28 small hemorrhages in the posterolateral thalamic region. Although the authors did not report side of lesion with respect to aphasia, 13 of 28 posterolateral lesions were in the left hemisphere. One patient with a small dorsal left thalamic hemorrhage also had a transient aphasia. Involvement of the pulvinar to at least some extent was consistent with all cases showing aphasia. The case of Papagno and Guidotti (1983) also had a posterior thalamic hemorrhage that could be consistent with involvement of the pulvinar. To summarize, if one takes the data of Kameyama (1976/1977), Ciemans (1970), Mohr et al. (1975), Crosson et al. (1983, 1986), Kawahara et al. (1986), and Papagno and Guidotti (1983) into account, these hemorrhagic cases would be consistent with an involvement of the pulvinar in language. This conclusion would be consistent with the high density of naming errors found in electrical stimulation of the anterior superior lateral pulvinar (Ojemann, 1977).

One further study since 1984 has relevence to both the issues of intrathalamic localization in hemorrhagic lesions and—indirectly— incidence. Cappa, Papagno, Vallar, and Vignolo (1986) described five cases of hemorrhage in the posterior portion of the dominant thalamus in which no aphasia occurred. Likewise, Hirose et al. (1985) failed to mention aphasia in two cases of posterior dominant thalamic hemorrhage, but cognitive disturbances were not the focus of their study. Cappa et al. (1986) noted that it was difficult to draw firm conclusions regarding intrathalamic localization and aphasia based on their data, given the contradictory indications in previous literature. Some data on thalamic infarcts (Graff-Radford et al., 1985), which will be discussed below, point more to anterior portions of the thalamus than the pulvinar, yet some data on hemorrhage does point to the pulvinar, as discussed above. The hemorrhages of Cappa et al. (1986) without aphasia undoubtedly included the dominant pulvinar.

The frequency of aphasia after dominant thalamic hemorrhage is also an issue of some interest. If the incidence is quite low, it would call the notion of thalamic aphasia into question. Crosson (1984) cited two studies in which incidence could be determined. Walshe, Davis, and Fisher (1977) reported aphasia in four of seven (57%) cases who survived dominant thalamic hemorrhage and were examined for language deficits. Cappa and Vignolo (1979) reported aphasia in seven of eight (88%) cases of dominant thalamic hemorrhage.

The issue of persistence of thalamic aphasia after dominant thalamic hemorrhage is also of some interest. Data reported on thalamectomy cases give the impression that aphasia after dominant thalamic lesion is a very transient phenomenon in an overwhelming majority of cases. Indeed, some authors have even referred to aphasia after dominant thalamic lesion in general as a transitory phenomenon (e.g., Benson, 1979). Fifteen of the hemorrhagic cases reviewed by Crosson (1984) were followed over at least a minimal time period. Aphasia persisted for at least 2 months and up to 32 months in 12 of 15 cases reviewed. Aphasia remitted in the other three cases. At 22 months postonset, Robin and Schienberg (1990) also reported persistence of severe impairment in naming, repetition, and writing with some improvement of other functions for their case of dominant thalamic hemorrhage.

It is probably true that cases of persisting aphasia are overreported in the literature compared to those that remit because the longer-lasting cases are more likely to catch the attention of clinicians and researchers. Thus, the figure of 13 of 16 cases of aphasia (81%) persisting is, in actuality, an over-estimate of the number of cases of aphasia that persist after dominant thalamic hemorrhage. Nonetheless, this figure is impressive enough to suggest that thalamic aphasia deserves serious attention as a long-term phenomenon.

To summarize: Aphasia after dominant thalamic hemorrhage does appear to cohere into a syndrome. The syndrome involves paraphasias predominantly of the semantic type, comprehension less impaired than verbal output, and minimally impaired repetition. The phenomenon is frequent but not invariably present after dominant thalamic hemorrhage, and some language deficit persists in many cases. Though aphasia is not always present after hemorrhage in the dominant pulvinar, available evidence points to the pulvinar as the nucleus involved in language.

However, some caution must be exercised in attempting to localize behavioral symptoms on the basis of hemorrhagic lesions, at least acutely. The intracerebral hematomas that acutely present as a result of intracerebral hemorrhages most likely exert pressure effects on structures surrounding the hematoma (Graff-Radford et al., 1984; McFarling et al., 1982). The effects on neighboring structures may alter symptom patterns. Thus, one cannot be certain whether symptoms are due to the primary effects of thalamic hematomas or secondary pressure effects on different structures, and this observation raises some question about the syndrome of thalamic aphasia based upon hemorrhage data. Since pressure effects dissipate as the hematoma is resorbed, this criticism is not so relevant to observations about the persistence of aphasia after dominant thalamic hemorrhage. In order to overcome this difficulty of pressure effects due to intracerebral hematomas, some investigators have turned to the examination of aphasia after dominant thalamic infarction.

Aphasia after Dominant Thalamic Infarction

With respect to the question of syndrome, dominant thalamic infarctions present a considerably more variable picture than dominant thalamic hemorrhages. Of the nine cases reviewed by Crosson (1984), only three met all four criteria for thalamic aphasia, and one additional case met three of his four criteria with no major contradictions of the criteria (see Table 3-3) (Archer, Ilinsky, Goldfader, & Smith, 1981; Cohen, Gelfer, & Sweet, 1980; Demeurisse et al., 1979; Graff-Radford et al., 1984; McFarling et al., 1982). Reasons for cases not fitting the

Table 3-3. How Cases of Infarction Fit Crosson's (1984) Criteria for Thalamic Aphasia

Source	Degree of fit		
	Good fit	Fair fit[a]	No fit
Cases reviewed by Crosson (1984)	3	1	5
Cases since 1984[b]	5	3	7

[a]Cases meeting three of four of Crosson's (1984) criteria for thalamic aphasia, with no major contradiction of the criteria.
[b]Bogousslavsky, Regli, & Assal (1986), Bruyn (1989), Fasanaro et al. (1987), Fensore, Lazzarino, Nappo, & Nicolai (1988), Gorelick, Hier, Benevento, Levitt, & Tan (1984), Mori, Yamadori, & Mitani (1986), Puel, Demonet, Cardebat, Berry, & Celsis (1989), Robin and Schienberg (1990), Tuszinski and Petito (1988)

syndrome included comprehension as impaired as output (four cases), predominance of phonemic paraphasias (one case), and an absence of paraphasias (one case—who also showed comprehension as impaired as output). Although these cases did not generally meet the four criteria for thalamic aphasia, it is worth noting that all nine cases had unimpaired repetition.

Several cases of thalamic infarction have been published since that time (Bogousslavsky, Regli, & Assal, 1986; Bruyn, 1989; Demonet et al., 1989; Fasanaro et al., 1987; Fensore, Lazzarino, Nappo, & Nicolai, 1988; Gorelick et al., 1984; Mori et al., 1986; Puel et al., 1989; Robin & Schienberg, 1990; Tuszynski & Petito, 1988) that contain enough detail to allow them to be examined for consistency with Crosson's (1984) criteria. Of the additional 15 cases (see Table 3-3), 5 met all four criteria for thalamic aphasia, and 3 cases met three of four criteria with no major contradictions. The reasons for not meeting the criteria in the other seven cases included comprehension as impaired as output (two cases), absence of paraphasias (two cases), nonfluent language (two cases—one of which had comprehension as impaired as output), impaired repetition (two cases), and predominance of phonemic paraphasias (two cases—one of which also had impaired repetition). Thus, it can be seen that cases of dominant thalamic infarction do not fit the 1984 definition of thalamic aphasia nearly as well as the cases of dominant thalamic hemorrhage. In particular, comprehension may be equally impaired to output; phonemic paraphasias occasionally predominate over semantic paraphasias, or a lack of paraphasias is reported; or language may be nonfluent. Regarding repetition, this function was unimpaired or minimally impaired in 12 of these 15 cases, less impaired than other language functions in one case, and as impaired as other language functions in 2 cases.

Table 3-4. Cases of Dominant Thalamic Infarction with Aphasia by Lesion Territory and by Fit with Thalamic Aphasia Criteria[a]

| | Degree of fit | | |
Artery	Good fit	Fair fit	No fit
Tuberothalamic	1	2	6
Paramedian	1	—	3
Geniculothalamic	1	—	—
Anterior choroidal	1	2	1
Posterior choroidal	—	—	—

[a]Four of the cases reported in Table 3-3 did not have localization precise enough to classify arterial distribution.

One of Robin and Schienberg's (1990) two cases of dominant thalamic infarction had impaired repetition, but in this case the lesion extended into the anterior and posterior limbs of the internal capsule. When viewed with their case of dominant thalamic hemorrhage, both cases of Robin and Schienberg with impaired repetition had extensions of the lesion into the anterior limb of the internal capsule. This extension may have been responsible for the impaired repetition.

The question of intrathalamic localization is of some interest. Table 3-4 shows the arterial territories of the cases reviewed above for which adequate data exists. (In some cases, the arterial territory involved was inferred from location of lesion.) Aphasia occurs more frequently after dominant thalamic infarction in the territory of the tuberothalamic (polar) artery than in other arterial territories. The tuberothalamic territory includes the ventral anterior nucleus and portions of the anterior, ventral lateral, and dorsal medial nuclei. Aphasia also occurs after infarction in the territory of the paramedian thalamic (interpeduncular profundus) artery. There is no apparent difference in the percentage of cases in either of these two territories that meet the 1984 definition of thalamic aphasia. The majority of cases (2/3) do not meet this definition. If the ventral anterior nucleus (tuberothalamic territory) and the intralaminar nuclei (paramedian territory) are indeed linked, either directly by fibers from the intralaminar nuclei to the ventral anterior nucleus or indirectly by projections to or from common cortical areas (see Chapter 1), then this similarity between the two in terms of pattern of aphasia is not surprising and may imply some functional relationship. Aphasia also can occur after infarctions in the territory of the anterior choroidal artery or the geniculothalamic arteries, but the reported number is not great enough to ascertain how they fit the 1984 definition of thalamic aphasia. As expected, the

Table 3-5. Cases of Aphasia with Infarctions in Different Territories of the Dominant Thalamus[a]

Tuberothalamic	7/7 (100%)
Paramedian	2/9 (22%)
Geniculothalamic	1/6 (17%)
Anterior choroidal	5/16 (31%)
Posterior choroidal	1/1

[a]Based on Bogousslavsky, Reglin, & Uske (1988), DeCroix, Graveleau, Masson, & Cambier (1986), Graff-Radford, Damasio, Yamada, Eslinger, & Damasio (1985). There were too few cases in the posterior choroidal arteries' distribution to give an accurate percentage of cases showing aphasia. Figures given in table represent the following: Number of cases with aphasia/Total number of cases (% of cases showing aphasia).

infarctions in the territory of the anterior choroidal artery include the posterior limb of the internal capsule and possibly portions of the globus pallidus (Archer et al., 1981; Gorelick et al., 1984; McFarling et al., 1982).

Three studies have been published that have relevance to the question of incidence of aphasia after thalamic infarction. Graff-Radford and colleagues (1985) and Bogousslavsky and colleagues (1988) both covered four of five arterial territories thought to supply the parts of the thalamus. Graff-Radford et al. did not cover the posterior choroidal arteries; Bogousslavsky and his colleagues did not cover the anterior choroidal artery. DeCroix, Graveleau, Masson, and Cambier (1986) covered anterior choroidal infarctions. All these three series apparently involved consecutive cases with no selection criteria; thus, they are excellent studies for looking at the incidence of aphasia after infarction of these different areas.

The cumulative number of patients from these three studies with aphasia and/or language impairment after infarctions is presented in Table 3-5. Cases have been separated by the arterial territories affected. No cases of aphasia after unilateral lesion of the nondominant thalamus occurred in these studies. One other facet is immediately apparent: all cases of dominant tuberothalamic infarction were reported to have aphasia. This finding was consistent with the predominance of tuberothalamic infarction in the thalamic aphasia cases listed in Table 3-4 above. (It should be noted that the cases of Graff-Radford et al. [1985] and two of the cases of Bogousslavsky et al. [1988] were included in Table 3-4 via previous previous reports.) The cases of aphasia after dominant paramedian thalamic artery infarction were at a lower frequency than might be expected in comparison to the cases detailed in Table 3-4. Further, the cases of aphasia and/or language impairment after dominant anterior choroidal infarction are more frequent than might be expected from the data in Table 3-4; however, Graff-Radford et al. (1985) did describe their three cases of language impairment after dominant anterior choroidal infarction as having "mild difficulties with some tasks of the Multilingual Aphasia Battery but not conforming to aphasic syndrome." Of interest is the fact that Bogousslavsky and colleagues' (1988) description of aphasia in the four dominant tuberothalamic artery infarctions included "hypophonia, reduced output, verbal paraphasias, moderate impairment of comprehension, and preserved repetition." This description more closely parallels Crosson's 1984 criteria of thalamic aphasia than Bogousslavsky and colleagues' (1986) description of two cases, where one case had greater phonemic than semantic paraphasias.

The persistence of language dysfunction after dominant thalamic infarction is also of some interest. Of the nine cases of dominant thalamic infarction presented in Crosson's 1984 review, seven had follow-up data. Aphasia persisted in all seven cases anywhere from 3 to 48 months. Of the 16 cases reviewed since that time, eight had follow-up data. Language dysfunction persisted from 3 to 12 months in six of these eight cases, though language generally was reported to have improved from the acute phase. In two cases, language dysfunction was noted to have remitted. As with hemorrhage, there may be some prejudice toward reporting cases in which language symptoms persisted. Nonetheless, persistence of language symptoms in 13 of 15 cases with follow-up data does suggest that aphasia after dominant thalamic infarction is often an enduring phenomenon.

To summarize: Aphasia after dominant thalamic infarction does not cohere as a syndrome like cases of aphasia after dominant thalamic hemorrhage. Output may be nonfluent, phonemic paraphasias occur at a greater frequency, and comprehension may be as impaired as other functions. However, repetition is usually minimally impaired similar to the hemorrhagic cases. As with hemorrhagic cases, symptoms often persist. Aphasia is most frequent and most severe after infarctions in the territory of the tuberothalamic artery, which includes the ventral anterior nucleus. This location is in contrast to the hemorrhage data, which were more suggestive of pulvinar involvement. Aphasia is always after infarction to the dominant thalamus as opposed to the nondominant thalamus. Frequency of aphasia after dominant thalamic infarction, particularly in the tuberothalamic territory, and persistence of symptoms indicate that serious attention must be given to a possible role for certain thalamic nuclei in language.

Deficits in Written Language after Thalamic Lesion

Deficits in reading and writing after dominant thalamic lesion have not been nearly so frequently reported as deficits in spoken language. Often, consideration of written language has been omitted from reports; at other times, it is mentioned primarily as an afterthought without much consideration to deficit patterns in reading and writing. In a notable exception, Deloche, Andreewsky, and Desi (1982) presented a case of thoroughly analyzed reading and writing abilities. Unfortunately, the lesion included cortical and white matter injury in addition to thalamic injury. The lesion was a choroid plexus angioma that invaded the pulvinar. Neurosurgical intervention was performed, and the postsurgical CT scan revealed lesions in the dominant temporal lobe as in well as the dominant pulvinar. With respect to reading, the patient was classified as a "surface dyslexic." In other words, he was overly dependent on grapheme to phoneme conversions in reading with some disturbance of more direct lexical access routes. Errors in oral reading frequently involved substituting alternative, more common pronunciations for certain letters or letter combinations. Similarly, errors in writing involved the erroneous selection of a grapheme from possible candidates. This pattern of performance on written language would be consistent with observations in many cases of spoken-language deficit with dominant thalamic lesion, where the abundance of semantic paraphasias indicates disruption of the semantic as opposed to the phonological aspects of language.

In the case of Crosson and colleagues (1986), a hemorrhagic infarction was confined to the left dorsal lateral thalamus and pulvinar. Results of reading and writing subtests from the Boston Diagnostic Aphasia Examination (BDAE) were given. In general, the patient performed poorly on the Reading Comprehension subtests, except that Comprehension of Oral Spelling was quite good. Likewise, the patient performed poorly on the Writing subtests, except that Spelling to Dictation was noticeably better than the other subtests. These patterns in reading and writing were consistent with the patient's performance in spoken language and imply that words were better accessed through routes related to phonological functions (i.e., phoneme-to-grapheme and grapheme-to-phoneme conversions). In a general way, these findings are also consistent with the results of Deloche et al. (1982), just discussed.

Glosser et al. (1982) also presented results of the BDAE subtests of written language in their case of subcortical aphasia. Their results were the opposite of Crosson et al. (1986). In the acute phase, Comprehension of Oral Spelling and Spelling to Dictation were among the worst written language subtests. Other poorly performed subtests included Word Recognition, Written Confrontation Naming, and Sentences to Dictation. This pattern is consistent with difficulty with phonologically related processing routes, such as grapheme-to-phoneme or phoneme-to-grapheme conversion. It is also consistent with their patient's large number of phonemic paraphasias seen in spoken language. However, it must be remembered that the effects of the lesion extended acutely beyond the thalamus. Indeed, the chronic CT scan showed a lesion in the putamen.

Robin and Schienberg (1990) reported mild impairment of reading comprehension in two of three cases of thalamic aphasia with severe impairment of reading comprehension in the third. Oral reading ranged from minimally impaired in one case to moderately impaired in the second case to severely impaired in the third case. Writing was minimally impaired in one case, severely impaired in one case, and not tested in one case. Deficits in written language were not described in enough detail to yield insights into the mechanism of impairment.

Thus, the study of written language after thalamic lesion has not been as extensive as study of spoken language. Some cases demonstrate parallels with deficits found in spoken language after thalamic lesion, that is, semantic access routes appear more impaired than routes dependent upon phonological processing. As would be expected in cortical aphasias, impairment of written language skills seems to accompany impairment of spoken language skills and is consistent in the pattern of deficit.

Studies of Cerebral Blood Flow or Metabolism and the Thalamus

As I noted in the last chapter, evolving techniques during the late 1970s and 1980s have allowed investigators to study cerebral blood flow or metabolism in various pathological and nonpathological conditions. One of the largest groups of relevant studies are the investigations reported by Metter and his colleagues. A number of their relevant findings relating to subcortical structures in general (as well as the basal ganglia specifically) were reviewed in Chapter 2. However, some of their findings are specifically relevant to the role of the thalamus in language. It will be recalled that this series of studies was performed in a resting state with eyes and ears unoccluded; (^{18}F)-fluorodeoxyglucose was used for PET studies.

One case of dominant thalamic hemorrhage with aphasia (Metter et al., 1986) showed distinct metabolic asymmetries (left < right) in the caudate head and thalamus. Metter et al. (1987) found greater metabolic asymmetries (left < right) in the thalamus, caudate head, and cortical areas for aphasic patients showing cerebellar metabolic asymmetries than for aphasic patients without cerebellar metabolic asymmetries. However, patients with cerebellar metabolic asymmetries also showed more structural injury to the thalamus and some of the other structures with metabolic asymmetries. Thus, structural injury to the thalamus (as opposed to metabolic changes in the absence of structural damage) probably was the factor dictating the relationship to cerebellar metabolic asymmetries.

The findings of the Metter et al. (1988) study are of particular interest because they give us insight into the relationship of subcortical nuclei to other structures in the language system for fluency (i.e., fluent vs. nonfluent output). As with damage to other subcortical structures, the degree of thalamic damage in aphasic patients was related to frontal glucose metabolism, which was in turn related to fluent output. Further, as with other subcortical structures, the thalamus may influence glucose metabolism in the temporal lobe via mediation of frontal metabolic activity. In other words, the thalamus may influence fluency of output and temporal lobe metabolism through its effects on the frontal lobe metabolism in a heterogenous sample of patients with aphasia.

Metter and colleagues' (1989) findings indicated that there may be some specificity between types of aphasia and metabolic asymmetries in cortical and subcortical structures. Patients with Broca's and Wernicke's aphasias both demonstrated significant metabolic asymmetries (left < right) in the thalamus, caudate head, and areas of the cortex. However, patients with Broca's aphasia demonstrated greater metabolic asymmetries in the thalamus, caudate head, and frontal cortex than patients with either Wernicke's or conduction aphasia. Again, though, one must look at the degree of damage to the different structures. Patients with Broca's aphasia also showed more damage to the thalamus and caudate head than did patients with Wernicke's or conduction aphasia.

Baron et al. (1986) studied cerebral metabolism in ten patients with vascular lesions of the thalamus using either (^{18}F)-fluorodeoxyglucose or $C^{15}O_2$–$^{15}O_2$ continuous inhalation and PET. Five of six dominant thalamic lesions produced aphasia or some form of language impairment. There were significant metabolic asymmetries in the cortex of the affected side in nine of ten patients. Since lesions were located in different parts of the thalamus and occupied different volumes, it is not surprising that no single pattern of cortical metabolic asymmetry was found. However, there was some trend for anterior thalamic lesions to accompany metabolic asymmetry in the fronto-parietal cortex and posterior thalamic lesions to accompany metabolic asymmetry in the temporo-occipital cortex. Four of ten subjects had repeat PET scans. These repeat scans indicated trends toward bilateral increases in metabolic rate and decreases in metabolic asymmetry, which paralleled clinical improvement. Findings of this study cannot be explained by inadequate blood supply in the same arterial distribution for two reasons. Some (6) of the lesions were hemorrhagic and not related to occlusion. Further, lesions were not consistently in the same arterial distribution as the cortical areas of metabolic asymmetry. In other words, some of the thalamic lesions were outside the distribution of the middle cerebral artery that supplies the affected cortical areas, and the explanation invoked by Olsen and colleagues (1986) for aphasia with ischemic lentiform lesions cannot be applied to Baron and colleagues (1986) study.

Demonet et al. (1989) reported one case of aphasia with dominant thalamic lesion that met his criteria for dissident aphasia as well as Crosson's (1984) criteria for thalamic aphasia. Regional cerebral blood flow was performed using SPECT and ^{133}Xe, and 11 regions of interest within each hemisphere were compared to mean hemispheric blood flow. Bilateral subcortical hypoperfusion, predominantly posterior, was noted.

Puel et al. (1989) described three right-handed patients with some degree of language dysfunction and left thalamic lesions. The first case showed a language deficit similar to the "dissident aphasia" described by Demonet et al. (1989). MRI scan showed the ischemic lesion to include the genu of the internal capsule, the ventral lateral nucleus, and the anterior ventral nucleus. The SPECT scan indicated decreased left hemisphere perfusion to the caudate head and the temporoparietal cortex, with some hypoperfusion located in the right parieto-occipital and lateral frontal regions. The second case showed an anomia and a mild reduction of spontaneous language. The MRI scan indicated a cavernous angioma in the left anterior nucleus of the thalamus, with prior hemorrhage. In the chronic state, there was bilateral hypoperfusion in the caudate head and thalamus, with some hypoperfusion of the right lateral frontal and insular cortex. The third case had relatively normal language testing but periodic incoherent jargon due to abundant paraphasia with some perseveration. The MRI scan indicated cavitation of the left pulvinar surrounded by hemosiderin from prior hemorrhage. SPECT images indicated hypoperfusion in the left central region, right lateral frontal cortex, and bilateral temporoparietal regions. Thus, the SPECT cerebral blood flow data were different between the cases of Puel et al. (1989) and probably related at least in part to the varying locations of the lesions.

Fasanaro et al. (1987) used ^{133}Xe and SPECT to study a case of aphasia with left thalamic infarction. These investigators found decreased cerebral blood flow in the left temporoparietal cortex. The site of lesion within the thalamus was not further delineated.

A couple of studies of cerebral blood flow in normals during performance of language tasks should be mentioned. Wallesch et al. (1985) compared narrative language conditions to resting and nonlanguage oral production conditions in six healthy volunteers. [133]Xe and SPECT were used. In addition to cortical and other subcortical structures, the left thalamic/pallidal region demonstrated increased cerebral blood flow during narrative language. The language study of Petersen et al. (1988, 1989) was not remarkable regarding subcortical functions except for an almost total lack of subcortical activation by their language-production tasks. These investigators used PET and [15]O labeled water to examine cerebral blood flow during various language-related activities. It should be noted that their tasks required the semantic generation, repetition, or passive observation of or listening to single words. The methodological differences between Wallesch et al. (1985) and Petersen et al. (1988, 1989) are too great to make detailed comparisons between the two studies. However, difference between generating words versus generating discourse could account for the subcortical activation in the Wallesch et al. study but not the Petersen et al. study.

Thus, studies of cerebral metabolism in aphasia suggest a role for the thalamus in language. One study in particular (Metter et al., 1988) suggests that the thalamus, as well as the basal ganglia, may have more direct effects on fluency than upon language comprehension. This finding is not consistent with data indicating that thalamic hemorrhage produces fluent output (see above discussion). After cases of vascular thalamic lesion, including those with aphasia, it is common for decreased metabolism or blood flow to occur in the cortex. It is not surprising that different areas of cortical dysfunction are seen in various patients since the location of the lesions within the thalamus varies. Changes in cortical blood flow and metabolism after thalamic lesion cannot be attributed to circulatory phenomena because the cortical areas and thalamic nuclei are generally supplied by different arterial distributions. It is more likely that decreases in cortical blood flow and metabolism after thalamic lesion reflect decreased synaptic activity in areas of the cortex receiving fibers from the damaged thalamic nuclei. Increases in dominant thalamic cerebral blood flow may occur during narrative language (Wallesch et al., 1985).

Synthesis and Conclusions

Several issues should be considered when attempting to derive some meaningful conclusions from the data just discussed concerning the thalamus and language. One issue is whether aphasia after dominant thalamic lesion persists long enough to deserve serious attention. If one considers only thalamectomy data from the 1960s and 1970s, one would conclude that aphasia after thalamic lesion ordinarily remits rapidly and is a curiosity as opposed to a bona fide phenomenon. But other evidence indicates that a significant number of aphasias after dominant thalamic hemorrhage or infarction do persist for periods of months or even years. If one considers all of the evidence carefully, the apparent discrepancy regarding the persistence of aphasic symptoms after thalamectomy versus after vascular lesion is easily resolved. The thalamectomy target in the ventral lateral thalamus is an area that affects motor function. It is unlikely that such a motor area also participates in complex cognitive functions such as language (even though the motor functions of this area are necessary for the final expression of language in speech). Crosson (1984) suggested that the ventral lateral nucleus itself, or at least that part of it ablated in thalamectomies, is not directly involved in language. Rather, the process of creating the lesion disrupts language function in neighboring areas of the thalamus that do participate in language function. This scenario would explain why vascular lesions of the dominant thalamus often cause lasting language disturbance while ventral lateral thalamectomies cause only temporary dysfunction.

A second issue concerns the syndrome of aphasia after dominant thalamic lesion. Several points should be made in this regard. Patients with dominant thalamic hemorrhage generally fit Crosson's (1984) criteria for thalamic aphasia better than patients with dominant thalamic infarction. Reasons for nonfit in cases of infarction include language comprehension more impaired than Crosson's criteria would indicate, greater phonemic than semantic paraphasias, and/or nonfluent output. The potential reasons for these discrepancies in syndrome between hemorrhage and infarction are many. One is that many cases of thalamic hemorrhage appeared earlier in the literature and depended upon clinical impression as opposed to standardized aphasia testing. Standardized aphasia testing has been more common in cases of infarction. Perhaps how impairments in functions like comprehension compare to impairments of other language functions is not obvious without standardized testing.

Another, similar problem is the varying definitions of some phenomena, for example, fluency and paraphasias. Unfortunately, some investigators have defined fluency versus nonfluency by using "word-fluency" tasks such as how many animals can be named in a minute or how many words beginning with a given letter can be generated in a minute. I have referred to such tasks as word-list generation. These word-list-generation tasks are affected by frontal lesions (Lezak, 1983), and at times may be unrelated to deficits in basic language functions such as those seen in aphasia. Definitions like the one provided in the original Boston Diagnostic Aphasia Examination (Goodglass & Kaplan, 1972) are more representative of true disorders of linguistic fluency. Those criteria included decreased length of word runs without interruption, decreased variety of grammatical forms in conversational speech, decreased articulatory agility, and lack of normal intonational patterns in conversational speech. Many patients with moderate-to-severe aphasia will have difficulty in word-fluency tasks, but are not necessarily nonfluent with respect to Goodglass and Kaplan's (1972) criteria. For example, this was strikingly the case during the first testing of the patient presented by Crosson and colleagues in 1986. This patient had a fluent aphasia with greater impairment on the word-fluency task (Animal Naming) than any other naming task.

Regarding paraphasias, most investigators do not say how they classify a substitution that is phonemically similar to the target word but is another real word. Is this a phonemic paraphasia or a semantic paraphasia? How this issue is resolved may affect the relative frequency of "phonemic" versus "semantic" paraphasias and the conclusions drawn regarding these frequencies. For example, the word substitutions in the case of Crosson et al. (1986) were semantically similar to the target in spoken-language tasks, but phonemically similar to the target in oral-reading tasks. These authors concluded that the patient was using a phonemic strategy to compensate for a semantic deficit in oral-reading tasks. Thus, the way in which investigators define or fail to define language characteristics such as fluency or paraphasias introduces some difficulties into the task of making comparisons between different studies and could affect the conclusions drawn.

Although results of the above review of the literature indicate that cases of thalamic infarction often do not meet even Crosson's (1984) relatively simple criteria for thalamic aphasia, the overwhelming majority of cases of dominant thalamic hemorrhage or infarction with aphasia do show one feature: minimally impaired or unimpaired repetition. There are at least two possible explanations for this phenomenon. The first was presented by McCarthy and Warrington (1984). These investigators showed that the repetition of conduction aphasics could be made better, and the repetition of a transcortical motor aphasic could be made worse, if they semantically loaded the repetition task. On the basis of these findings, McCarthy and Warrington suggested two routes to spoken language, one semantic and one phonological. Actually, as noted by the authors, this separation of phonological versus semantic routes to speech had been suggested much earlier by Lichtheim (1885). In simple repetition tasks, McCarthy and Warrington implied that output could be processed primarily through a phonological route without the need for extensive semantic processing. This phonological route is relatively intact in the transcortical motor aphasic and accounts for repetition being less impaired than other language functions. However, when a semantic component is loaded into the repetition task, the transcortical motor aphasic faltered because the semantic route to language production was damaged. It has been suggested that intact repetition in cases of aphasia with dominant thalamic lesion is performed through such a phonological processing mechanism (Crosson, 1981, 1985). This explanation would be consistent with the observation of greater semantic than phonemic paraphasias in many cases of thalamic aphasia and also consistent with the resulting conclusion that there is a semantic deficit in such cases (e.g., Cappa & Vignolo, 1979; Crosson et al., 1986). However, this explanation for intact repetition does not account for cases of thalamic infarction with aphasia in which repetition is relatively intact, but phonemic paraphasias seem to dominate (Bogousslavsky et al., 1986; Cohen et al., 1980). This may indicate that an intact phonological system is not necessary for relatively intact performance of repetition tasks.

This leads us to a second possibility. In their study of akinesia, Heilman and Watson (1989) noted a difference between movements that are generated primarily in response to an external stimulus (exo-evoked movement) and movements that are generated based upon motivations internal to an organism (endo-evoked movement). Goldberg (1985) has also reviewed similar phenomena relating to the supplementary motor cortex, though he used different terminology. It could be that repetition is exo-evoked language and the thalamus is primarily involved in endo-evoked language. (This explanation will be further analyzed in Chapter 8.) Hopefully, future studies of repetition in cases of thalamic aphasia will address the mechanism accounting for intact repetition. This will require detailed descriptions of how semantic and phonemic paraphasias are separated; use of tasks that semantically load repetition, such as those of McCarthy and Warrington (1984); and use of tasks other than repetition that are phonological in nature, such as rhyming.

The problem of intrathalamic localization of lesions causing aphasia is also an important issue. Exploration of intrathalamic localization with respect to aphasia may even shed some light on the topic of syndrome. As noted in Chapter 1, various thalamic nuclei are distinctly connected to the different cortical and subcortical centers that may be involved in language. These patterns of connection have implications for intrathalamic localization: logically, one would expect thalamic nuclei connected to cortical language areas to be involved in language and thalamic nuclei not connected to cortical language areas not to be involved in language functions. Implications of cortico-thalamic and thalamo-cortical connections for syndromes of aphasia exist but are not uncomplicated. For example, the ventral anterior nucleus has connections with both frontal and parietal regions, and the pulvinar has both frontal and temporoparietal connections.

Even though cases of hemorrhage in the posterior dominant thalamus without aphasia can be found (e.g., Cappa et al., 1986), cases of hemorrhagic lesions and aphasia do tend to favor involvement of the pulvinar in language (Ciemans, 1970; Crosson et al., 1986; Kameyama, 1976/1977; Mohr et al., 1975). A focus in the pulvinar is supported by studies of retrograde degeneration of the thalamus in cases of aphasia after cortical damage (Van Buren, 1975; Van Buren & Borke, 1969). These authors found retrograde degeneration in the anterior superior pulvinar in three of five cases with persistent aphasia due to cortical lesion. Electrical stimulation data (e.g., Ojemann, 1977) also implicates the anterior superior lateral pulvinar in anomia. Detracting from the hypothesis of dominant pulvinar involvement in language are the studies of pulvinar ablation without changes in language (Brown et al., 1971; Vilkki & Laitinen, 1976). However, it should be noted that surgical lesion of the pulvinar may not include the margins of this nucleus, such as the anterior superior lateral pulvinar, which was implicated in language by Ojemann (1977) and Van Buren and Borke (1969).

Studies of dominant thalamic infarction lead to a different conclusion. Examination of these studies clearly indicates infarction in the territory of the tuberothalamic artery (i.e., anterior portions of the dominant thalamus) to most frequently lead to aphasia (Bogousslavsky et al., 1988; Graff-Radford et al., 1985). The involvement of the ventral anterior, ventral lateral, and/or anterior ventral nuclei is supported by the studies of Schaltenbrand (1965, 1975) during which language was elicited from electrical stimulation in these nuclei. Aphasia is less frequent and milder with infarcts that may involve the dominant pulvinar (Graff-Radford et al., 1985).

One possible reason for the discrepancy in hemorrhage versus infarction data is that hemorrhage and infarction may affect different thalamic areas in different ways. For example, if one inspects the sketches of arterial distribution drawn by Graff-Radford et al. (1985), it is apparent that there may be some overlap in the arterial supply of the anterior superior lateral pulvinar from the anterior choroidal and geniculothalamic arteries. Such overlap might leave the area of the pulvinar critical for language at least partially functional after cases of occlusive infarction. Such selective sparing of the anterior superior lateral pulvinar would not be the case with posterior dominant thalamic hemorrhage. This explanation would be consistent with the fact that the pulvinar is often involved in cases of hemorrhagic lesion with aphasia but is less frequently represented in cases of infarction. Furthermore, this hypothesis might be a partial explanation for why cases of hemorrhage meet criteria for thalamic aphasia (Crosson, 1984) better than cases of infarction. It may be that lesions that incapacitate the anterior superior lateral pulvinar are more prone to show the thalamic aphasia syndrome than lesions that incapacitate other areas of the thalamus.

Unfortunately, one cannot unequivocally accept this hypothesis regarding different types of lesions. First, it must be recognized that whether the anterior choroidal distribution reaches the thalamus is a controversial issue (Bogousslavsky et al., 1988; Percheron, 1973). Second, cases of hemorrhage that include the dominant pulvinar but do not produce aphasia do exist (Cappa et al., 1986). Thus, alternative hypotheses regarding the discrepancy between infarct and hemorrhage data must be entertained.

One such hypothesis is that pressure effects of hematomas resulting from intracerebral hemorrhage may affect surrounding structures. This explanation, however, is unconvincing for two reasons. First, cases of medial thalamic hemorrhage in which memory but not language is affected do exist (e.g., Choi et al., 1983). In other words, if pressure effects are so prominent, then why do hemorrhages of the medial thalamus not cause aphasia through their pressure effects? Second, pressure effects are most likely to be transmitted to nearby structures, such as the posterior limb of the internal capsule and the globus pallidus. These structures are closely related to the thalamus (at least the ventral anterior, ventral lateral, dorsal medial, and intralaminar nuclei) in that the globus pallidus projects to the thalamus through the posterior limb of the internal capsule and nearby white matter tracts.

A second alternative hypothesis is simple. It states that individual differences may to some degree be responsible for differences in location and/or syndrome seen between different cases. This explanation would account for the fact that some cases of posterior dominant thalamic hemorrhage show aphasia while others do not (Cappa et al., 1986). Yet, this explanation does not account for the fact that hemorrhage but not infarction cases meet the criteria for thalamic aphasia. It is probable that some combination of all these hypotheses will be necessary to account for all the phenomena discussed above.

Before summarizing, I should note that some investigators (Bogousslavsky et al., 1989; Brown, 1975) favor involvement of the dominant dorsal medial nucleus in language. The cases summarized in Table 3-5, including those of Bogousslavsky et al. (1988), however, do not strongly favor this hypothesis. Further, the involvement of the dorsal medial nucleus in language is not necessarily supported on the basis of lesions in the territory of the paramedian thalamic artery that show aphasia. It is possible that damage to the central median nucleus, which is also in the distribution of this artery, could be responsible for aphasic symptoms when they do occur.

In summary: When considered together, electrical stimulation, thalamectomy, and vascular lesion data all support a role for the dominant thalamus in language. When aphasia does occur with thalamic lesion, it occurs almost exclusively with lesions in the dominant thalamus. The syndrome of semantic paraphasias sometimes deteriorating into jargon, less severely affected auditory-verbal comprehension, and relatively preserved repetition fits cases of dominant thalamic hemorrhage well, but not cases of dominant thalamic infarction. Yet, relatively preserved repetition does exist in a vast majority of aphasias due to thalamic lesion, both for hemorrhage and infarction. Future studies should carefully explore the reason for preservation of this function. Data on dominant thalamic hemorrhage lean toward involvement of the pulvinar, but infarction data strongly implicate nuclei in the territory of the tuberothalamic artery. The reasons for this apparent discrepancy are most likely complex and multiple, but the nuclei in the territory of the tuberothalamic artery and the pulvinar are the most likely candidates for involvement in language.

4

Theories of Subcortical Functions in Language

Data regarding the relationship of language to subcortical structures is important to facilitate our understanding of how brain systems produce the phenomena we know as language. Only in the relatively recent past has a significant amount of attention been paid in neurobehavioral literature to the role of subcortical structures in language. Although proponents of subcortical participation in language can be found over a century ago, only since the 1970s has a more widespread interest in the topic been shown. In part, this situation is due to limits in the technology and techniques available to localize subcortical lesions prior to the 1970s. Thus, the invention of the computerized tomography (CT) scan and, more recently, the magnetic resonance (MR) scan, was a necessary condition to make widespread study of the topic possible.

The number of cases of subcortical aphasia studied since the mid-1970s has confirmed a smaller number of earlier autopsied cases of subcortical aphasia. Stimulation and lesion studies performed during thalamectomies for movement disorders or, less commonly, for chronic pain have also supported the role of subcortical structures in language. The phenomena from all these types of studies demand explanation for students of the neurobehavioral basis of language. Resulting theoretical positions have varied from the nonparticipation of subcortical structures in language phenomena proper (e.g., Alexander et al., 1987; Luria, 1977) to complex systems involving subcortical structures (e.g., Crosson, 1985; Wallesch & Papagno, 1988).

111

The purpose of this chapter is to explore theoretical perspectives regarding subcortical functions in language. I will briefly discuss perspectives from the late 1800s and the early 1900s. Next, the chapter will address unitary theories of thalamic function. Unitary-function theories suggest that thalamic nuclei are involved in a single function that directly or indirectly affects language. Although few unitary theories of basal ganglia functions in language have been set forth in recent decades, I will also address the applicability of other theories to linguistic behavior. Then, I will critique and contrast more complex systems theories. Finally, discussion will turn to the implications of subcortical language models for understanding other cognitive systems. The reader should note that all the theoretical systems presented in this chapter have flaws. Nonetheless, such theories can serve the heuristic function of guiding future research that will eventually lead to more accurate models.

Perspectives from the Late 1800s and the Early 1900s

Wallesch and Papagno (1988) traced the concept of subcortical aphasia as far back as Broadbent (1872). Broadbent believed that the basal ganglia (caudate nucleus, putamen, globus pallidus) were the structures in which words were generated as motor acts. Kussmaul (1877; cited in Wallesch & Papagno, 1988) held the opposing view that the functions of the basal ganglia were entirely motor in nature. In the case of speech and language production, the latter author assumed the basal ganglia only to be involved in articulation. It is of interest that the more recent work of Alexander (Alexander, 1989; Alexander et al., 1987) reflects somewhat similar themes.

Carl Wernicke (1874), to whom modern aphasiology owes a great deal, thought destruction of the left lenticular nucleus caused aphasia. He ascribed this aphasia to the convergence of frontal fibers upon the basal ganglia (cited in Wallesch & Papagno, 1988). However, in the classical aphasia theory derived from the work of Wernicke (e.g., Geschwind, 1972), the emphasis regarding "subcortical" pathways was on the fibers connecting different cortical areas (i.e., cortico-cortical fibers). Again, this emphasis on pathways can also be seen in the work of Alexander (Alexander et al., 1987). Many other more recent works focus on the gray structures to the exclusion of the important fiber systems connecting them. It is clear that both subcortical tracts and the cortical areas and subcortical nuclei they connect must be carefully studied if we are truly to understand the phenomenon of subcortical aphasia.

Marie (1906) believed that the structures involved in language included the quadrilateral zone that extended into the deepest portions of the left hemisphere (cited in Wallesch & Papagno, 1988). Marie's student, Moutier (1908), described three cases of subcortical aphasia, all with nonfluent aphasia. Although this effort represents one of the first attempts to systematically study cases of subcortical aphasia (cited in Wallesch & Papagno, 1988), Marie's view of aphasia as a unitary disorder is not widely accepted today (Benson, 1985).

Thus, some early discussions of aphasia did make reference to the participation of subcortical structures in language. Many of the themes articulated over 100 years ago are echoed in more modern studies. The evolution of more complex approaches to the role of subcortical structures in language, however, was dependent upon the development of brain-imaging techniques that could confirm the involvement of the dominant thalamus and basal ganglia in cases of aphasia.

Single-Function Theories of Thalamic Participation in Language

Surgical and autopsy studies did afford some hints of thalamic involvement in language prior to the widespread use of CT scans. Frequently, the theoretical speculations based upon such data posited a single function for the subcortical structures. Crosson (1984) reviewed such models concerning the thalamus and considered them to be at an early stage of development at that time.

He noted that nonspecific theories emphasized the numerous connections between the thalamus and the cortex, but did not propose a role unique to the thalamus. Riklan and Levita (1965) suggested that subcortical lesions affected language at a diffuse and unlateralized stage. Information processing in other modalities is disrupted as well. The overwhelming lateralization of thalamic aphasias to the dominant hemisphere (discussed in Chapter 3) highlights the problems with this line of thought.

Several authors have emphasized a role for the thalamus in cortical arousal. For the purposes of this chapter, the term *arousal* is used to refer to tonic changes in the level of cortical activity that are necessary for maximal efficiency in cortical processing of information. Horenstein et al. (1978) suggested that aphasia in their thalamic hemorrhage cases was due to cortical inactivation, and noted a diffuse slowing of the EEG. Riklan and Cooper (1975) and McFarling et al. (1982) hypothesized that higher-level language functions required greater diffuse energizing from thalamic centers. Similarly, both

Cooper et al. (1968) and Samra et al. (1969) believed the dominant thalamus to direct activation important for the modulation and integration of speech and language. Such activating influences might be more specific than tonic-arousal mechanisms. Although Luria (1977) considered language disturbance after dominant thalamic lesion to be caused by disruption of vigilance mechanisms specifically related to language, he did not consider this type of deficit to be a true aphasia.

Crosson (1984) pointed out that theories proposing the thalamus to have a role in the generalized arousal of cortical language structures could not account for the specificity of language symptoms in thalamic aphasia. In other words, the relative sparing of repetition in the context of impairment in semantic production aspects of language can not be explained by the generalized arousal hypothesis. If there was a generalized deficiency in arousal of cortical language mechanisms, one would expect repetition and the phonological aspects of language to be as impaired as the semantic aspects. In contrast, arousal explanations specific to semantic encoding for language or to a semantic feedback mechanism more closely fit the data.

Penfield and Roberts (1959) were among the first to suggest that the dominant thalamus played a role in the integration of language. Ojemann et al. (1968) also considered this a probability. Botez and Barbeau (1971) thought that cortico-thalamo-cortical circuits were under the control of brain stem and basal attention mechanisms. These circuits performed the final matching or understanding of verbal messages as well as the formation of new motor patterns for spoken language. Access to semantic-memory stores was the common denominator in these activities. Reynolds et al. (1979) also emphasized that dominant thalamic participation in language processes involved verbal memory. These authors hypothesized an attention mechanism gating both storage and retrieval for verbal memory. Cappa and Vignolo (1979) emphasized that the linguistic role of the dominant thalamus was related to the use of words as meaningful units. This latter explanation could be viewed as consistent with the proposals of Botez and Barbeau (1971) and Reynolds et al. (1979).

The reader will recall that Schaltenbrand (1965, 1975) elicited words, phrases, or short sentences irrelevant to the experimental context when he stimulated the more anterior segments of the thalamus. Based upon this observation, Schaltenbrand (1975) proposed that the thalamus controlled the release or inhibition of preformed "speech" patterns and the temporal ordering of "speech." Crosson (1985) arrived at a similar conclusion in examining the data of both Schaltenbrand and Van Buren (Van Buren, 1963, 1966; Van Buren et al., 1966). I shall discuss this elaboration shortly.

In a different approach to the topic of subcortical structures in language, Schuell, Jenkins, and Jimenez-Pabon (1965) proposed that prior to verbal execution of language, the language system received feedback from the auditory system about the adequacy of the output. The contradiction between this hypothesis and Schuell's theoretical position on language was that Schuell, similar to Marie (1906), perceived language to be a unitary system in which functions are not differentiated among structures. If all language processing is accomplished by such a single, unified system, then there would be no outside system or subsystem capable of providing objective feedback about the adequacy of output from the language system.

Crosson (1981) also suggested that the thalamus was involved in semantic feedback. Unlike Schuell, however, he saw pre- and retrorolandic language areas as playing significantly different roles in language. Pathways using thalamic nuclei conveyed language from the anterior to the posterior language cortex so that the posterior language cortex could monitor the formulations of the anterior cortex. This position does not explain the variation in degree or type of language symptoms after thalamic infarct.

In summary: Single-function theories of thalamic participation in language proposed that the thalamus was involved in nonspecific arousal or specific activation of language cortex, in integrative functions linking language to other systems, or in semantic feedback processes. No single-function theory can account for the variations of syndromes seen in thalamic aphasia; therefore, multiple-function theories must be considered.

Basal Ganglia Models of Behavior and Applicability to Language

Theories concerning the participation of the dominant basal ganglia in language have not been as prolific as hypotheses related to thalamic functions. However, more general theories of basal ganglia function can be considered in terms of their implications for language. In an earlier work, Crosson et al. (1988) reviewed more general theories of basal ganglia function as they applied to language. The following paragraphs expand upon this discussion.

For example, some believe the basal ganglia are involved in triggering actions or complex action plans. Wing and Miller (1984) thought that the basal ganglia played a role in the activation of preplanned movement. Similarly, Marsden (1984) suggested that the basal ganglia are involved in automatically running the sequence of motor programs that make up a motor plan. Although the actual motor programs might be stored in the cortex, the initiation and execution of the sequence of movements in a complex motor program would be determined by the basal ganglia. These hypotheses would be consistent with the earlier suggestion of Watson, Valenstein, and Heilman (1981) that basal ganglia lesions could cause unilateral akinesia. Indeed, Laplane, Baulac, Widlocher, and DuBois (1984) described a bilateral "psychic" akinesia after bilateral lesions in and around the globus pallidus.

The triggering of motor programs is similar to Schaltenbrand's (1975) hypothesis about the thalamus. As mentioned above, he felt that the thalamus controlled the release or inhibition of predetermined speech and sequences in speech. Given the projections of the striatum to the globus pallidus, and the projections of the globus pallidus to the ventral anterior and ventral lateral nuclei of the thalamus, it is certainly possible that the basal ganglia and thalamic nuclei are linked in performing the release of cortically generated language segments. This latter hypothesis is consistent with the fact that language has been elicited at the offset of caudate stimulation (Van Buren, 1963, 1966; Van Buren et al., 1966) as well as from thalamic stimulation (Schaltenbrand, 1965, 1975). As I will discuss momentarily, the participation of both the basal ganglia and the thalamus in the release of preformed language segments for motor programming was one of the major tenets of Crosson's (1985) theory.

It is also possible that there may be a parallel for akinesia in the language system. Such a parallel dysfunction might involve difficulty initiating and maintaining language output. As noted in Chapter 2, this type of dysfunction can be seen after subcortical lesion. It may be due to a failure of release mechanisms for language.

Nonetheless, Mink and Thach (1987a, 1987b) disagreed with the notion that the basal ganglia were involved in the initiation of movement. In ballistic movements they found that an overwhelming majority of pallidal neurons began to change firing rates after the earliest agonist muscle changes, suggesting that the basal ganglia were not involved in the initiation of the fast movements that happen too rapidly to be adjusted by sensory feedback. Rather, they thought that the basal ganglia were involved in turning off postural holding responses that would impede movements. It should be noted, however, that for slower, visually guided movements, a greater number of pallidal neurons did begin to change firing rates before the earliest agnonist EMG changes. Thus, the explanation for ballistic movements may not apply to movements that are guided by corrective feedback.

Another set of investigators has suggested an integrative role for the basal ganglia in cognition. The reader will recall that the striatum receives input from a broad range of neocortical and limbic regions, perhaps leaving it in a position to integrate divergent inputs. Both Iversen (1984) and Stern (1983) have hypothesized that the caudate nucleus and putamen play a role in integrating sensory input with motor output. As we shall see below, Wallesch and Papagno (1988) agreed with this conceptualization of the basal ganglia for language and included internal motivations as aspects of behavior integrated by the basal ganglia.

Penney and Young (1983, 1986) put forth a more complicated model of basal ganglia functioning in movement. Their 1986 version is an excellent theoretical work, and it has received support from recent work on experimental chorea (Mitchell, Jackson, Sambrook, & Crossman, 1989). A detailed description of the Penney and Young model is beyond the scope of this chapter. For current purposes, it should suffice to say that the authors saw the cortico-striato-pallido-thalamo-cortical loop as playing a central role in movement, along with a cortico-thalamo-cortical loop, a striato-nigro-striatal loop, and a lateral pallido-subthalamo-medial pallidal subloop. Brunner et al. (1982) were among the first to suggest the importance of the former loop in language. This type of cortico-striato-pallido-thalamo-cortical loop plays a role in the theories of both Crosson (1985) and Wallesch and Papagno (1988).

In summary: A number of roles have been suggested for the basal ganglia in movement that can be applied to language. The release of preformulated motor programs may be parallel to the release of preformulated language segments. The basal ganglia may be involved in the integration of sensory input with motor output for both movement and language. If the basal ganglia are indeed involved in language, it is likely that they play their role through cortico-striato-pallido-thalamo-cortical loops.

Recent Theories of Subcortical Functions in Language

I will spend most of the remainder of this chapter discussing, comparing, and contrasting three recent theoretical positions regarding subcortical functions in language. These theoretical positions can be distinguished from those discussed above in that they take into account many of the complexities of language as a cognitive system and/or they focus on anatomical data to explain lesion phenomena. The first is derived from the work of Alexander, Naeser, and their colleagues and is most clearly explained in the study of Alexander, Naeser, and Palumbo (1987). These authors take the position that nonthalamic subcortical lesions cause aphasia primarily because they interrupt cortico-cortical pathways traversing subcortical space. The second theory was developed by Wallesch and his colleagues and is most clearly explained in a chapter by Wallesch and Papagno (1988). Wallesch and Papagno take the position that the striatum and other subcortical structures are involved in lexical decision making between cortically generated alternatives. The third theory was developed by Crosson and his colleagues. This theory was originally expressed in Crosson's (1985) article, with some clarifications in subsequent works (Crosson, 1989; Crosson & Hughes, 1987; Crosson et al., 1988). A more extensive revision of the theory is currently in progress (Crosson & Early, 1990). Crosson has maintained that cortico-striato-pallido-thalamo-cortical loops are involved in regulating the release of cortically formulated segments, that the thalamus is involved in tonic arousal of anterior language cortex, and that cortico-thalamo-cortical pathways serve to transfer information from anterior to posterior language cortex and vice versa.

The purpose of this discussion is heuristic in nature. It is not meant to resolve the current questions regarding subcortical functions. Rather, comparison of the three positions should help to focus attention on the important issues and help to generate questions for future consideration. All the models must be considered viable to some degree, though it appears likely that our eventual understanding of subcortical phenomena in language may involve quite different concepts than some or all of these models postulate.

The Subcortical Pathways Model

The two main tenets of Alexander and colleagues' model were stated in the 1987 study (Alexander et al., 1987). The first is that the striatum is minimally involved in language. The basis for this assumption is that the authors found isolated lesions in the striatum to cause, at most, mild word-finding difficulty or hesitancy in verbal output. Because these deficits do not constitute aphasia (according to the authors' own definition), they assume the striatum to be minimally involved in language. Since the authors believe that the striatum is minimally involved in language, they also assume that damage to subcortical white matter pathways must cause aphasia in nonthalamic subcortical lesions. Thus, Alexander et al. (1987) emphasized the involvement of white matter pathways in language.

The model of Alexander and colleagues does not provide a complete description of language comprehension or language output at this time, primarily for two reasons. First, many more severe and/or lasting language deficits may be caused by combined lesions to two or more pathways (e.g., see Naeser et al., 1989). Second, not all the important pathways contained in the various white matter areas are well mapped at this time.

With respect to language production, Alexander et al. (1987) suggested that lesions in the connections between the supplementary motor area and Broca's area was the minimal lesion necessary for transcortical motor aphasia. This hypothesis was based on the fact that this pathway is embedded in the anterior-superior periventricular white matter, and the authors observed a patient with an infarct primarily in this region who exhibited a mild transcortical motor aphasia. This suggestion is consistent with the claims of some investigators that damage to the supplementary motor area causes transcortical motor aphasia (Ardila & Lopez, 1984; Tijssen, Tavy, Hekster, Bots, & Endtz, 1984). Additional damage to the anterior limb of the internal capsule or callosal fibers to or from the right hemisphere might make the syndrome worse.

According to the 1987 article, white matter pathways involved in speech output include the superior periventricular white matter and the genu of the internal capsule through which corticobulbar fibers descend. The more anterior portions of the periventricular white matter and the anterior limb of the internal capsule may also be involved in speech output. These are the pathways through which fibers from the motor association cortex to the contralateral cerebellum descend and through which the fibers from the ventrolateral thalamus to the motor cortex ascend. As the reader may recall, this position was expanded upon by Naeser et al. (1989), who found that patients with Broca's aphasia were differentiated from patients with no speech output or automatisms only by lesions in both the middle one-third of the periventricular white matter and the medial subcallosal fasciculus for the group with greater impairment of output. The latter pathway carries fibers from the anterior cingulate area and the supplementary motor area to the caudate nucleus. Since Naeser et al. were dealing mainly with speech output (i.e., motor output as opposed to linguistic elements), this finding does not contradict their proposal that the striatum is not involved in language.

Alexander (1989) further explored the speech versus language aspects of fluency, and he concluded that nonthalamic subcortical lesions caused nonfluent speech (i.e., disturbed intonation and articulatory agility) but minimal changes in the language aspects of fluency (i.e., number of words in an uninterrupted run and variety of grammatical forms). But, in his 1989 paper, Alexander does seem to admit that some aspects of disturbed initiation in nonthalamic subcortical lesions may be linguistic in nature. Further, he did not extensively discuss the word-finding difficulty in these cases.

Alexander et al. (1987) also noted two pathways potentially to be involved in auditory-verbal comprehension deficits in subcortical aphasia. The first is the pathway between the left medial geniculate nucleus and the primary auditory cortex in the dominant temporal lobe, which in turn is connected to temporal association areas involved in language comprehension. The second is the transcallosal pathway connecting the auditory association cortex of the right hemisphere to the auditory association cortex of the left hemisphere. Concurrent damage to both pathways would have a particularly severe affect on auditory-verbal comprehension since the cortex responsible for this function could no longer receive auditory information.

Finally, with respect to repetition, Alexander et al. (1987) noted fibers in the external or extreme capsules or the fibers of the arcuate fasciculus to be important. Damage to these fiber systems leads to conduction aphasia (i.e., aphasia with disproportionately impaired repetition). Phonemic as opposed to semantic paraphasias are more common in this variety of aphasia.

The model of Alexander and colleagues is summarized for purposes of comparison to other models in Figure 4-1. (It should be noted that Alexander et al. might consider this type of diagram an overspecification of their model.) Fibers from the supplementary motor area to Broca's area are important in linking the limbic system to the language system to provide the motivation for language. Damage to these fibers causes transcortical motor aphasia. Corticobulbar, cortico-cerebellar, thalamo-cortical, and cortico-striatal fibers are important to speech, but are minimally involved in language. Input to the language-comprehension areas of the dominant temporal lobe from the medial geniculate nucleus of the thalamus via the primary auditory cortex, and from the auditory association cortex of the right hemisphere, are important to language comprehension. Damage to these fiber tracts keeps auditory information from reaching the cortex responsible for auditory-verbal comprehension. Fibers connecting Broca's area to posterior left-hemisphere areas are important for repetition.

There are several positive aspects to the theoretical perspective of Alexander, Naeser, and their colleagues. First, their perspective focuses attention on the subcortical white matter pathways of the left

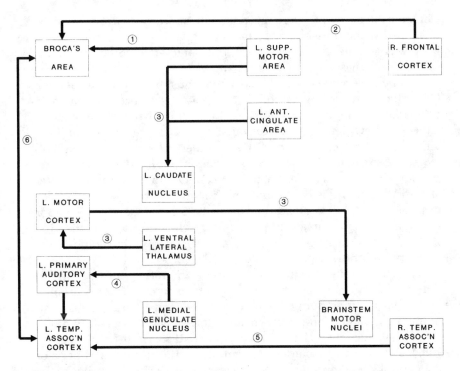

Figure 4-1. Model of Alexander, Naeser, & Palumbo (1987) for subcortical aphasia. The following pathways are depicted: (1) Pathway conveying motivation to Broca's area. (2) Secondary transcallosal pathway possibly capable of conveying motivation to Broca's area. (3) Pathways important in speech (i.e., motor output). (4) Primary auditory relay from left medial geniculate nucleus to left temporal lobe. (5) Secondary input to left temporal auditory-verbal comprehension area from right temporal association area. (6) Long posterior to anterior left hemisphere pathways. This diagram is more specific than most likely intended by Alexander et al. (1987); however, it has been done for purposes of comparison to other models. One pathway from Naeser, Palumbo, Helm-Estabrooks, Stiassny-Eder, & Albert (1989) has been added.

hemisphere as important to language. Cramon (1989) noted a tendency to focus too much attention on gray structures and not enough on the pathways connecting them. Damage to the pathways between the gray structures can be just as disruptive to behavior and cognition as damage to the gray structures themselves. Second, the work of this group is based upon some of the most consistent and careful anatomical and image analyses of the language system done to date. Their tracing of some the pathways likely to be involved in language is an important contribution. Third, they have shown how at least some elements of aberrant language after left subcortical lesion may be explained without invoking the basal ganglia. Thus, their model must be given serious consideration as one alternative for nonthalamic subcortical aphasia.

Nonetheless, their model, like others, must be critically examined. One criticism regarding its explanatory power is its incompleteness. In particular, the model does not lead to a comprehensive explanation either of how language is formulated and expressed or of how language is comprehended. Do Alexander, Naeser, and their colleagues mean to invoke classical explanations for language production phenomena (e.g., see Geschwind, 1972)? Or do they wish to alter classical assumptions based upon their studies? They have failed, for example, to take a stand on the anterior versus the posterior formulation of language. Indeed, one might question whether the group has too uncritically accepted and operated within some of the assumptions of the classical model of aphasia.

Another problem is their failure to incorporate serious consideration of thalamic language functions into their model. The reader may recall that the most serious and consistent language deficits occur in dominant thalamic infarction when the infarct is in the territory of the tuberothalamic artery (Bogousslavsky et al., 1988; Graff-Radford et al., 1985). This territory includes the ventral anterior nucleus and parts of the ventral lateral nucleus. These nuclei receive a primary output of the basal ganglia via the medial globus pallidus. Although it appears that there are additional reasons why tuberothalamic infarcts cause severe language deficits, at least part of the reason is most likely the fact that they receive this input from the basal ganglia. In other words, it appears unlikely that the basal ganglia are totally uninvolved in language.

Perhaps the symptoms of difficulty in initiation and word-finding deficits noted by Alexander (1989) hold the key to this participation. This line of thinking has not been well developed in the works of Alexander, but future works may address the problem. Further, Alexander's division between the speech and language aspects of fluency may need further revision. In particular, one might question whether agrammatism truly belongs to the realm of nonfluency, or whether it deserves attention as a separate phenomenon. The fact that larger, more anterior lesions cause agrammatism which coincides with nonfluent language and speech does not mean that agrammatism must be considered as an element of nonfluent language. It may be that the initiation and continuation of more extended language productions are the essential elements of fluency for the language domain, and agrammatism is not a component of nonfluent language. Consideration of Alexander's (1989) data in this light indicates that language fluency might be more impaired in his subcortical patients than he realized from his perspective.

Finally, it has been noted that small cortical lesions do not generate serious, long-lasting language deficits (Brunner et al., 1982). This being the case, it is not totally unexpected that small lesions confined to one area of the striatum do not cause serious or lasting aphasia. Indeed, Brunner et al. (1982) found that combined cortical-subcortical lesions caused more severe and long-lasting deficits than cortical or striatal lesions alone. Further, the subtlety of acute nonthalamic subcortical lesions may be an indication either that they play a role in language different from the thalamus or the cortex, or that the functions in which the basal ganglia participate can be partially performed through alternative routes when the basal ganglia are damaged.

To summarize: Alexander and colleagues make an important contribution by focusing attention upon subcortical pathways that may contribute to language and by questioning the participation of the striatum in language. Up to this point in time, they have not provided a comprehensive model for language production or comprehension, and they have failed to integrate thalamic mechanisms into their consideration of basal ganglia mechanisms. They have not accounted for those language symptoms that do occur with nonthalamic subcortical gray matter lesions, and they may have placed undue emphasis on the lack of language symptoms with small striatal lesions. Yet their theoretical perspective must be considered as a viable alternative. Further iterations on their model are likely to be important contributions to our understanding of subcortical and cortical language functions.

The Lexical Decision Making Model

The writings of Wallesch contain a model of striatal functioning that is in many respects at the opposite pole from the minimal-participation assumption of Alexander and his colleagues. One of the first suggestions of the participation of cortico-striato-pallido-thalamo-cortical loops in language can be found in the work of Brunner et al. (1982), in which Wallesch participated. He was more explicit regarding his ideas in a 1985 study of several patients with subcortical aphasia, but the most complete rendering of his theoretical constructs (in English) is found in the 1988 chapter by Wallesch and Papagno.

Wallesch's works exhibit several contrasts the works of Alexander. First, Wallesch does integrate the ventral anterior and ventral lateral thalamic nuclei into his model, a feature largely absent from

Alexander's discussions. Second, Wallesch emphasizes information-processing capacities and decision-making capabilities at the level of the basal ganglia, or possibly even in structures downstream from the basal ganglia in the cortico-striato-pallido-thalamo-cortical loop. Third, Wallesch does take a stand regarding classical language assumptions, suggesting that lexical alternatives are posteriorly generated and conveyed both to the striatum and the anterior language cortex. Fourth, Wallesch's model includes a more complete description of the processes necessary for language production.

A diagram of the anatomical assumptions regarding the cortico-striato-pallido-thalamo-cortical loop in the model (Wallesch & Papagno, 1988) is shown in Figure 4-2. Wallesch and Papagno emphasized input to the striatum from limbic and related cortex, from the posterior language cortex, from the anterior language cortex, and from

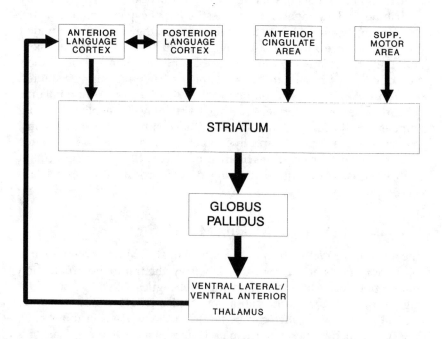

Figure 4-2. Model of Wallesch and Papagno (1988) for subcortical language functions. Note that inputs from limbic, language, and motor cortex are assumed to communicate within the subcortical portions of the loop. The collation of information from these different sources is assumed ultimately to lead to selection of the best lexical alternative among multiple cortically generated choices.

non–language cortex. This model necessitates the interaction of these inputs either at the level of the striatum, or downstream in the loop from the striatum. The projection back to the anterior language cortex from the loop is also emphasized.

Wallesch (1985) suggested that the subcortical structures in the cortico-striato-pallido-thalamo-cortical loop were involved in choosing the response "eventually executed from among a number of cortico-cortically" generated response alternatives that are processed in parallel. A more detailed description of the model can be found in Wallesch and Papagno (1988). In the latter work, the authors stated that competing responses are processed in parallel modules that are transmitted from posterior to anterior language cortex. Borrowing from Eccles (1977) and Goldman-Rakic (1984), these authors proposed that inhibition of parallel modules governs behavior by survival of the fittest potential response. The anterior cortex could further combine and recombine modular inputs, providing for flexibility of response.

The role of the subcortical portions of the loop is integrative. These structures monitor cortical processing of the parallel modules and integrate situational and motivational constraints. The lexical alternative (in the module) that is most appropriate to the internal goal and the external constraints is then selected and gated to output channels. External constraints are monitored through input to the striatum from the language and non–language areas of the cortex. Inputs from the anterior cingulate area and supplementary motor area act to convey information about motivations internal to the organism. Information concerning the status of parallel modules, of course, is conveyed to the striatum through connections with the language cortex.

Ultimately, the gating of the most suited alternative is a function of the influence of the ventral thalamus (ventral lateral, ventral anterior) on the anterior cortex involved in language. These nuclei control gating in the anterior cortex by exciting inhibitory cortical interneurons. A lesion in this part of the thalamus results in semantic paraphasias because of the admission of less-than-optimal lexical alternatives into language-output channels. In other words, there is a failure of gating mechanisms regulated by thalamic input. Normally, the thalamic input acts to dampen the less-than-optimal alternatives by activating the inhibitory cortical interneurons.

Ordinarily, the globus pallidus exercises an inhibitory influence on the ventral thalamic nuclei which acts to control thalamic gating, as just noted. Pallidal lesions are presumed to cause transcortical motor aphasia because such lesions would lower inhibition of the ventral thalamic nuclei which, in turn, would lead to unselective excitation of the inhibitory cortical interneurons. The increased activity of the inhibitory cortical interneurons would uniformly dampen the anterior component of all cortico-cortical modules, causing difficulties in language initiation and lexical selection. However, repetition remains intact because the constraints provided by an external model during repetition cause all cortico-cortical modules to come up with the same alternative and there is no competition between modules. This lack of competition between modules means that there is no need for subcortical gating during repetition. Finally, the authors noted that the ultimate excitatory versus inhibitory influence of the striatum on the ventral thalamus (via the globus pallidus) is not yet understood.

According to Crosson and Early (1990), this model puts the striatum in a supraordinate position with respect to the cortex, that is, it regulates which among several cortically generated alternatives is expressed. It further demands a high level of information-processing capacity at the level of the striatum, and perhaps beyond in the loop. This information-processing capacity is necessary to monitor various cortical inputs and make the selection as to which module contains the most appropriate lexical alternative. In short, the striatum is a decision-making organ with a high information-processing capacity.

Finally, Wallesch and Papagno (1988) indicated that possible alternatives to the cortico-striato-pallido-thalamo-cortical loops for gating lexical alternatives exist. Specifically, thalamo-frontal and fronto-thalamic connections may allow for the loop through the basal ganglia to be bypassed. Thus, the authors emphasized the plasticity of the frontal cortex with respect to its ability to reroute information-processing and selection functions through other subcortical structures.

The Wallesch model has several strong points. First, Wallesch does integrate thalamic and basal ganglia functioning to consider a cortico-striato-pallido-thalamo-cortical loop as important in language. In general, the concept of such a loop is consistent with the recent influential review of Alexander et al. (1986) concerning such loops. Second, the consideration of the striatum as involved in complex information processing is consistent with the ideas of Divac (Divac, 1984; Divac, Oberg, & Rosenkilde, 1987) that the striatum operates on the basis of patterned neuronal output. According to Divac, patterned (as opposed to quantitative) neuronal output conveys coded information and is disrupted by both electrical stimulation and lesion. Thus, the capacity to handle patterned neuronal activity would be necessary for complex information processing. Third, the Wallesch model has some explanatory value for some symptoms of subcortical aphasia. According to this model, semantic paraphasias would be the result of an inability to select the most appropriate cortically generated lexical alternative. The nonfluency sometimes seen in speech and/or language after nonthalamic subcortical lesion can be accounted for by the disinhibition of thalamo-cortical neurons that excite inhibitory cortical interneurons.

Some difficulties with this theoretical perspective must also be noted. For example, the model of Wallesch and Papagno (1988) requires the integration of inputs to the striatum from the limbic system, the language system, and non–language cortex. Presumably, such integration would take place at the level of the striatum or further downstream in the subcortical components of the cortico-striato-pal-lido-thalamo-cortical loop. While the notion of this type of loop participating in language is generally consistent with the concepts of Alexander et al. (1986), the specifics as outlined by Wallesch and Papagno are not consistent with the review of Alexander et al. The primary problem is that the different loops, particularly the dorsal lateral prefrontal loop, the anterior cingulate loop, and the motor loop (projecting to the supplementary motor area) were anatomically distinct from one another at all levels from the cortex through the basal ganglia and the thalamus. Thus, if one accepts the conclusions of Alexander et al. (1986), then one must also conclude that the type of integration suggested by Wallesch and Papagno (1988) is unlikely to take place in the subcortical structures of the left hemisphere.

With such an important role, which implies high information processing capabilities, one would predict that basal ganglia lesions would regularly lead to rather drastic deterioration in language. Yet Alexander (1989) described varying degrees of word-finding problems with initiation problems as the only language deficits found with many cases of nonthalamic subcortical aphasia. Further, the more complicated and specialized is the function ascribed to a structure, the harder it will be to compensate for the loss of the structure. Wallesch and Papagno (1988) attributed a highly complex and specialized role to the striatum, but they also suggested that cortico-thalamo-cortical connections could replace that role.

Finally, Wallesch and Papagno (1988) seem to imply that the generation of lexical alternatives is a function of the posterior cortex, with the cortico-subcortico-cortical loop and anterior language cortex acting upon the alternatives that are generated. This suggestion mirrors the implication from classical aphasia theory that language is generated posteriorly and conveyed forward to the anterior cortex which performs motor programming. To date, there is no good evidence for such a model of language generation.

The Response-Release/Semantic-Feedback Model of Language

Crosson (1985) proposed a model for subcortical functions that, unlike the model of Alexander et al. (1987), includes a role for the striatum in language. However, it attributes a less ambitious role to the striatum than the model of Wallesch and Papagno (1988). The role that Crosson attributed to the striatum and other components of the cortico-striato-pallido-thalamo-cortical loop was one of regulating the release of preformulated language segments. According to this earliest version of the model, this loop is also involved in maintaining the proper level of arousal for the anterior language cortex. A third function, which includes a pathway through the pulvinar (Crosson & Hughes, 1987; Crosson et al., 1988), is a semantic feedback loop between the anterior and the posterior language cortex.

According to Crosson (1985)[1] language is formulated in the more anterior zones of the left hemisphere's language cortex. This formulation is done in segments of phrase or short-clause length. Each formulated segment is monitored for semantic accuracy by the same posterior language cortex that is responsible for semantic decoding of incoming language (see Figure 4-3[A]). Language segments are conveyed from the anterior formulation centers to the posterior semantic-decoding centers by a pathway from the anterior cortex to the pulvinar to the posterior cortex. If a semantic inaccuracy is found during monitoring, information about the needed correction is conveyed from the posterior language cortex to the pulvinar to the anterior language cortex. If no semantic inaccuracies are found during monitoring, then the language segment is released for motor programming.

The release of a language segment for motor programming (see Figure 4-3[B]) takes place through a cortico-striato-pallido-thalamo-cortical loop associated with language. According to the 1985 model, the release mechanism operates as follows: The dominant temporal lobe normally maintains an inhibition over the dominant caudate head. This results in a low level of activity in the inhibitory link between the caudate head and the medial pallidal segment. Consequently, the inhibition of the ventral anterior thalamus by the medial pallidal segment is normally high, which limits the amount of excitation conveyed from the ventral anterior thalamus to the anterior language cortex.

---

1. Data supporting the 1985 version of the model were reviewed in the original article. Considerations of time and space do not allow for in-depth consideration of the supporting data; the interested reader is referred to the original manuscript.

A. SEMANTIC MONITORING PATHWAY

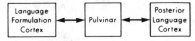

B. MECHANISM FOR RELEASE OF FORMULATED LANGUAGE

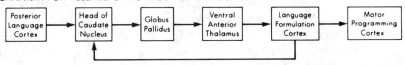

C. PHONOLOGICAL MONITORING MECHANISM

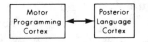

D. MECHANISM FOR RELEASE OF MOTOR PROGRAMS

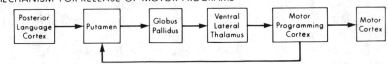

Figure 4-3. Neural pathways and mechanisms for: (A) semantic monitoring, (B) release of formulated language, (C) phonological monitoring, and (D) release of motor programs.

A formulated language segment is held in a buffer in the anterior cortex until semantic confirmation of the segment has taken place. Once semantic verification has been accomplished, the dominant temporal cortex releases the dominant caudate head from inhibition. This increases the inhibitory influence of the caudate head over the medial globus pallidus. The result is a dampening of pallidal inhibition of the ventral anterior thalamus, which leads in turn to increased excitatory transmission from the ventral anterior thalamus to the anterior language cortex. This increase in thalamo-cortical excitation serves as an impetus to release the formulated language segment in the anterior buffer for motor programming. When motor programming is complete, fronto-striatal pathways help to reestablish the normal temporal lobe inhibition over the caudate head, and the cycle can begin again.

This cortico-striato-pallido-thalamo-cortical loop was also thought to be involved in controlling the tonic-arousal level of the anterior language cortex. The anterior language cortex could increase or decrease its own tonic-arousal level through its connection with the caudate head depending upon external demands. The caudate head, then, could gate tonic excitation from the ventral anterior thalamus to the cortex through its connection with the globus pallidus. Tonic excitation from the midbrain reticular formation is conveyed to the ventral anterior thalamus through the thalamic intralaminar nuclei, and it is this tonic influence that is gated to the anterior cortex by pallidal inhibition. Thus, a phasic (fast-acting, time-limited) change in excitatory input to the anterior language cortex from this loop is responsible for the release of verified language segments for motor programming. A tonic (slow-acting, extended) change in levels of excitatory input to the anterior language cortex changes the readiness of the anterior language cortex to respond to internal or external demands for language output.

A similar set of mechanisms (see Figure 4-3[C] and 4-3[D]) was proposed for motor programming. Motor programming was monitored for phonological accuracy by the posterior cortex, which normally phonologically decodes incoming language, via the arcuate fasciculus. The response-release mechanism included the putamen and ventral lateral thalamus instead of the caudate head and the ventral anterior thalamus.

Figure 4-4 indicates how language might be produced in a narrative format. Note that the processing is sequential within a language segment, but parallel between segments. Within the language segment, language is formulated, then monitored for semantic accuracy. Once semantically verified, it is released for motor programming. The motor program is monitored for phonological accuracy and released for motor execution once it is phonologically verified. After the first segment is formulated and while it is being monitored for semantic accuracy, formulation of the second segment can begin. When the first segment reaches motor programming and the second segment reaches semantic monitoring, the third language segment can be formulated, and so on. Note that a semantic correction must take place in segment 3 of the diagram (see Figure 4-4), and segment 4 is held in the semantic buffer until the correction is completed. Thus, further processing of segment 4 is delayed until the semantic correction on segment 3 is finished.

According to the model, symptoms caused by lesions of dominant subcortical structures follows from their function, including the nature of their output (i.e., excitatory versus inhibitory) to other structures. According to the model, lesion of the ventral anterior thalamus or its connections to the cortex would lead to nonfluent language output because of decreased tonic arousal to the anterior cortex along with interruption of the response-release mechanism. Lesion of the globus pallidus would cause a fluent aphasia because the ventral anterior thalamus would be released from tonic inhibition and too much

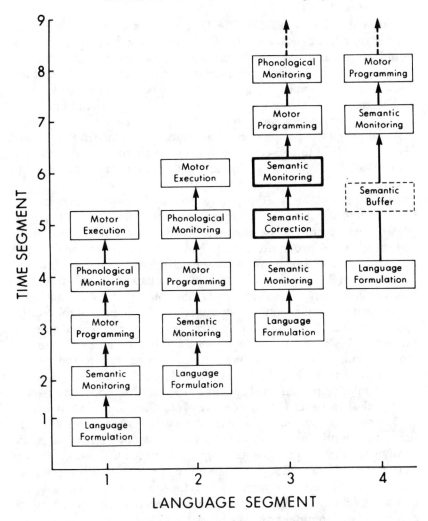

Figure 4-4. Language is processed serially within segments, but in a parallel fashion between segments. Once one language segment has been formulated and has proceeded to the semantic monitoring stage, the ensuing segment can then be formulated. This parallel processing allows for the smooth flow of language in discourse.

excitation would be passed on to the anterior language cortex. The response-release mechanism would still be interrupted, but in contrast to ventral anterior lesion, the model suggests the anterior language cortex to be left in a state of tonic hyperarousal as opposed to tonic hypoarousal. Dysfunction in the head of the caudate nucleus or its striato-pallidal fibers would prevent the caudate nucleus from inhibiting the globus pallidus. The response-release mechanism would be interrupted, and, as with the ventral anterior dysfunction, the cortex would be left in a tonic state of hypoarousal because of increased pallidal inhibition of the ventral anterior thalamus. Disruption of the connections between the temporal cortex and the caudate head would lead to tonic hyperarousal because of a release of the caudate head from inhibition, and extraneous segments would be admitted into the chain of language production as a result. Lesion of fronto-caudate fibers would lead to perseveration because of an inability to terminate the release of the formulated segment in the anterior cortical language buffer.

Crosson and Early (1990) have described several flaws in this theory. First, consistent with the criticism of Wallesch and Papagno (1988), they pointed out that the cortico-striato-pallido-thalamo-cortical loop was proposed to participate in two separate functions: a tonic-arousal and a response-release mechanism. These two different functions might require different neuroanatomical substrates to function efficiently. Further, Jones (1985) noted that the intralaminar nuclei send fibers through the ventral anterior thalamus to the frontal cortex, but these fibers do not give off collaterals to the ventral anterior thalamus. It is therefore unlikely that the intralaminar nuclei convey tonic excitation from the midbrain reticular formation to the ventral anterior nucleus, as suggested by Crosson (1985). Second, lesions to the ventral anterior nucleus in tuberothalamic infarcts do not cause the predicted disturbance (Bogousslavsky et al., 1986; Graff-Radford et al., 1985). The model predicts decreased fluency, but characteristics of both fluent and nonfluent output are observed. The nonfluent chacteristic involves decreased spontaneous language output; the fluent character-istic involves semantic paraphasias so prolific that output can degenerate into semantic jargon. Third, Crosson's (1985) model would predict an inhibitory neurotransmitter between the temporal language cortex and the dominant caudate head, but evidence (e.g., Kocsis et al., 1977; Spencer, 1976) suggests that the cortico-striatal neurotransmitter is glutamate, which has an excitatory influence on the striatal neurons. Fourth, although Yeterian and Van Hoesen (1978) suggested overlap-ping cortico-striatal projections from reciprocally connected cortical areas which would accomodate the model, the work of Goldman-Rakic and Selemon (1986) suggests that the terminal fields of such cortical areas in the striatum are adjacent, not overlapping.

Crosson and Early (1990) reasoned that the mechanisms proposed in Crosson's (1985) model were viable, but that the neuroanatomical substrates needed reconsideration. The new concepts of the neu-roanatomical systems have been depicted in Figures 4-5 and 4-6. The cortico-striato-pallido-thalamo-cortical loop is the same as proposed in the 1985 paper, but the revised model suggests that it is only involved in the response-release mechanism for language. The tonic-arousal mechanism conveys tonic arousal from the intralaminar nuclei directly to the cortex, not via the ventral anterior nucleus. Nonetheless, the fibers to the frontal cortex from the thalamic intralaminar nuclei (see Figure 4-5) do pass through the ventral anterior nucleus, as noted by Jones (1985). (The intralaminar nuclei, of course, receive input from the midbrain reticular formation.)

The anterior-to-posterior, cortical, semantic-feedback loop still takes place through the pulvinar as suggested in later explanations of the original Crosson model (Crosson & Hughes, 1987; Crosson et al., 1988). As the reader will remember from Chapter 1, Jones (1985) had questioned previous evidence (e.g., Bos & Benevento, 1975; Trojanowski & Jacobson, 1974) that the pulvinar projected to frontal cortex. He suggested that these previous studies had confused fibers originating from the posterior intralaminar nuclei as belonging to the pulvinar. However, Asanuma et al. (1985) have demonstrated that fibers from

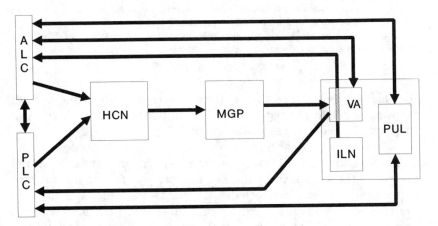

Figure 4-5. Crosson and Early's conceptualization of three subcortical systems affecting language. (1) *Arousal* of the anterior language cortex (ALC) is accomplished by the intralaminar nuclei (ILN) which receive input from the midbrain reticular formation. Fibers from the intralaminar nuclei to the anterior language cortex pass through the ventral anterior thalamus (VA). (2) *Semantic feedback* occurs between the anterior language cortex and posterior language cortex (PLC) through the pulvinar (PUL). (3) *Response release* for verified language segments occurs through a cortico-striato-pallido-thalamo-cortical loop. This loop includes the anterior language cortex, the posterior language cortex, the head of the caudate nucleus (HCN), the medial globus pallidus (MGP), and the ventral anterior thalamus. The loop is partially closed by projection from the ventral anterior thalamus to the anterior language cortex.

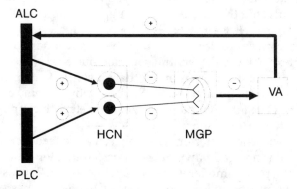

Figure 4-6. Crosson and Early's conceptualization of the cortico-striato-pallido-thalamo-cortical loop in language. Fibers from anterior and posterior language cortices converge upon adjacent areas of the striatum, which act to convert patterned input to quantitative output. Spatial summation of this quantitative output from adjacent striatal areas occurs in disc-shaped dendritic fields within the medial globus pallidus. This spatial summation is inhibitory and decreases the inhibitory output from the globus pallidus to the ventral anterior thalamus, resulting in greater excitation of the anterior language cortex by the ventral anterior thalamus. Normally, a balance in lateral inhibition within the striatum prevents high levels of inhibition over the pallidum by the striatum. However, this lateral inhibition is overcome during release of a language segment by focused input from the cortex. Pluses and minuses in circles indicate excitatory and inhibitory neurotransmitters, respectively.

the medial pulvinar projecting to frontal cortex actually comingle with neurons projecting to parietal cortex and that neurons projecting to these two locations are separate neurons.

Figure 4-6 is a conceptual representation of the cortico-striato-pallido-thalamo-cortical loop. In the revised model, the striatal component acts to convert patterned neuronal input from the cortex to a quantitative output in which the patterned aspects of neuronal firing are irrelevant (Crosson, 1989). During times when the person is not engaged in speech, a relatively equal input to the striatum from cortical language areas keeps lateral inhibition balanced within the striatum, thereby limiting striatal outflow (after Groves, 1983). This leaves pallidal inhibition of the ventral anterior thalamus high, limiting the excitatory outflow from the ventral anterior nucleus to the anterior language cortex. When a language segment is formulated, a focused input from the frontal cortex to the caudate head increases striatal inhibition of the globus pallidus within the disc-shaped dendritic fields of specific pallidal neurons (see Chapter 1). However, this increased inhibition is not enough by itself to change pallidal outflow. When a language segment has been semantically verified, increased excitation of an adjacent striatal area by the posterior language cortex increases the inhibitory outflow of this adjacent striatal area. When spatial summation of these inhibitory inputs occurs within the disc-shaped pallidal dendritic fields, pallidal outflow to the ventral anterior thalamus is decreased significantly. This allows for the temporary increase in thalamo-cortical excitation to cause release of the formulated segment for motor programming. When motor programming is complete, the excitation of the fronto-striatal connections decreases, inhibitory outflow from the caudate head to the globus pallidus decreases, and the higher inhibition of the ventral anterior nucleus by the globus pallidus resumes. After verification of the ensuing language segment, the cycle of the response-release mechanism begins again.

Because it is not available elsewhere in the literature, the reasoning and data supporting this revision of the model are worth exploring in greater detail. First, I will discuss some data regarding the semantic-feedback loop. Then, I will explore the data and reasoning behind the revised conceptualization of the response-release mechanism. Subsequently, I will note the separation of tonic-arousal from response-release mechanisms. Finally, I will undertake an evaluation of the current version of the model.

The Semantic Feedback Loop

The semantic-feedback loop has been a consistent feature of this model. Although the pulvinar was not picked as the most likely thalamic participant in this loop in the original model (Crosson, 1985), later explanations of the original model (Crosson & Hughes, 1987; Crosson et al., 1988) did suggest the loop to include the pulvinar as the sole thalamic site participating in this cortico-thalamo-cortical feedback mechanism. The inclusion of the pulvinar in semantic processing is supported by the fact that some patients with vascular lesions including the pulvinar show semantic deficits (e.g., Ciemans, 1970; Crosson et al., 1986; Puel et al., 1989) and the fact that pulvinar stimulation causes anomia (e.g., Ojemann, 1977).

Since the model dictates that semantic feedback must occur prior to spoken language, activity in the pulvinar must precede the motor programming of the language segment that is being monitored. There is no evidence supporting such activity prior to spoken segments in language. However, if such a mechanism were to exist for language, then one might expect such a mechanism to exist in phylogenetically older systems. For example, one might wonder if the pulvinar might monitor segments of movement for their internal consistency with a plan of action. Some data in the literature do actually suggest that the pulvinar may play a role in monitoring some aspects of movement. For example, cells in the monkey pulvinar show changes in firing rate related to specific aspects of movement (e.g., Magariños-Ascone, Buño, & Garcia-Austt, 1988). More importantly, Cudeiro, Gonzalez, Perez, Alonso, and Acuña (1989) have reported a small population of cells in the pulvinar (probably about 1%) that increase firing rates well in advance of the earliest changes in the motor cortex. The activation of these cells appeared unrelated to the metrics of movement, but more related to the intention to move. The authors hypothesized that these cells were somehow informing motor cortex "about the immediate execution of intentional movement independent of its metrics" (p. 369). Thus, cells in the pulvinar are active prior to changes in the motor cortex in some types of movement, suggesting that they could be involved in monitoring some aspects of the planned movement, and such a mechanism also might apply to language.

The Response Release Mechanism

As noted above, the response-release mechanism is now hypothesized to work on a significantly different basis than in the previous version of the model. In the current version, activity in the anterior language cortex is presumed to project to a limited set of neurons in the caudate head. When a language segment has been formulated in the anterior language cortex, the excitatory influence of this anterior activity on caudate neurons causes them to overcome the normally balanced lateral inhibition within the caudate head, resulting in an increase in inhibitory outflow to the globus pallidus. After semantic verification of the language segment, temporoparietal projections into the caudate nucleus activate a specific set of caudate neurons in a region adjacent to that activated by anterior input, also resulting in increased inhibitory output to the pallidum. When the inhibitory influences from the caudate head excited by frontal and temporoparietal cortical input are spatially summated within the same disc-shaped dendritic fields within the pallidum, the combined inhibitory input is enough to cause a decrease in inhibitory pallidal output to the thalamus. This results in increased firing from the ventral anterior thalamus to the cortex, activating the release of the monitored language segment for motor programming.

As noted above, this mechanism implies a regulatory role for the cortico-striato-pallido-thalamo-cortical loop in language. Such a regulatory role could be carried out on the basis of quantitative as opposed to patterned neuronal activity. This distinction between types of neuronal activity has been made by Divac et al. (1987). *Quantitative activity* can involve either the rate of firing of a neuron or the number of neurons in a cluster with increased or decreased firing rates. In general, quantitative outputs serve to modify the activity level or other aspects of the target structure's neural activity. *Patterned activity*, on the other hand, involves the coding of specific information. Patterned functions can involve the pattern of firing within a single neuron or the temporal relationships in firing between neuron pairs or multiple neurons.

The behavioral effects of electrical stimulation and lesion differ for quantitative versus patterned neuronal activity. According to Divac et al. (1987), lesions will reduce or eliminate quantitative activity, and electrical stimulation will increase quantitative activity. Thus, from a behavioral standpoint, stimulation and lesions have opposite effects. In contrast, both stimulation and lesions disrupt patterned functions. Stimulation probably does so because the information-carrying patterns have been replaced or disrupted by the pattern of stimulation and the indiscriminate activation of multiple neurons.

One important conclusion can be drawn about stimulation: if stimulation evokes a complex behavior, such as a segment of language, it is likely that the stimulation is doing so through its effects on quantitative neuronal activity. Stimulation is unlikely to evoke complex behaviors as a direct result of its effects on patterned activity because it can only interfere with patterned activity. It is unlikely that stimulation of a given amplitude, wave form, and frequency will mimic any complex patterns of neural activity. But stimulation can affect the rate of firing or number of neurons firing in areas close to the stimulation. In short, the evocation of complex behaviors like language is most probably related to the quantitative rather than the patterned aspects of neural output.

This postulate seems to be borne out if one examines the effects of cortical stimulation on language. Schaltenbrand (1965) himself noted that cortical stimulation never leads to the production of words or sentences. Penfield and Roberts (1959) and Ojemann (1983) concur that language production during cortical stimulation is at best a rare phenomenon. Thus, the generation, reception, or transfer of information through patterned neural firing, concepts consistent with our general understanding of cortical function, seem only to be interrupted and not facilitated by cortical stimulation. Further, given that cortical output seems to be patterned in nature, it also seems likely that input to the striatum from the cortex is patterned.

On the other hand, the fact that language can be evoked by electrical stimulation–induced changes at the level of the caudate head (Van Buren, 1963, 1966; Van Buren et al., 1966) leads to the conclusion that output from the caudate head may influence language through quantitative mechanisms. The case can be made even more clearly regarding the ventral anterior nucleus, where language is evoked during stimulation (Schaltenbrand, 1965, 1975). The fact that language can be evoked in a significant percentage of cases during stimulation or stimulation offset at these two structures, and the fact that these two structures are linked via the pallidum, imply that they are linked in some regulatory function for language that uses quantitative firing as a mechanism.

If cortical input to the striatum is patterned in nature, but the output of the striatum is quantitative, then the striatum may act to convert patterned input from the cortex to quantitative output to the globus pallidus (Crosson, 1989). The possibility of pattern-to-quantity converters in the brain was mentioned by Divac et al. (1987). Divac (1984) himself has suggested that striatal output is patterned in nature. Nonetheless, the evocation of language from stimulation-induced changes in striatal activity is difficult to explain from a patterned model of striatal output. According to the current model, the quantitative output from adjacent striatal areas driven by the anterior and posterior language cortices, respectively, is summated within the disc-shaped dendritic fields of the pallidum. Anterior cortical input sets up the readiness to respond, but it takes additional input from the posterior cortex to the striatum to activate the response-release mechanism.

Some electrocorticography data can be interpreted as consistent with the suggested roles of the cortex in the response-release mechanism. Fried, Ojemann, and Fetz (1981) demonstrated a slow-wave potential for anterior language cortex during silent naming. It started at onset of the stimulus to be named and reached maximum at about 750 msec. The potential was found in the premotor, motor, and posterior inferior frontal cortices. At temporal and parietal sites, there was a flattening of the electrocorticogram with suppression of rhythmic activity, resembling the desynchronization observed in the electroencephalogram during arousal. At one site, the desynchronization began after a negative potential with a mean latency of 160 msec and lasted about 800 msec. Ojemann, Fried, and Lettich (1989) confirmed statistically significant desynchronization in left temporal and parietal sites related to naming, occurring most often in the 700 to 1200 msec post-stimulus-onset epoch. This activity at both anterior and posterior sites during silent naming, and the temporal relationship between the activity with anterior sites apparently becoming active first, are both consistent with the hypothesized roles of the cortex in language formulation.

A final question to be answered is why spontaneous language

during striatal stimulation experiments seems to occur at stimulation offset as opposed to during stimulation (Van Buren, 1963, 1966; Van Buren et al., 1966). The reason for this phenomenon may relate to a lateral inhibitory network formed by GABA-ergic collaterals of striatal spiny I neurons. When electrical stimulation is applied directly to the caudate head, it is not only stimulating potential striatal output mechanisms but also stimulating mechanisms that inhibit the same output mechanisms. The net result may be no striatal output during stimulation. However, when the stimulation ends, the sudden termination of inhibition may cause a rebound effect, leading to rapid depolarization and an efferent volley from the striatum, resulting in activation of the response release mechanism for language.

Separation of Response-Release and Tonic-Arousal Mechanisms

As noted above, the model now separates the response-release mechanism, a function of the cortico-striato-pallido-thalamo-cortical loop, and the tonic-arousal mechanism, a function of the intralaminar nuclei. However, since fibers from the intralaminar nuclei to the anterior cortex course through the ventral anterior nucleus, an infarction in the territory of the dominant tuberothalamic artery would cause disruption of both the response-release and the tonic-arousal mechanisms. Interference with the response-release mechanism at this level leaves the ventral anterior thalamus unable to convey temporary increases in excitation to the anterior language cortex, which would normally release formulated segments for motor programming. The result is difficulty initiating spontaneous language. This initiation problem would probably be more pronounced except for the second effect of ventral anterior lesions, disruption of the fibers from the intralaminar nuclei to the anterior language cortex. There is some evidence (Gentilini, De Renzi, & Crisi, 1987) that disruption of the more posterior components of the thalamic intralaminar nuclei bilaterally will produce confusion, that is, a disorganization of cognition. Likewise, disruption of the pathway coursing through the dominant ventral anterior nucleus from the intralaminar nuclei is hypothesized to cause a disorganization of language. This accounts for the paraphasic output degenerating into jargon. Thus, the lack of spontaneous language and the paraphasic output seen in dominant tuberothalamic infarction (Bogousslavsky et al., 1986; Graff-Radford et al., 1985) are the result of disruption of the response-release mechanism for language segments and disruption of pathways subserving tonic arousal of the language cortex, respectively.

Although these mechanisms are hard to separate at the level of the thalamus because of anatomical considerations, they should be more easily separated at the level of the basal ganglia. Lesions to the caudate head would disrupt the response-release mechanism by failing to overcome pallidal inhibition of the ventral anterior thalamus at the appropriate time. Thus, there would be difficulty in initiating language output, consistent with the observations of Alexander (1989). In contrast, lesions of the pallidum would interfere with the response release mechanism not by a failure to lower inhibition of the ventral anterior nucleus at the proper time, but by the absence of such inhibition. This results in an overexcitation of the anterior language cortex, allowing unmonitored and extraneous segments to be released into the language-production chain. This would result in fluent, paraphasic language (e.g., Gorelick et al., 1984).

A lesion to the posterior language cortex would result in reduced excitation of lateral inhibition, leading to a normally higher level of striatal inhibition of the globus pallidus from the striatal area connected to posterior language cortex. Although this higher inhibition of pallidal neurons alone would not be enough to produce increased pallidal output, when language segments are formulated and excitation of striatal output from anterior input also occurs, this striatal output combined with the higher striatal output from the loss of lateral inhibition in striatal segments related to posterior language cortex would cause language segments to be released before monitoring. This result would be similar to effects of pallidal lesion: fluent paraphasic language. Lesion to the anterior cortex would lead to failures in language formulation, irrespective of effects on the subcortical mechanisms, but damage to fronto-caudate connections without damage to the anterior language cortex would lead to perseveration because of an inability to signal an end to motor programming and clear the language buffer. Thus, dysfunction in the pathways into or out of the caudate head might cause perseveration, difficulty initiating language, or admission of extraneous segments into language, depending upon which pathway is injured, consistent with Mehler's (1988) observations.

Evaluation of the Respose-Release/Semantic-Feedback Model

One strength of this revision is that it brings the model into line with several sources of data that were in conflict with previous versions of the model: (1) The model now fits better data about the effects of thalamic infarction on language (Bogousslavsky et al., 1988; Graff-

Radford et al., 1985). (2) Further, it is now in line with data indicating that the cortico-striatal neurotransmitter is excitatory in nature (e.g., Kocsis et al., 1977; Spencer, 1976). (3) The model now takes into account microhistological aspects of striatal structure discussed by Groves (1983), and it also takes into account similar microhistological considerations for the globus pallidus, as detailed by Yelnik et al. (1984) and discussed by Alexander et al. (1986). (4) Thalamic neuroanatomy as defined by Jones (1985) and Asanuma et al. (1985) is more consistent with the current version as opposed to the past version of the model. (5) Further, the roles of the striatum (pattern-to-quantity conversion), the globus pallidus (spatial summation), and ventral anterior thalamus (gating excitation to anterior language cortex) are better defined than in the original discussion of the model. (6) The fact that the revision no longer proposes both tonic and phasic excitatory mechanisms for the cortico-striato-pallido-thalamo-cortical loop is also an improvement.

Nonetheless, this model must also be critically reviewed. One potential problem for the model is the role proposed for the intralaminar nuclei. Watson, Valenstein, and Heilman (1981) suggested that the intralaminar nuclei play a role in the initiation of action. This hypothesis was in part based on an earlier study by Watson, Miller, and Heilman (1978) that indicated unilateral akinesia was associated with unilateral lesion of the intralaminar nuclei. With respect to language, Crosson and Early (1990) have proposed such a role for the basal ganglia, not the intralaminar nuclei. It should be noted that Watson et al. (1981) also proposed a role for the basal ganglia in the initiation of movement. However, the hypothesis that the intralaminar nuclei play a role in initiation is contradictory to Crosson and Early's hypothesis that the connections between the intralaminar nuclei and the anterior cortex subserve arousal and that hypoarousal leads to confused language. The resolution to this issue may lie in noting that the intralaminar nuclei have a major output to the striatum and may play some role in the tonic arousal of striatal as well as cortical mechanisms. Thus, a lesion to the intralaminar nuclei might cause akinesia because of the influence on the basal ganglia, not the cortex. If only the connections between the intralaminar nuclei and the anterior language cortex are affected, such as in tuberothalamic infarction, cortical but not striatal mechanisms might be selectively affected.

Another problem with Crosson and Early's revision is that its verifiability is limited, at least by lesion methods that are most commonly used to study the neural substrates of language. This problem is clearest in examining the effect of a lesion on a structure that receives a strong inhibitory influence from another structure (Crosson, 1989). If the lesion is placed so as to damage the incoming fibers without damaging the part of the structure from which the critical output originates, the effect will be the opposite from a lesion that affects the critical output from the structure. Take the case of Gorelick et al. (1984), for example. The authors attributed the fluent aphasia to the thalamic lesion which included the ventral lateral and ventral anterior nuclei. However, it must be noted that the globus pallidus and the posterior limb of the internal capsule were damaged; thus, input to the ventral lateral and ventral anterior nuclei was also affected and could have been responsible for language symptoms if a critical portion of the ventral anterior nucleus was intact. In other words, one wonders whether the input or the output of the ventral anterior nucleus was affected. The model of Crosson and Early has two inhibitory links (striato-pallidal, pallido-thalamic) that would require such fine distinctions in anatomy. Yet, such distinctions are nearly impossible to make on the basis of our imaging techniques or our neuroanatomical knowledge.

A related issue is that the complexities of micro- and macrohistology and neurotransmitter functions are such that, given enough thought and creativity, one might be able to justify almost any position, no matter how wrong it might be. This is no trivial criticism. The danger is that a bogus theory might be uncritically accepted and could hamper discovery of more valid principles and bias inquiry. Thus, it is best in the area of subcortical functions to maintain some skepticism about any theoretical approach.

To summarize: Crosson and Early's revisions of Crosson's (1985) model bring the model more into line with current knowledge regarding subcortical structure and function. One significant question that remains to be addressed is the role of the thalamic intralaminar nuclei in the initiation versus the organization of language. One profitable direction would be to explore similarities and differences to attentional and intentional functions, such as those addressed by Heilman's work (e.g., Heilman, Bowers, Valenstein, & Watson, 1987) and Watson and colleagues' (1981) model. Resolution of the difficulties in the use of structural images (CT, MR) after lesion of subcortical structures may never be adequate to test this theory. Perhaps innovations in PET or SPECT techniques will add to our knowledge in these areas. Thus, it may take one or two more revisions before this model can be either deemed as a useful approximation of language production or discarded for another alternative that provides a better accounting of the data.

Implications of Subcortical Models of Language Function

Models of subcortical functions in language should not be considered only in isolation but also must be compared and contrasted to subcortical models of other functions. Eventually, such comparisons should lead to a better understanding of the parallels, the differences, and the points of overlap between language and other cognitive systems. For example, Watson et al. (1981) discussed the difference between *attentional systems*, which allocate resources for the processing of incoming information, and *intentional systems*, which allocate resources for the planning and execution of actions. The intentional system was thought to include the basal ganglia, the ventral lateral thalamus, and the intralaminar nuclei. Since the models of Wallesch and Papagno (1988) and Crosson and Early (1990) deal primarily with language production, they are more similar to Watson and colleagues' intentional system. The suggested anatomy is very similar between the two language models and the 1981 intentional model. Nonetheless, some differences in the way in which Watson et al. (1981) and Crosson and Early (1990) have conceptualized the intralaminar nuclei exist. These differences were discussed in the previous section. The relationship between intention and language should be further explored in future studies.

Another system in which overlap and parallels might be important is the memory system. Many have referred to the distinction between *procedural* (skills) and *declarative* (facts) learning. According to the work of Squire, Butters, and others (e.g., Cohen & Squire, 1980; Martone, Butters, Payne, Becker, & Sax, 1984; Squire, 1987), diencephalic structures are involved in establishing declarative memory while basal ganglia structures are involved in establishing procedural memory. What relationship declarative memory might have to the semantic aspects of language, and what relationship syntax might have to procedural memory, is not entirely clear. However, it seems that declarative memory might be dependent, in many cases, on intact semantic processing when the facts to be learned are presented verbally. Learning the rules of syntax may be a type of procedural memory. Further exploration of the links between language and verbal memory systems is warranted. Other potential parallels between memory and language systems will be explored in Chapter 8, after a more in-depth consideration of memory systems.

Schizophrenia is another area for which subcortical language theories have some relevance. Alexander et al. (1986) described an anterior cingulate cortico-striato-pallido-thalamo-cortical loop. This loop would be parallel to the loop suggested by Crosson (1985) and Crosson and Early (1990) as involved in language and includes components of the cortico-striato-pallido-thalamo-cortical circuitry discussed by Wallesch and Papagno (1988). Swerdlow and Koob (1987) have invoked the anterior cingulate loop to explain schizophrenia, mania, and depression. Their hypothesis was that dopamine *excess* in the connections between the ventral tegmental area and the nucleus accumbens (ventral striatum) accounted for psychosis. Conversely, Early et al. (1989a, 1989b) suggested that a dopamine *deficiency* in the nucleus accumbens of the left hemisphere accounted for the thought disorder, hallucination, and ideas of control in schizophrenia. This hypothesis was in part based on the work of Early, Reiman, Raichle, and Spitznagel (1987) which showed increased blood flow to the left globus pallidus in never-medicated schizophrenics.

One explanation given for schizophrenic thought disorder is an inability to hold language segments in a buffer in the anterior language cortex (Crosson & Hughes, 1987; Early et al., 1989b; Patterson, Spohn, Bogia, & Hayes, 1986). This deficiency would cause an inability to reference later segments in a chain of communication back to earlier segments, which in turn would lead to disjointed thought and communication (i.e., thought disorder). This explanation, of course, is entirely consistent with the language theory of Crosson and Early in that they have suggested that language segments are held in a buffer in the anterior cortex. It seems quite possible that the anterior cingulate might have something to do with this buffering process.

The continued development of models of subcortical language functions will have a definite impact on our understanding of subcortical functions in other aspects of cognition such as memory and attention. There could even be some impact on schizophrenia research. Work on these models, then, can be seen as very important for increased understanding of a broad range of phenomena in the behavioral neurosciences.

Conclusions

This chapter has reviewed theories of what subcortical structures do in the language system as a whole. Many different perspectives have been proposed. Early (1950s, 1960s, 1970s) hypotheses regarding the thalamus have included general attentional mechanisms, attentional mechanisms specific to language, gating material from long-term memory stores, gating the release of preformed language sequences, and integration of language. Hypotheses regarding the basal ganglia were not as prolific at that time.

Later theories (Crosson, 1985; Crosson & Early, 1990; Wallesch & Papagno, 1988) have proposed that cortico-striato-pallido-thalamo-cortical loops are involved in language. Wallesch and Papagno suggested that this loop was involved in monitoring and selecting from multiple lexical alternatives originating in the posterior language cortex of the left hemisphere and transmitted forward to the anterior language cortex in a modular fashion. Crosson has suggested that this loop triggers the release of language segments at the appropriate time, after semantic monitoring. Thus, for Crosson, the loop plays a regulatory function vis-à-vis the cortex, a function that requires less of an information-processing capacity than that suggested by Wallesch and Papagno. Crosson and Early have further suggested that the thalamus is involved in tonic arousal of the anterior language cortex (intralaminar nuclei) and in transmitting semantic segments for monitoring from the anterior to the posterior cortex (pulvinar). Alexander and colleagues (Alexander, 1989; Alexander et al., 1987) have suggested a third point of view: the basal ganglia are involved in speech functions but minimally involved in language functions.

The continued development of such theories is important for the behavioral neurosciences, not only for language theory, but also for the understanding of other cognitive processes. Yet, one impediment to the development of subcortical language theories is the inability to develop appropriate animal models. Since complex communication with spoken and written symbols, particularly including high levels of abstraction, is a uniquely human function, it is difficult to establish an animal model that could help to advance the study of language. Such models have been particularly useful in memory (e.g., Mishkin, 1982) and have been the basis for determining the neuroanatomic origin of human memory problems after medial thalamic lesion (e.g., Cramon, Hebel, & Schuri, 1985; Graff-Radford et al., 1990). It should be further noted that since complex spoken and written symbolic communication is uniquely human, many of the evolutionary advances noted in man may be related to this communication function. Thus, it may be that interspecies differences related to evolution are particularly relevant to language. For this reason, we must be cautious in applying models developed in animals for other behaviors to language.

It is more likely that functional imaging techniques such as PET and SPECT may eventually provide more information regarding subcortical language functions in normals. The spatial resolution of these devices has limited their utility to some degree; nonetheless, some studies have added important data regarding subcortical mechanisms in language. Wallesch et al. (1985), for example, found subcortical activation during narrative language of neurologically normal subjects, but Petersen et al. (1988, 1989) failed to find such activation during a semantic word generation task. Metter and his colleagues (e.g., Metter et al., 1983, 1986, 1988) have found relationships between cortical and subcortical glucose metabolism, subcortical damage, and language in patients with aphasia. Hopefully, such future research will become more theory oriented and can advance our understanding of subcortical language mechanisms.

II

SUBCORTICAL STRUCTURES IN MEMORY

5

Subcortical Neuroanatomy and Memory

Understanding subcortical neuroanatomy is just as important for the eventual understanding of memory functions as it is for the understanding of language. The way in which structures interact to perform the necessary operations for memory depends upon the structures available for this task and how they are connected. Since memory is a relatively complicated cognitive process, the neural system for memory is likely to be complex. If the only important issue regarding memory was determining where memories are stored, the task of understanding memory would be rather simple. However, the investigation of patients with profound memory deficits has taught us that the questions regarding memory are much more complicated. Many of these so-called amnesics have relatively intact stores of old memories (at least for some past periods), but they are unable to place new information into long-term memory storage. Thus, disruption of the ability to store new memories does not necessarily imply the disruption of all old memories. Understanding the process of how memories are stored in the brain, and what structures are involved in the process of storage, has been the focus of many studies of the neurological amnesias.

This chapter, of course, will focus on those subcortical structures thought to be involved in various memory processes. As in Chapter 1, which covered subcortical structures in language, I will place some emphasis on how the various structures are connected to one another. I will not discuss evidence regarding the participation of these structures in memory in detail until later chapters of the book. Instead,

149

this chapter will endeavor to provide a road map of the structures critical for memory and the pathways between them.

The dorsal medial nucleus of the thalamus (e.g., McEntee et al., 1976; Speedie & Heilman, 1982, 1983; Victor, Adams, & Collins, 1971), the anterior nuclei of the thalamus (e.g., Aggleton, 1986; Cramon et al., 1985; Graff-Radford et al., 1990), and the basal ganglia (Butters et al., 1987; Butters et al., 1986; Levin, Llabre, & Weiner, 1989; Martone et al., 1984) have all been implicated in memory functions. Since I covered these structures in some detail in Chapter 1, I will touch on them only briefly in this chapter. But several structures thought to be involved in memory that were not mentioned in Chapter 1 will be discussed in detail below.

One such structure is the midline nuclei of the thalamus, which were briefly mentioned by Mishkin (1982). According to Mishkin, this set of thalamic nuclei are involved in a system that helps to consolidate visual representations in visual association cortex. Another set of structures implicated in memory is the mammillary bodies, which technically are a part of the hypothalamus. Until the work of Victor et al. (1971), damage to these structures alone was thought sufficient to produce severe recent memory disturbance such as that seen in alcoholic Korsakoff's syndrome. Although Victor and his colleagues maintained that the mammillary bodies were not involved in this type of memory disturbance, more recent thinking has suggested that damage to the mammillothalamic tract is a prerequisite for severe diencephalic amnesia (Cramon et al., 1985; Gentilini et al., 1987; Graff-Radford et al., 1990).

A third set of structures implicated in memory are located in an area known as the basal forebrain. The most critical structures in this area as far as memory is concerned are probably the substantia innominata, the medial septal nucleus, and the nucleus of the diagonal band of Broca. Since these basal forebrain structures are strongly interconnected with other structures involved in establishing new memories, it is not surprising that recent evidence has shown memory deficit after they are damaged (e.g., Damasio et al., 1985a; Damasio et al., 1985b; Phillips et al., 1987).

White matter pathways between the structures involved in memory are better analyzed than white matter pathways potentially involved in language. This situation is in part due to the ability to establish animal models for memory (e.g., Aggleton, 1986; Bachevalier et al., 1985; Mishkin, 1982) that have strongly influenced subsequent human investigations (e.g., Cramon et al., 1985; Graff-Radford et al., 1990). One of the best papers tracing the pathways potentially involved in memory is that of Cramon (1989), which will be cited in this chapter.

The fornix (the main output of the hippocampal formation), the ventral amygdalofugal pathway, and the mammillothalamic tract all appear to be critical to memory.

The interconnection between structures involved in memory, of course, allows them to act as a system. I will address two well-known attempts at describing systems that may be relevant to memory, Papez' circuit (Papez, 1937) and Mishkin's model (1982). The original description of Papez' circuit suggested that system was involved in emotion, and it was only later that others implicated it in memory. Mishkin's work was always focused on memory. Some of the pathways and structures in Mishkin's model overlap with those of Papez. After exploring neural systems that may be involved in memory, I will draw a few conclusions regarding the neuroanatomical substrates of memory.

As in Chapter 1, I need to say a few words regarding how to read this chapter before embarking upon detailed neuroanatomical descriptions. For the neuroanatomically less experienced reader, it is probably enough to familiarize oneself with the major nuclei and their connections. For example, a general familiarity with the mammillary bodies and their connections is sufficient for further reading. While some knowledge of the subnuclei of the mammillary bodies could be useful, it is not required to understand ensuing chapters. As with Chapter 1, Chapter 5 can be treated as a reference to which the reader can return as the information it contains becomes important. The reader who finds the level of neuroanatomc detail unsatisfying is referred to more extended neuronatomic texts, such as Nauta and Fiertag (1986) or Carpenter and Sutin (1983).

Additional Diencephalic Structures Potentially Related to Memory

The *diencephalon* is a term used for a group of related structures that have some proximity to the third ventricle. According to Carpenter and Sutin (1983), the diencephalon can be divided into four parts: the thalamus, the hypothalamus, the epithalamus, and the subthalamus. For the most part, the nuclei of the thalamus that are relevant to memory (anterior nuclei, dorsal medial nucleus) were discussed in Chapter 1; however, because of their mention in the work of Mishkin (1982), the midline thalamic nuclei will be introduced in this chapter. The hypothalamus, beneath the anterior portions of the thalamus, plays a role in secretion of hormones from the pituitary gland, the maintenance of body temperature, feeding, drinking, mating, and aggression. The mammillary bodies are the portion of the hypothalamus that have a bearing upon memory. These unique divisions of the hypothalamus lie at its inferior posterior border. I will cover the mammillary bodies after discussing the midline thalamic nuclei.

The Midline Thalamic Nuclei

Carpenter and Sutin (1983) describe the midline thalamic nuclei as the periventricular gray matter in the dorsal half of the wall of the third ventricle and in the interthalamic adhesion. (The interthalamic adhesion is a structure not present in all humans that connects the two thalami across the third ventricle.) Carpenter and Sutin further state that these nuclei are small and difficult to delimit in humans. Indeed, many neuroanatomy texts minimize or ignore these structures. The approximate location of the midline nuclei in relationship to the interthalamic adhesion can be seen in Figure 5-1. According to

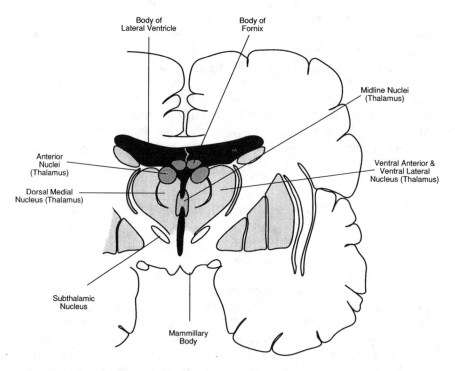

Figure 5-1. A frontal section through the interthalamic adhesion, showing the midline nuclei (after Carpenter & Sutin, 1983). According to Carpenter and Sutin, the interthalamic adhesion is present in 80% of human brains and absent in the other 20%. (Drawings are composed to indicate relationships between structures but are not meant to be anatomically precise.)

Carpenter and Sutin, the midline thalamic nuclei include the paraventricular nuclei, the nucleus reuniens, the paratenial nucleus, the rhomboid nucleus, and the median central nucleus, but agreement as to which structures should be considered midline nuclei is not unanimous.

Indeed, Jones (1985) does not honor the "midline nuclei" as a division of the thalamus. He includes the paratenial nucleus and the nucleus reuniens as a part of the medial nuclear complex along with the dorsal medial nucleus. In his schema, the anterior and posterior paraventricular nuclei are a part of the epithalamus, and the rhomboid nucleus is grouped with the intralaminar nuclei. Since the rhomboid nucleus receives input from the midbrain reticular formation and projects to the striatum, it does seem to belong more with the intralaminar nuclei. Because our interest in the so-called midline nuclei arises partly from reference to them in the work of Mishkin (1982), I will honor the distinction of the midline nuclei, minus the rhomboid nucleus. The reader should keep in mind, however, that this distinction has been challenged.

If one peruses Jones (1985) for the nuclei that Carpenter and Sutin (1983) include in the midline thalamic nuclei, one can get some idea of the connections of this group of structures. Table 5-1 lists the afferents and efferents of the midline nuclei. The afferents include limbic structures: the amygdala, the hippocampal gyrus (via the fornix), and the septal nuclei. The hypothalamus and raphe nuclei may also contribute fibers to midline nuclei. Efferents include most of the mesial cortex, including the cingulate gyrus, the parahippocampal gyrus including the entorhinal cortex, and the hippocampus. The inferior

Table 5-1. Afferent and Efferent Connections of the Midline Thalamic Nuclei and the Mammillary Bodies

Brain structure	Afferents	Efferents
Midline Thalamic Nuclei	Amygdala Parahippocampal gyrus (via fornix) Septal nuclei Hypothalamus Raphe nuclei	Amygdala Parahippocamal gyrus & hippocampus Cingulate gyrus Inferior mesial frontal cortex Nucleus accumbens
Mammillary Bodies	Hippocampal formation (via fornix) Ventral tegmental area Midbrain reticular formation	Anterior nuclei of thalamus Ventral tegmental area Midbrain reticular formation

frontal cortex and/or the nucleus accumbens are probably also targets of the paratenial nucleus. Carpenter and Sutin (1983) list the amygdaloid nuclear complex as receiving fibers from the midline thalamic nuclei.

Mammillary Bodies

At the base of the forebrain, posterior to the optic chiasm and the pituitary gland but anterior to the emergence of the third cranial nerve, are two small rounded protuberances called the mammillary bodies. They are on either side of the midline and can be seen without dissection at the junction of the forebrain and the brain stem (see Figure 5-2). Technically, the mammillary bodies are a part of the hypothalamus, constituting the most inferior and posterior portion of this structure. Yet, unlike other parts of the hypothalamus, the nuclei of the mammillary bodies have few interconnections with other hypothalamic nuclei (Nauta & Feirtag, 1986). Each of the mammillary bodies can be divided into a medial, an intermediate, and a lateral nucleus.

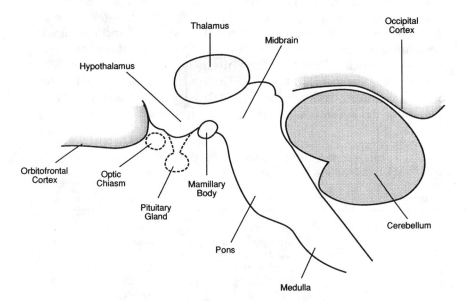

Figure 5-2. A saggital section through the forebrain and the brain stem slightly lateral to midline shows the mammillary bodies. The optic chiasm and pituitary, which are in the midline, are shown in broken lines (Carpenter & Sutin, 1983; Haines, 1987). (Drawings are composed to indicate relationships between structures but are not meant to be anatomically precise.)

Afferents to and efferents from the mammillary bodies are listed in Table 5-1. The hippocampal formation sends fibers to the medial mammillary nucleus via the fornix. The midbrain reticular formation contributes afferents to the lateral mammillary nucleus via the mammillary peduncle, and the ventral tegmental area sends fibers through the same route. Apparently, inputs to the intermediate mammillary nucleus are not well understood (Carpenter & Sutin, 1983).

The anterior nuclei of the thalamus are one target for efferent fibers of the mammillary bodies. Through the mammillothalamic tract, fibers from the medial mammillary nucleus reach the ipsilateral anterior ventral and anterior medial nuclei. The lateral mammillary nuclei contribute outputs to the anterior dorsal nuclei bilaterally. Inputs to the lateral mammillary nucleus from the midbrain reticular formation and the ventral tegmental area are reciprocated by outputs to these structures (Carpenter & Sutin, 1983).

Basal Forebrain Structures Potentially Involved in Memory

The *basal forebrain* is a term applied to a set of subcortical structures that surround the inferior tip of the frontal horn of the lateral ventricle, or that are inferior to the head of the caudate nucleus, the anterior limb of the internal capsule, or the anterior portion of the globus pallidus. As I will discuss below, structures of the basal forebrain can be considered a part of the limbic system, since they are closely interconnected with various limbic structures, including the amygdala and the hippocampus. Given the involvement of the latter two structures in memory (e.g., Cramon et al., 1985; Graff-Radford et al., 1990; Mishkin, 1982), it should not be surprising that lesions in the basal forebrain region can cause severe memory disturbance (e.g., Damasio et al., 1985a, 1985b; Phillips et al., 1987). The basal forebrain can be considered important to memory both for the nuclei it holds and the fibers that traverse it.

The basal forebrain can be considered to consist of the nucleus accumbens, the septal nuclei, the substantia innominata, and the diagonal band. The latter three entities will be discussed in the paragraphs to follow. Because it can be considered a part of the striatum, the nucleus accumbens was discussed in Chapter 1 and will not be addressed below. One potentially important factor regarding the basal forebrain is that it provides the major source of cholinergic output to the cerebral cortex.

Substantia Innominata

According to Nauta and Feirtag (1986), the substantia innominata is the gray and white matter separating the globus pallidus from the inferior surface of the forebrain. Interspersed within the substantia innominata is a constellation of large neurons referred to as the nucleus basalis of Meynert (see Figure 5-3). Some of these cells even extend into the medullary lamina of the globus pallidus, which divide the medial and lateral globus pallidus and the two portions of the medial globus pallidus (Carpenter & Sutin, 1983). In its anterior extent, the substantia innominata is superior and lateral to the optic chiasm. Its most medial portions approach the medial forebrain bundle at this level. In its more posterior portion, the medial extent nears the lateral hypothalamus (Ranson & Clark, 1959). The more lateral portions of the substantia innominata apparently lie beneath the globus pallidus and extend to the amygdala. Most modern neuroanatomy texts have devoted little attention to this cluster of cells in the basal forebrain; according to Nauta and Feirtag (1986), the area is not well understood.

However, one important aspect regarding the tracts traversing the substantia innominata is that the ventral amygdalofugal pathway runs through this area (Nauta & Feirtag, 1986). While this important pathway carries reciprocal fibers between the amygdala and the hypothalamus, it also contains fibers running from the amygdala to the dorsal medial nucleus of the thalamus. The most definitive works regarding this pathway into the dorsal medial thalamus and its role in memory are those of Mishkin (e.g., Bachevalier et al., 1985a; Mishkin, 1982), Cramon et al. (1985), and Graff-Radford et al. (1990). These works will be discussed in detail later in this chapter or in subsequent chapters. While the importance of the ventral amygdalofugal pathway has been discussed regarding its route through the thalamus (e.g., Cramon et al., 1985; Graff-Radford et al., 1990), its journey through the basal forebrain has been largely ignored in studies of memory deficit after basal forebrain lesion. Although the tract from the amygdala to the dorsal medial thalamus departs the ventral amygdalofugal pathway before reaching the most medial extent of the substantia innominata, lesions affecting the more lateral extent of the substantia innominata would impinge upon the connections between the amygdala and the dorsal medial thalamus (see Graff-Radford, 1990). While many if not most basal forebrain lesions miss this portion of the ventral amygdalofugal pathway, the likelihood of a lesion impinging on this important pathway should at least be mentioned in such studies. It is quite likely that disruption of this

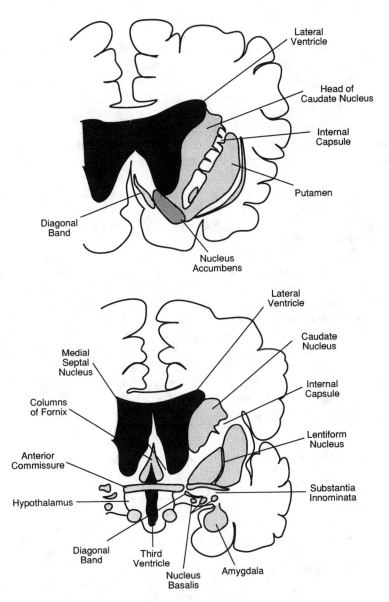

Figure 5-3. Two frontal sections through the basal forebrain. The top, more anterior section shows the nucleus accumbens and the diagonal band in its more medial, vertical position. The bottom, more posterior section shows the septal nuclei, the substantia innominata (with the nucleus basalis), and the diagonal band in its more lateral, horizontal position (as it merges into the substantia innominata). Note that the ventral amygdalofugal pathway enters the substantia innominata before fibers bound for the inferior thalamic peduncle depart. The inferior thalamic peduncle is posterior to this section (Carpenter & Sutin, 1983; Haines, 1987; Nauta & Feirtag, 1986). (Drawings are composed to indicate relationships between structures but are not meant to be anatomically precise.)

pathway, whether at the level of the thalamus or at the level of the basal forebrain, can have an impact on memory.

Afferents to the substantia innominata (i.e., the nucleus basalis) are listed in Table 5-2. The known inputs to this structure are primarily from structures considered to be a part of the limbic system or closely related to it. Both the septal region and the amygdala send fibers to the substantia innominata (Nauta & Feirtag, 1986). Further, there are afferents to the substantia innominata from the dorsal medial nucleus of the thalamus (Nauta, 1962). The reader will remember that the dorsal medial nucleus is thought to be a part of the anterior cingulate loop through the basal ganglia and that the entorhinal and anterior cingulate cortex both project into this loop via the nucleus accumbens (Alexander et al., 1986).

Efferents from the substantia innominata include reciprocal fibers to the septal region (Nauta & Feirtag, 1986), the amygdala (Nauta & Feirtag, 1986), and the dorsal medial thalamus (Carpenter & Sutin, 1983; Nauta, 1961). An equally important type of efferent fiber from the nucleus basalis is its projections to the cerebral cortex. There is an orderly projection from this nucleus to virtually every part of the neocortex. It is widely accepted that these projections use acetylcholine as their neurotransmitter, and there has been some speculation that deterioration of the large cholinergic cells in the nucleus basalis and the rest of the basal forebrain contributes to the symptoms of senile dementia of the Alzheimer's type (Nauta & Feirtag, 1986).

Table 5-2. Afferent and Efferent Connections in the Basal Forebrain

Brain structure	Afferents	Efferents
Nucleus basalis	Septal nuclei Amygdala Dorsal medial thalamus	Septal nuclei Amygdala Dorsal medial thalamus Neocortex
Nucleus of the diagonal band	Hippocampus Amygdala Pyriform cortex	Hippocampus

Medial septal nucleus	Nucleus basalis
	Amygdala
	Hippocampal
	  formation (via fornix)
	Midbrain reticular
	  formation
	Olfactory tubercle
		Nucleus basalis
		Amygdala
		Hippocampal
		  formation
		Midbrain tegmentum
		Hypothalamus
		Habenula

Nucleus of the Diagonal Band

Similar to the substantia innominata, the diagonal band contains both white matter pathways and cell bodies. Just anterior to the anterior commissure and the optic chiasm, the diagonal band begins in the most medial portion of the cerebral hemispheres, medial to the inferior tip of the frontal horn of the lateral ventricle (see Figure 5-3). As one proceeds posteriorly, the diagonal band turns inferiorly and laterally toward the amygdala. However, the diagonal band does not reach the amygdala; rather, it merges into the substantia innominata. The fibers of the diagonal band form a white band on the medial basal surface of the brain from which the structure derives its name (Nauta & Feirtag, 1986). The cells interspersed within the diagonal band constitute the nucleus of the diagonal band (Larsell, 1951).

Again, the diagonal band is a structure about which little is known. The white matter of the diagonal band bridges the substantia innominata with the septal region, carrying reciprocal fibers between these two structures (Nauta & Feirtag, 1986). One might safely assume that many facts remain to be discovered about the afferents and efferents of the nucleus of the diagonal band. However, known connections are listed in Table 5-2. Nauta and Feirtag have noted both fibers from the hippocampal formation to the nucleus of the diagonal band, and fibers from the nucleus of the diagonal band to the hippocampal formation. Like the projections from the nucleus basalis to the cortex, the efferents from the nucleus of the diagonal band to the hippocampal formation are cholinergic, originating in large cells within this nucleus. The nucleus of the diagonal band also receives fibers from the pyriform cortex in the anterior medial temporal lobe via the ventral amygdalofugal pathway (Carpenter & Sutin, 1983).

The Medial Septal Nucleus

As noted above, the medial septal nucleus has also received attention as a part of the basal forebrain. The septum (or septum pellucidum) is a thin band of gray matter separating the two frontal horns of the lateral ventricles. As the septum proceeds inferiorly toward the column of the fornix, a small amount of gray matter passes laterally to the fornix, between the inferior portion of the frontal horn and the column of the fornix. This gray matter is the medial septal nucleus (see Figure 5-3). Just posterior to the medial septal nucleus is the anterior commissure, and anteriorly, the medial septal nucleus is continuous with the diagonal band. The lateral septal nucleus is just lateral to the medial septal nucleus, lying inferior and lateral to the most inferior tip of the lateral ventricle's frontal horn (Carpenter & Sutin, 1983; Haines, 1987).

Of the basal forebrain nuclei discussed in this chapter, perhaps the most is known about the connections of the medial septal nucleus. The medial septal nucleus receives afferents from a number of sources (see Table 5-2). As noted above, there are afferents from one other basal forebrain nucleus, the nucleus basalis (Nauta & Feirtag, 1986). It is noteworthy that the medial septal nucleus also receives fibers from both the hippocampus and the amygdala. In fact, this is one area where the projections from the amygdala and the hippocampus overlap. Other sources of afferents include the olfactory tubercle and the midbrain reticular formation (Carpenter & Sutin, 1983). Thus, the medial septal nucleus is closely related by its inputs to the limbic system.

Indeed, fibers from the amygdala are reciprocated by efferents from the medial septal nucleus, and fibers from the hippocampus are reciprocated by fibers in the opposite direction which traverse the fornix (Carpenter & Sutin, 1983). Fibers are also sent back to the substantia innominata (Nauta & Feirtag, 1986). Other targets of projections from the medial septal nucleus include the hypothalamus (via the medial forebrain bundle), the habenular nucleus, and the midbrain tegmentum (Carpenter & Sutin, 1983). Again in the efferents of the medial septal nucleus, connections with limbic system structures can be seen.

Major White Matter Pathways in Memory

One characteristic of the subcortical-memory literature is a relatively careful consideration of the white matter pathways involved in memory. As previously noted, this is in part because adequate animal models for memory have been explored (e.g., Aggleton, 1986; Bachevalier et al., 1985; Graff-Radford et al., 1990; Mishkin, 1982). According to the work of Mishkin and his colleagues, there are two important temporal lobe structures for memory: the amygdala and the hippocampal formation. Earlier studies in his series of experiments (e.g., Mishkin, 1978; Mishkin & Oubre, 1977) showed that severe memory dysfunction did not occur in monkeys unless both the amygdala and the hippocampal formation were damaged. This view has come to be accepted as valid for human memory as well. Further, it is not simply these two temporal lobe structures but also their projection systems that are important for memory. The major projection of the hippocampal formation is the fornix, and one major projection system from the amygdala is the ventral amygdalofugal pathway.

Two other subcortical white matter structures are of interest for memory. First, the mammillary bodies have long been considered a part of Papez' circuit (Papez, 1937: see below). Although the original application of this circuit was to emotion, subsequent suggestions that the circuit is involved in memory have been made. In particular, the mammillary bodies have been implicated in memory, and their connection with the anterior nucleus of the thalamus has been emphasized, particularly in recent memory literature (e.g., Cramon et al., 1985; Gentilini et al., 1987; Graff-Radford et al., 1990). This connection is made through a pathway called the mammillothalamic tract. Second, inputs to the parahippocampal gyrus, and thus the hippocampus, pass through a structure recently named the collateral isthmus. Cramon and his colleagues (1988) have maintained that these parahippocampal inputs passing through the collateral isthmus are important for memory.

Cramon and others assert that an understanding of all these pathways is essential for understanding the system of structures important for laying down new memories. I shall continue to develop this theme in this and subsequent chapters of this book. Therefore, it is worth spending the time now to acquaint ourselves in some detail with these pathways.

The Fornix

As noted above, the fornix (see Figure 5-4) is the major output system of the hippocampal formation. It is composed of fibers originating in the hippocampus proper and the subiculum. (The subiculum is the medial and superior portion of the parahippocampal gyrus which transitions into the hippocampus. It has an archicortical structure like the hippocampus.) The fornix contains approximately a million fibers, making it comparable in size to the optic tract (Nauta & Feirtag, 1986). Fibers from the subiculum and hippocampus spread themselves over the lateral and superior surface of the hippocampus and converge at the medial surface to form the fimbria. The fimbria becomes thicker as it proceeds in a posterior direction. As the posterior hippocampus begins to curve superiorly and before reaching the splenium of the corpus callosum, the fibers break away from the hippocampus to form the crus of the fornix (Carpenter & Sutin, 1983).

The crus arches superiorly under the splenium, and the two crura begin to converge medially toward each other. In this region, there is a thin sheet of fibers that depart from each crus to cross to the opposite side, forming the hippocampal commissure. The two crura then

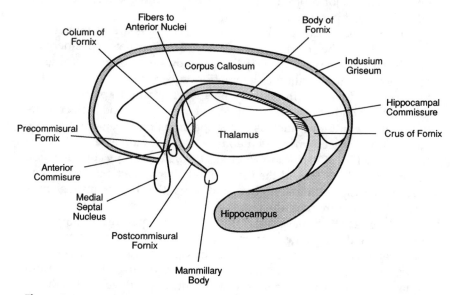

Figure 5-4. The fornix, the major output pathway from the hippocampus and subiculum. Note connections of the precommissural fornix with the medial septal nucleus, connections of the postcommissural fornix with the mammillary bodies, and the departure of fibers from the fornix to the anterior thalamic nuclei (Carpenter & Sutin, 1983; Haines, 1987; Nauta & Feirtag, 1986). (Drawings are composed to indicate relationships between structures but are not meant to be anatomically precise.)

converge to form the body of the fornix, which proceeds anteriorly beneath the corpus callosum. At the anterior margin of the thalamus, the fiber bundles separate from each other again and turn inferiorly to become the anterior columns of the fornix (Carpenter & Sutin, 1983). The anterior thalamic nuclei receive as many direct fibers from the fornix as they do from the mammillary bodies (Carpenter & Sutin, 1983).

After the body of the fornix becomes the anterior columns, the fibers of this pathway approach the anterior commissure from a superior position. As each anterior column nears the anterior commissure, it splits into two branches. The postcommissural fornix passes behind the anterior commissure, proceeding in an inferior and posterior direction. After the postcommissural fornix passes the anterior commissure, it gives off fibers that progress superiorly to the anterior thalamic nuclei. The postcommissural fornix then traverses the rest of the hypothalamus in order to reach the mammillary bodies, terminating primarily in the medial mammillary nucleus. Some postcommissural fornix fibers descend past the hypothalamus to terminate in the midbrain reticular formation (Carpenter & Sutin, 1983).

The second branch is the precommissural fornix, which passes in front of the anterior commissure. It is a less compact bundle than the postcommissural fornix. It is the means by which fibers from the hippocampal formation reach the septal nuclei, the lateral preoptic area, the nucleus of the diagonal band, and the anterior portion of the hypothalamus. Some of the precommissural fibers continue inferiorly into the central gray matter of the midbrain (Carpenter & Sutin, 1983).

There is a small component of the fornix that progresses above the corpus callosum along with the portion of the hippocampus known as the indusium griseum. Here there are two fiber bundles that are called the medial and lateral longitudinal striae. They are imbedded in the indusium griseum. It is not known if this portion of the hippocampus participates in memory (Cramon, 1989).

In summary: The fornix is a complex fiber system, distributing fibers from the hippocampus and subiculum to numerous structures. The evidence for participation of the fornix in memory has been mixed. However, Cramon (1989) has pointed out that whether memory deficits appear after injury to the fornix most likely depends upon where the fornix is injured. This evidence will be reviewed in greater detail in Chapter 6.

The Mammillothalamic Tract

The mammillothalamic tract provides a second means by which the hippocampal formation can access the anterior thalamic nuclei, mediated by the mammillary bodies. Efferent fibers emerge from the mammillary bodies coursing in a superior direction. Soon thereafter, this fiber bundle divides into one segment projecting to the midbrain tegmentum and the mammillothalamic tract. As it proceeds superiorly into the thalamus, both Carpenter and Sutin (1983) and Nauta and Feirtag (1986) show the mammillothalamic tract passing through the ventral anterior nucleus. As we shall see in Chapter 6, this location is felt to be important in evaluating the presence or absence of severe memory deficit after lesions to the dorsal medial thalamus.

The Ventral Amygdalofugal Pathway

The ventral amygdalofugal pathway is one projection from the amygdala which is considered to arise from both the basolateral amygdaloid nuclei and the pyriform cortex of the temporal lobe. (The pyriform cortex is the cortex in the most anterior portion of the mesial temporal lobe, just posterior and mesial to the temporal pole. It projects to the amygdala, as well as to the nucleus of the diagonal band, lateral preoptic area, and entorhinal cortex.) Soon after it emerges from the superior medial amygdala and pyriform cortex, the ventral amygdalofugal pathway turns medially, passing into the substantia innominata and becoming a part of the white matter beneath the lentiform nucleus. After coursing medially, fibers from this pathway enter the septal region, the lateral preoptic area, the hypothalamus, and the nucleus of the diagonal band.

However, some of the fibers bypass the preoptic region and the hypothalamus after emerging from the substantia innominata and turn in a more superior direction to enter the inferior thalamic peduncle. From the inferior thalamic peduncle, these fibers project into the magnocellular division of the dorsal medial nucleus of the thalamus (Carpenter & Sutin, 1983). According to Graff-Radford et al. (1990), the fibers from the ventral amygdalofugal pathway take a position just lateral to the mammillothalamic tract in the ventral anterior nucleus as they approach the dorsal medial nucleus. It is also worth noting that projections from the nucleus basalis probably enter the inferior thalamic peduncle via the substantia innominata and project to the magnocellular division of the dorsal medial nucleus, along with fibers from the amygdala (Carpenter & Sutin, 1983). Thus, a lesion of the inferior thalamic peduncle would deprive the dorsal medial nucleus of inputs both from the amygdala and the nucleus basalis.

The Collateral Isthmus

Although cortico-cortical connections generally are not the focus of this book, it is worth briefly mentioning an area of white matter dubbed the "collateral isthmus" by Cramon, Hebel, and Schuri (1988). The collateral sulcus is a fissure on the basal surface of the temporal lobe that separates the parahippocampal gyrus from the occipitotemporal gyrus. At the posterior portion of the parahippocampal gyrus, a number of fibers from various association cortices run through the bottleneck between the superior extent of the collateral sulcus and the temporal horn of the lateral ventricle. This bottleneck is the collateral isthmus. Fibers to and from the frontal, temporal, and occipital neocortical association areas form a horizontal fan at the level of the collateral isthmus. These fibers arise from and terminate upon the posterior parahippocampal gyrus in a topographic fashion (Cramon, 1989). Lesions in the territory of the left posterior cerebral artery that include the collateral isthmus and the parahippocampal gyrus cause verbal-memory deficits (Cramon et al., 1988). As noted by Cramon (1989), it remains to be seen if lesions of the collateral isthmus alone can cause memory deficit. The suspicion is that such a discrete lesion could cause memory disturbance by interrupting the input to the parahippocampal gyrus, thereby severing communication between the hippocampal formation and the frontal, temporal, and occipital association cortices.

Systems and Subsystems Potentially Involved in Memory

To this point, I have mainly discussed some of the pieces of the puzzle of the system for laying down new memories. While I have mentioned the connections between various components, I have not discussed systems or subsystems that potentially are involved. It is necessary to understand the relationship between the various components of a system in order to decipher its operation as a whole.

Two potentially important sets of interconnections have been mentioned in Chapter 1 and will be addressed only briefly here. First, the basal ganglia have been implicated in at least some forms of memory, a topic I will discuss at greater length in Chapter 7. If one explores the connections of the basal ganglia, then it is not a large leap to suspect that cortico-striato-pallido-thalamo-cortical loops may be involved in memory. Second, the dorsal medial thalamus has been implicated in memory, a topic I will explore in greater length in Chapter 6. In considering this proposition, it does not take too much imagination to conjecture that of the bidirectional connections of the dorsal medial thalamus with the entire prefrontal cortex, some may have functions important to memory.

Most of the attention in the following paragraphs, however, is focused upon two systems that are most likely involved in memory and that have not yet been mentioned. The first is Papez' circuit (Papez, 1937) from which many modern notions about the limbic system have been derived. The second involves the two efferent systems of the temporal lobes, discussed by Mishkin (1982) and mentioned in passing above.

Papez' Circuit

In 1937, Papez described a circuit between limbic-system structures that is frequently mentioned even in current texts. (It should be noted that the term *limbic system* was not widely accepted then [Nauta & Feirtag, 1986].) This circuit is diagramatically represented in Figure

5-5. Papez' circuit (as it has come to be known) began with the hippocampus and its projections, via the fornix, to the medial mammillary nucleus. The mammillary bodies then project to the anterior nuclei of the thalamus. As determined since the proposal of Papez, the medial mammillary nucleus, to which the hippocampal formation projects, sends fibers to the ipsilateral anterior ventral and anterior medial nuclei within the anterior nuclear group. The lateral mammillary nucleus projects bilaterally to the anterior dorsal nuclei (Carpenter & Sutin, 1983). According to Carpenter and Sutin, the anterior ventral nucleus projects to the middle third and the posterior third of the cingulate gyrus while the anterior medial nucleus projects to the entire length of the cingulate gyrus with a heavier emphasis on the anterior third of the cingulate gyrus. The anterior dorsal nucleus sends fibers to the posterior portion of the cingulate gyrus, including the retrosplenial area. The cingulum is a massive fiber bundle derived primarily from cells of the cingulate cortex. The cingulum projects to the entorhinal cortex and the subiculum, though not directly to the hippocampus. The circuit of Papez' is closed by a massive projection from the entorhinal cortex to the hippocampus. Since some fibers of the fornix are derived from the subiculum, the circuit can also be considered to be closed by projections of the cingulum to the subiculum. In fact, it is probably fibers from the subiculum, as opposed to the hippocampus, which reach the mammillary bodies via the fornix (Carpenter & Sutin, 1983).

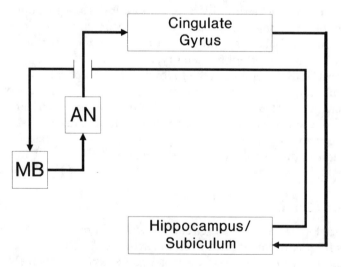

Figure 5-5. A diagrammatic representation of Papez' (1937) circuit.

Prior to Papez (1937), the structures of this circuit, especially the hippocampus, were considered to be involved in olfaction. After reviewing the evidence, however, Papez concluded that there was no evidence to support this view. Rather, he cited extensive evidence that these structures were involved in the experience and expression of emotion. Since Papez, it has become obvious that some of these structures, especially the hippocampus, are involved in memory. Papez (1937) did mention memory, but only with respect to the cingulate gyrus. Of the components of Papez' circuit, the cingulate gyrus has probably received the least attention with respect to memory, though it is not totally without mention in the memory literature. For example, on the basis of a case study, Lhermitte and Signoret (1976) hypothesized that the cingulate gyrus might be involved in memory-retrieval processes. Valenstein and his colleagues (Bowers, Verfaellie, Valenstein, & Heilman, 1988; Valenstein et al., 1987) and Cramon (1989) have presented evidence that the retrosplenial cortex may be involved in memory. If one thinks in terms of larger systems that might be involved in memory, then Papez' circuit is a primary candidate for future theoretical constructs and further investigation.

On the other hand, Nauta has noted that other limbic loops may exist (Nauta & Feirtag, 1986). For example, the septal nuclei project to the hippocampus, and the hippocampus projects back to the septal nuclei. The same is true of the midbrain reticular formation and the mammillary bodies, and of the ventral tegmental area and the mammillary bodies (Carpenter & Sutin, 1983). As mentioned above, the medial septal nucleus also maintains bidirectional connections with the nucleus basalis (Nauta & Feirtag, 1986) and the amygdala (Carpenter & Sutin, 1983). The amygdala maintains bidirectional connections with the nucleus basalis (Nauta & Feirtag, 1986) as does the dorsal medial thalamus (Carpenter & Sutin, 1983; Nauta, 1961, 1962). The role of all these reciprocated connections is uncertain at this time. It is certainly possible that some of these loops play a modulatory role in the activity of limbic structures. Through modulatory roles on one limbic structure, the effects might be felt broadly in the limbic system because of prolific interconnection of the components. Given the probable role of the limbic system in memory, it seems likely that at least some of these latter loops are involved in memory processes.

The Efferent Systems of the Mesial Temporal Lobe

In 1982, Mishkin revealed his concepts regarding visual-recognition memory in monkeys. The behavioral details regarding this work will be covered in Chapter 6, but the anatomical details will be explored below. Mishkin's model is graphically demonstrated in Figure 5-6. According to the model, visual information is distributed from the primary visual cortex (area OC) in the mesial occipital lobe to visual association cortex (areas OB, OA, TEO) in the occipital and posterior inferior lateral temporal lobe. Within the visual association cortex, the information is further distributed for purposes of "submodality processing." In other words, different aspects of the visual information are analyzed in these visual association areas. Then, information is reintegrated in the final visual association area (area TE) in the inferior lateral anterior temporal lobe.

After the visual information is reintegrated in the final link of the chain of visual association cortex (area TE), area TE activitates either of two mesial temporal structures: the amygdala or the hippocampus. When the amygdala is activated, it in turn activates the magnocellular division of the dorsal medial nucleus of the thalamus. The dorsal medial nucleus, because of its bidirectional connections with the amygdala, can feed activation back to the amygdala. In response to this input from the dorsal medial nucleus, the amygdala can in turn activate area TE. In this way, the activation of area TE can be extended in time by the temporo-amygdalo-thalamo-amygdalo-temporal loop. This continuation of activation allows the convergent inputs to area TE to be stored as representations of external visual stimuli, that is, as visual

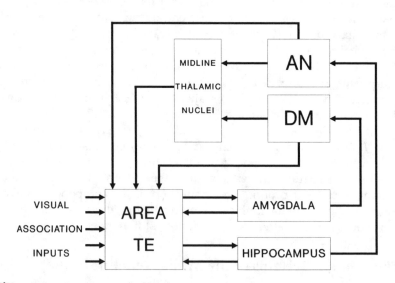

Figure 5-6. A diagrammatic representation of the efferent pathways from the temporal lobe implicated in memory by Mishkin (1982).

memories. According to the model, the amygdala also can sustain activation of area TE through its direct reciprocal connections. It is worth noting that the projections of the dorsal medial nucleus back to the amygdala may not exist; Carpenter and Sutin (1983) noted that the projections of the amygdala to the magnocellular division of the dorsal medial nucleus are not reciprocated.

Mishkin (1982) also hypothesized that sustained activation of area TE by the dorsal medial thalamus might be mediated by the midline thalamic nuclei. As noted above, the midline nuclei are distinct cell groups located on the wall of the third ventricle or in the interthalamic adhesion. There is indeed evidence that the midline nuclei project to the amygdala, the parahippocampal gyrus, and the hippocampus, but evidence of direct projections to visual association cortex are apparently lacking (Carpenter & Sutin, 1983). Jones (1985) noted that efferents from the nucleus reuniens to medial cortex come into relation with projections from the dorsal medial nucleus and the anterior nuclei, but no projections from either the dorsal medial nucleus or the anterior nuclei to the nucleus reuniens were mentioned.

It should be noted briefly at this point that Yakovlev (1948) described a limbic circuit involving the amygdala that differs somewhat from Mishkin's (1982) description. This circuit begins with projections from the amygdala via the ventral amygdalofugal pathway to the dorsal medial thalamus. The dorsal medial thalamus, in turn, projects to orbitofrontal cortex, and orbitofrontal cortex projects to the temporal pole via the uncinate fasciculus. The temporal pole completes the circuit by projecting to the amygdala. Given the probable involvement of the amygdala and the dorsal medial thalamus in memory, this circuit should also be given consideration when one discusses the neuroanatomy of memory.

It is also of some interest to review other projections into the magnocellular division of the dorsal medial thalamus. According to Carpenter and Sutin (1983), sources of input to this division in addition to the amygdala include the pyriform cortex of the temporal lobe, orbitofrontal cortex, and the olfactory tubercle. The projection to the orbitofrontal cortex is consistent with the observation of Alexander et al. (1986) that the magnocellular division of the dorsal medial thalamus is part of the orbitofrontal loop that also includes the ventral medial head of the caudate nucleus and the medial dorsomedial segment of the medial globus pallidus. Other cortical inputs to this loop include the superior temporal gyrus, the inferior temporal gyrus, and the anterior cingulate area. Thus, there may be some possibility of interaction between memory circuits and the cortico-striato-pallido-thalamo-cortical loop for the orbitofrontal cortex.

The other mesial temporal structure activated by area TE is the hippocampus. As previously noted, the hippocampus is connected to the anterior thalamic nuclei both directly through the fornix and indirectly with mediation via the mammillary bodies. According to the model, the anterior nuclei can feed activation back to the hippocampus, and the hippocampus can in turn project activation back to area TE. A review of Jones (1985) does indeed indicate projections from the anterior nuclei to the presubiculum and the parasubiculum. Thus, the hippocampus and related structures can provide a second mechanism for sustaining activation of area TE, allowing for storage of visual representations in area TE.

Other connections of the anterior nuclei (see Chapter 1) are also of interest. For example, the anterior nuclei have bidirectional connections with the cingulate cortex (via the anterior limb of the internal capsule), including the retrosplenial cortex (Carpenter & Sutin, 1983). As noted in the discussion of Papez' circuit, this connection would allow the anterior nuclei an alternative, less direct access to the hippocampus, through the cingulate gyrus, which projects (via the cingulum) to the entorhinal cortex. The latter structure then projects to the hippocampus. Connections of the retrosplenial cortex have been reviewed by Valenstein et al. (1987).

To summarize Mishkin's (1982) position: Visual analyses of various types are compiled into a visual object representation in area TE of the anterior inferior lateral temporal lobe. Upon compiling the visual representation, area TE can activate two mesial temporal structures (amygdala and hippocampus), which in turn can activate the diencephalic structures with which they are connected (magnocellular dorsal medial thalamus and anterior thalamic nuclei, respectively). These deep temporal and diencephalic structures can prolong the activation of area TE, allowing for storage of the visual representation. There is some evidence that concepts from both Papez' circuit and Mishkin's model may be needed to explain phenomena related to diencephalic amnesia, and possibly even basal forebrain amnesia. These matters will be discussed in Chapters 6 and 7, respectively.

Conclusions

According to Nauta and Feirtag (1986), the modern crtierion for inclusion in the limbic system is the relationship of the structure in question to the hypothalamus. Limbic structures are either directly connected to the hypothalamus, or connected to an intervening structure that is connected to the hypothalamus. By this standard, most of the structures that are involved in memory belong to the limbic system. The hippocampus, for example, provides direct inputs to the mammillary bodies of the hypothalamus via the fornix. The amygdala projects to other hypothalamic structures. The anterior nuclei of the thalamus are directly linked to the mammillary bodies by the mammillothalamic tract. Other structures that might be included in the limbic system are related to these three entities that all have a direct relationship with the hypothalamus.

The cingulate gyrus, for example, has connections both with the anterior nuclei of the thalamus and the hippocampal formation. Structures of the basal forebrain also could be included in the limbic system by the above criterion. The nucleus basalis is connected to the amygdala, and the nucleus of the diagonal band and the medial septal nucleus are related to both the amygdala and the hippocampus. The dorsal medial thalamus has a direct relationship with the amygdala. The nucleus accumbens, mentioned in Chapter 1, is sometimes referred to as the limbic striatum because of its connections with the hippocampal formation and the cingulate gyrus. The entorhinal cortex and other parts of the parahippocampal gyrus might also be included in the limbic system because of their direct input into the hippocampal formation or the fornix.

In addition to memory, the limbic system seems to subserve emotion and motivation. At present, the exact relationship between emotion and motivation on the one hand and memory on the other is unclear. However, Nauta and Feirtag (1986) speculated that the hippocampus assigns a degree of meaningfulness to passing events or objects and that this assignment of meaningfulness participates in making the events or objects memorable. The assignment of meaning-fulness to thoughts and events, of course, would be a function of emotion and motivation. The relationship of these processes and their underlying neurologic substrate to memory will undoubtedly be the subject of future investigations.

Important cortical limbic structures for memory encompass the cingulate cortex (including the retrosplenial cortex), the hippocampus, and the parahippocampal gyrus. Since these structures are technically cortical, they will not be a main focus of this work, except as they relate to subcortical structures. The amygdala, a deep temporal lobe structure, also will not be a major topic for this work. Instead, emphasis will be placed on various components of the diencephalon (i.e., dorsal medial thalamus, anterior nuclei of the thalamus, mammillary bodies of the hypothalamus); members of the basal forebrain (nucleus basalis, nucleus of the diagonal band, medial septal nucleus); and the basal ganglia (striatum, pallidum). Emphasis will also be placed on the major white matter pathways that connect the various structures involved in memory. These includes the fornix, the ventral amygdalofugal pathway, and the mammillothalamic tract. Diencephalic structures and memory will be covered in Chapter 6; the basal forebrain and basal ganglia will be covered in Chapter 7.

In summary: The complexities of subcortical involvement in memory is potentially greater than the complexity of subcortical participation in language. Not only are thalamic and basal ganglia structures potentially involved in memory, but structures in the hypothalamus and basal forebrain may also play a role in memory processes. In order to begin to understand the role played by all the subcortical components of the memory system, it will first be necessary to discuss various memory processes. This discussion will be included as a section of the next chapter, which focuses on the role of diencephalic structures in memory.

6

The Diencephalon in Memory

Studies regarding the participation of diencephalic structures in memory are concerned with two general topics: which diencephalic structures participate in memory, and what role diencephalic structures play in memory processes. These topic areas provide a convenient structure for the current chapter. Dividing the review in this way will also provide a foundation for the discussion of memory systems in Chapter 8. Consistent with the direction of this work, Chapter 8 will explore how subcortical structures participate together with cortical structures in memory processes.

The first general issue I will address in the present chapter is the anatomical one: Which diencephalic structures are involved in memory? Some historical progression in this area is present, and this progression presents a convenient organization for my discussion. A view prominent earlier in this century (e.g., Gamper, 1928) highlighted the mammillary bodies as the critical diencephalic structure for memory. Later, as noted in Chapter 5, Papez (1937) emphasized the mammillary bodies as part of a circuit concerned with emotion. Since Papez, this circuit (hippocampal formation to mammillary bodies, mammillary bodies to anterior thalamic nuclei, anterior thalamic nuclei to cingulate gyrus, cingulate gyrus to hippocampal formation) has been regarded as a likely candidate for involvement in memory processing. However, the influential work of Victor et al. (1971) helped turn attention to the dorsal medial thalamus as the primary candidate for diencephalic participation in memory. Even as attention was shifting toward consideration of the dorsal medial thalamus as critical in memory, Mishkin and colleagues' work with monkeys (e.g., Aggleton, 1985; Bachevalier et al., 1986; Mishkin, 1982) indicated that diencephalic structures related to both the amygdala and the hippocampal formation were involved in memory. More recent studies have extended Mishkin's work to cases of vascular and other lesions in the diencephalon and represent the latest thinking regarding thalamic participation in memory. Thus, current thinking is that both the mammillary bodies and medial thalamic nuclei are involved in establishing new memories. Finally, one must consider what diencephalic structures participate in the attentional processes that influence what material is processed for memory storage.

The section on structural issues will be followed by the section on the memory processes in which diencephalic structures are involved. Alcoholic Korsakoff's syndrome has frequently been used as a model for diencephalic amnesia. In spite of numerous problems with the alcoholic Korsakoff's literature, I will consider it in some detail. Although this literature does not provide definitive answers regarding diencephalic amnesia, its focus on processes of memory defines issues important in the study of amnesias that do have a discrete diencephalic focus and highlights certain issues regarding the conceptualization of memory processes. Subsequently, I will review memory processes after other forms of diencephalic lesion. In this discussion, the reader should remember that cases of infarction are less likely to cause pressure effects to surrounding structures than cases of tumor or hemorrhage. I will end the chapter by offering a few conclusions regarding the diencephalic structures involved in memory and the processes related to these diencephalic structures.

Diencephalic Anatomy and Memory

The study of diencephalic structures involved in memory has been greatly influenced by the type of cases available for study and the anatomical localization technique. Many of the early studies were based upon Wernicke-Korsakoff or tumor cases that had come to autopsy and implicated the mammillary bodies. With the advent and common availability of the CT scan, investigators have been able to study in-vivo structural changes in diencephalic structures, and some attention shifted toward the dorsal medial thalamus. Greater accuracy in localization was aided by the application of stereotactic atlases to the study of deep lesions (e.g., Archer et al., 1981). With the use of "stereotactic" localization, attention again shifted, this time to diencephalic white matter pathways involved in memory. The clarity of magnetic resonance imaging for some deep structures is giving a new generation of investigators increasing confidence regarding localization statements.

In spite of improving technology, one problem with the literature on anatomic localization and diencephalic amnesia should be mentioned. Investigators have generally focused on profound memory loss after diencephalic lesion, and they have seen mild to moderate memory losses as inherently uninteresting. A recent study by Mennemeier and colleagues (Mennemeier, Fennell, & Valenstein, 1990; Mennemeier, Fennell, Valenstein, & Heilman, 1990) emphasized the importance of studying anatomic relationships in cases of milder memory loss after diencephalic lesions. In order to provide a more complete understanding of the anatomy of memory, such studies of mild to moderate memory loss should continue.

As noted above, in this section of Chapter 6, I will first explore studies implicating the mammillary bodies in memory. Following that discussion I will offer a subsection regarding evidence for involvement of the dorsal medial thalamus in memory. The third topic I will cover is studies implicating diencephalic structures related to both the amygdala and the hippocampal formation in memory. Thus, discussion progresses toward the more recent conclusion that the mammillary bodies and possibly the anterior nuclei (both anatomically related to the hippocampal formation) and medial thalamic structures (anatomically related to the amygdala) all play a role in establishing new memories. Prior to making a few concluding remarks, I will discuss the role of thalamic structures in attentional processes that subserve memory.

Evidence Supporting the Role of the Mammillary Bodies

For some time, prevailing thought dictated the mammillary bodies as the probable locus of disturbance in diencephalic amnesia. Gamper's (1928) work was widely cited in this regard (e.g., Kahn & Crosby, 1972; Sprofkin & Sciarra, 1952; Williams & Pennybacker, 1954). Sprofkin and Sciarra (1952) noted that Gamper considered the mammillary bodies to be the most commonly involved structure in Korsakoff's syndrome and in Wernicke's encephalopathy (the acute state of alcoholic Korsakoff's syndrome). However, the thalamus and the brain stem were also noted to be involved. Gamper cited other investigators who found damaged mammillary bodies in cases of severe amnesic syndrome.

Sprofkin and Sciarra (1952) themselves reported two autopsied cases of tumor with extreme memory impairment, including confabulation. Only one case involved the mammillary bodies, and the authors felt their data to be inconclusive regarding the participation of the mammillary bodies in the amnesic syndrome. However, it should be noted that both cases involved the columns of the fornices and the septal region. Both these structures have implications for memory which I will discuss shortly (fornix) or in the next chapter (septal region). Both cases also included the corpus callosum, and the caudate nuclei and thalami were involved in the case with intact mammillary bodies.

Williams and Pennybacker (1954) also were conservative in their approach to localization. They noted that tumors in proximity to the third ventricle, as opposed to tumors in other areas, tended to cause amnesic syndromes, but they did not further delineate which structures in this area were related to the gross failure in memory.

Kahn and Crosby (1972) described five cases of craniopharyngioma in which patients developed amnesic syndrome with confabulation either before or after surgery for the removal of the tumors. In four cases, the symptoms disappeared within several days after removal of the tumor; the 5th case expired from bilateral pulmonary embolism postoperatively. In all cases, the craniopharyngiomas impinged upon the mammillary bodies, and the authors concluded that disruption of activity of the mammillary bodies may have caused the memory deficits because of interruption of Papez' circuit.

Mair, Warrington, and Weiskrantz (1979) presented detailed postmortem evaluation of the brains of two patients with the usual profound memory deficits associated with alcoholic Korsakoff's syndrome. There were two common defects for both patients: first, there was severe gliosis, shrinkage, and discoloration of the medial mammillary nuclei bilaterally; and second, a thin band of gliosis was interposed between the wall of the third ventrical and the dorsal medial nucleus. Some comparison to the anatomic findings of Victor et al. (1971) in alcoholic Korsakoff's syndrome were made. The thalamic lesions were generally medial to the area of damage described in the dorsal medial thalamus by Victor et al. (see below), with the cases of Mair et al. involving more the midline nuclei. Because of this difference, the authors leaned toward the hypothesis that damage to the mammillary bodies was the critical factor in the amnesic syndrome. They suggested that severe damage to the mammillary bodies may be sufficient to cause amnesic syndrome, but less severe damage at that site would be insufficient to cause amnesic syndrome without the involvement of other structures.

The hippocampal formation has, of course, been implicated in memory. Since a major output of the hippocampus is to the mammillary bodies via the fornix, the status of memory after damage to the fornix is of interest. Nonetheless, Cairns and Mosberg (1951) described section of one or both anterior columns of the fornix during removal of colloid cysts of the third ventricle. In their nine long-term survivors, no amnesic syndromes were reported, though mild effects on memory could not be entirely excluded. Because of the relationship of the fornix to the hippocampus, interruption of hippocampal input to the mammillary bodies by section of the anterior columns of the fornix without amnesic syndrome casts doubt on the proposition that damage to the mammillary bodies alone can cause amnesic syndrome.

This work of Cairns and Mosberg (1951) is sometimes cited as evidence that damage to the fornix can cause memory disturbance. They did report memory disturbance and/or dementia in two cases in which the colloid cyst impinged on the portion of the fornix above the cyst. In one case, operative intervention restored memory. It should be noted that impingement on the fornix in these two cases was at a point where not only hippocampal input to the mammillary bodies was affected, but input to the anterior thalamus from the fornix was likely affected as well. Of course, hydrocephalus often causes many of the symptoms associated with colloid cysts, and memory decrement is often associated with hydrocephalus. Thus, one must view data regarding memory and the fornix with some skepticism when the source of the data is the dysfunction caused by the colloid cyst itself.

Section of the fornix is one technique used for treatment of epilepsy. In such surgeries, Garcia Bengochea, de la Torre, Esquivel, Vieta, and Fernandez (1954) described no unfavorable sequela. The description of their approach leads one to believe they sectioned the anterior portions of the fornix. Umbach (1966) reported unilateral destruction of the fornix in 20 cases and bilateral destruction of the fornix for epilepsy in 5 cases. Even after bilateral destruction, no lasting disturbance of memory was found. The point at which the fornix was destroyed was described as at the "posterior margin of the anterior commissure." This point is near the departure of fibers to the anterior thalamic nuclei, perhaps leaving them intact. It appears that this lesion would leave fibers to the septal region intact.

Woolsey and Nelson (1975) showed chronic destruction of the fornix resulting from metastatic lesion in a single case. The fornix was destroyed bilaterally at the columns and "proximal portions of the body." No memory deficits generally were noted. The episodic confusion shortly before the patient expired was thought to be due to fever from pulmonary disease and metabolic disturbances. In this case, fibers from the fornix to the anterior thalamic nuclei probably were damaged, unlike the cases discussed above.

On the other hand, Heilman and Sypert (1977) found severe amnesic disturbance after a tumor invaded the posterior fornix bilaterally. Grafman, Salazar, Weingartner, Vance, and Ludlow (1985) reported moderately severe memory deficit after a penetrating head injury severed the anterior body of the fornix bilaterally. The point of interruption was anterior to the superior-most levels of the thalamus. This site would interrupt fibers from the fornix to the anterior nuclei.

As noted in Chapter 5, Cramon (1989) reviewed the literature regarding fornix lesions. He concluded that lesions that interrupted the anterior columns of the fornix after departure of fibers to the anterior thalamic nuclei did not cause severe memory disturbance. Although such lesions sever Papez' circuit, they leave an alternative route from the hippocampal formation to the anterior thalamus intact. However, Cramon noted that lesions of the fornix prior to the departure of fibers to the anterior thalamus do cause memory deficits because both sources of input to the anterior thalamic nuclei (i.e., fornix to mammillary bodies to anterior nuclei, fornix to anterior nuclei) are severed. With the exception of Woolsey and Nelson's (1975) case, Cramon's observations are consistent with data discussed above.

In summary: The literature regarding the involvement of the mammillary bodies and the fornix in memory fail to support the concept that the destruction of the mammillary bodies alone causes profound memory deficits. Most, if not all, studies implicating the mammillary bodies in memory have also involved damage to other structures. Further, severing Papez' circuit at a point that interrupts hippocampal input to the mammillary bodies but not hippocampal input to the anterior thalamic nuclei does not cause profound memory deficit. Nonetheless, this analysis of the data should not be taken to mean that the mammillary bodies are unimportant in memory. It does suggest, however, that profound memory disturbance requires the disruption of other structures in addition to the mammillary bodies. Further evidence for this view will be developed in the discussion that follows.

Evidence Supporting the Role of the Dorsal Medial Nucleus

Some impetus for giving the dorsal medial thalamus serious consideration as the critical site for diencephalic amnesia began with the book of Victor et al. (1971). This work described their extensive study of Wernicke-Korsakoff syndrome. At autopsy, they examined the relationship between atrophy of the mammillary bodies and the dorsal medial nuclei in 43 cases. In five cases, the mammillary bodies were affected, but there was no chronic amnesia. Since in all cases of chronic amnesia both the mammillary bodies and the dorsal medial thalamus were damaged, the authors concluded that the dorsal medial nuclei, and not the mammillary bodies, were responsible for memory processes at the diencephalic level. As will be seen in the next section, these data are subject to the alternate interpretation that both the mammillary bodies and the dorsal medial nuclei must be involved to produce diencephalic amnesia.

McEntee et al. (1976) found an amnesic syndrome with significant signs of retrograde amnesia in a patient who exhibited bilateral metastatic tumor invasion of the dorsal medial thalamus. There was no involvement of the mammillary bodies or of the mammillothalamic tract. The authors concluded that severe memory deficits could exist in the presence of dorsal medial thalamic destruction without involvement of the mammillary bodies. However, areas outside the diencephalon were involved in this case, and other cognitive deficits were present. The other areas of the brain involved included the head of the left caudate nucleus, the septum pellucidum at the level of the anterior commissure, the occipital lobe, and the midbrain and pons along the aqueduct of Sylvius. Since the floor of the left temporal horn of the lateral ventricle was involved, the left hippocampal formation may have been affected. At least for the left hemisphere, then, structures related to both the hippocampal formation and the amygdala (i.e., dorsal medial thalamus for the latter) may have been involved. Other diencephalic structures also involved included the centre median nuclei, the medial pulvinar, the habenular nuclei, and the stria medullaris. Thus, while it is likely that the dorsal medial lesions contributed to the amnesic syndrome in this case, damage to other structures may also have played a role.

Squire and Moore (1979) attributed the greater verbal than nonverbal memory deficit in their patient N.A. to his lesion in the left dorsal medial thalamus. The lesion had been created by a stab wound from a miniature fencing foil, and the appearance of the CT scan and etiology led the authors to assume the lesion had been hemorrhagic. However, a subsequent report of the case (Squire, Amaral, Zola-Morgan, Kritchevsky, & Press, 1989) casts considerable doubt on the idea that N.A.'s memory deficit could be attributed to the dorsal medial lesion alone. The more accurate localization provided by the MR scans revealed damage to the left postcommissural fornix, mammillothalamic tract, internal medullary lamina, anterior and posterior intralaminar nuclei, and left and right mammillary bodies in addition to the left dorsal medial damage. All these structures have been implicated in memory. Additionally, the left ventral anterior and ventral lateral nuclei were involved. Lesion of the right temporal pole, amygdala, and entorhinal cortex in addition to the right mammillary body did not cause as severe an impairment of visual as of verbal memory.

Speedie and Heilman (1982) demonstrated greater impairment of verbal than nonverbal memory in a right-handed patient with a left dorsal medial thalamic infarction. Although the patient had a history of paranoid schizophrenia, the onset of memory problems was sudden and coincidental with the thalamic infarction. In 1983, the same authors noted greater visual- than verbal-memory impairment in a right-handed man with right medial thalamic infarction. In this latter case, the lesion included the dorsal medial nucleus, with encroachment on the adjacent anterior, posterior lateral, and pulvinar nuclei. In both reports, the authors noted that the dorsal medial nucleus receives direct input from temporal lobe structures such as the amygdala and indirect input from Papez' circuit via the septal region. Thus, they emphasized the importance of the dorsal medial nucleus in the memory disturbance.

Choi et al. (1983) found severe memory deficits in three cases of intracerebral hemorrhage. All cases impinged upon the medial thalamus, and the authors attributed memory deficits to medial thalamic involvement, though they stopped short of specifying the dorsal medial nucleus as the important component. Similarly, Karabelas, Kalfakis, Kasvikis, and Vassilopoulos (1985) implicated bilateral medial thalamic infarction in severe memory disturbance, but they did not analyze the lesions carefully enough to specify which structures other than the dorsal medial nucleus might be involved.

Some work done in monkeys has also implicated the dorsal medial thalamus in memory. For example, Schulman (1964) used radioactive implants to destroy the dorsal medial thalamus in monkeys that had been trained in a spatial-delayed-response task. Postlesion performance was severely impaired compared to prelesion performance in all monkeys for whom 100% of the dorsal medial thalamus was destroyed bilaterally. Performance was variable in animals in which this nucleus was incompletely destroyed, but some deficit was usually noticed. The author attributed the memory deficits to lesions in the dorsal medial thalamus. However, it should be noted that the implants destroyed other structures within and outside of the thalamus, including the centre median nucleus and/or other intralaminar nuclei in all animals, the ventral posterior medial nucleus in some animals, the anterior nuclei in some animals, the mammillothalamic tract in some animals, portions of the pulvinar in some animals, the habenula or related structures to some degree in all animals, the posterior commissure in some animals, the posterior corpus callosum in one animal, and the fornix to some degree in all but one animal. Given the potential involvement of the anterior nuclei, the mammillothalamic tract, and the fornix in memory, it is hard to agree with the author's emphasis on the dorsal medial nucleus alone as critical for memory.

Zola-Morgan and Squire (1985) seemed to show that lesions to the posterior dorsal medial nucleus in monkeys was sufficient to cause severe memory deficits in a delayed-nonmatching-sample task similar to that used in Mishkin's lab. (See discussion of Mishkin's work, below.) Animals lesioned in the posterior dorsal medial nucleus showed significantly greater deficits on this task than control animals. There were no differences between groups in a pattern matching task which the authors compared to procedural learning in humans. (See discussion of procedural memory, below.) It is worth noting that the fornix as well as the habenula was damaged in all experimental animals. Although the authors' arguments that damage to the fornix did not cause the memory deficits were convincing, they did not take into account the possibility that combined damage to the posterior dorsal medial thalamus and the fornix may have been necessary to produce the amplitude of memory deficit observed. This interpretation would be consistent with Mishkin's (1982) suggestion that damage to both temporal lobe systems involved in memory must be present to cause severe memory deficit in monkeys. These systems are Papez' circuit and the amygdala-dorsal medial thalamus system. The latter interpretation is also consistent with the data I shall examine momentarily.

In summary: Data that the dorsal medial thalamus alone is the site of diencephalic memory function are little more convincing than data regarding the mammillary bodies. In many studies, other structures potentially important for memory are damaged along with the dorsal medial nuclei. In other studies, insufficient data were provided to rule out damage to structures close to the dorsal medial nucleus, such as the mammillothalamic tract and the ventral amygdalofugal pathway. The use of stereotactic atlases to more closely specify the extent of lesions has yielded some insight into involvement of these structures in memory. Many of the studies reviewed in the next section have used such localization techniques.

Relationships with Temporal Fugal Systems

In 1982, Markowitsch's extensive review of the literature on the dorsal medial nucleus and memory suggested that severe memory deficit resulted from dorsal medial damage only when other structures were also involved. But it was the work of Mishkin that provided one impetus to consider the proposition that damage to both the dorsal medial and anterior thalamic nuclei, or damage to mesial temporal inputs to both structures, was needed to cause severe memory disturbance. Mishkin studied memory functions in monkeys using recognition-memory tasks. In his early studies (e.g., Mishkin, 1978), he found memory performance to be impaired by removal of both the amygdala and the hippocampus, but not by removal of either structure alone. In a later study (Bachevalier et al., 1985), findings were extended to the major output systems of these temporal lobe structures. Separate lesions of the amygdalofugal pathways and the bodies of the fornix (prior to departure of fibers to the anterior thalamus) did not cause severe memory disturbance, but combined destruction of these pathways did. Aggleton (1986) extended these findings to the level of the diencephalon. Lesions to the anterior medial thalamus, the posterior medial thalamus, or medial mammillary nuclei alone produced only mild memory deficits. But, combined lesion to the anterior and posterior medial thalamus produced profound memory deficit. Aggleton concluded that both the diencephalic target of hippocampal projections (i.e., the anterior nuclei) and the diencephalic target of amygdala projections (i.e., the dorsal medial nucleus) must be damaged to produce severe amnesia. Mishkin's work was one reason why investigators began to look at the course of the mammillothalamic tract and the ventral amygdalofugal pathway within the thalamus to help explain diencephalic amnesias.

Before considering this issue further, however, I must be allowed one digression regarding circulation of the medial thalamus. One aspect of paramedian thalamic artery circulation is the not infrequent absence of a tuberothalamic (polar) artery. In such cases, paramedian infarcts will extend into the ventral anterior and neighboring nuclei because the paramedian artery supplies much of the territory of the missing tuberothalamic artery. In cases where the tuberothalamic artery is present, infarcts may be limited to a more posterior area. The implications of more posterior versus more anterior paramedian infarcts was first explored by Cramon and colleagues (1985), as we shall see shortly. Another aspect of paramedian circulation is that infarcts in the territory of the paramedian thalamic artery are often bilateral. This sometimes happens because the paramedian artery of both sides is supplied by a single pedicle emerging from one posterior cerebral artery just after the bifurcation of the basilar artery into the two posterior cerebral arteries. However, an occlusion extending from the basilar artery minimally into both posterior cerebral arteries may also block both paramedian arteries even when they have separate origins (see Castaigne et al., 1981).

Cramon et al. (1985) were one of the first groups to apply the works of Mishkin and colleagues to the realm of human memory impairment after thalamic infarction. Four of their six patients with paramedian thalamic artery infarctions had significant memory dysfunction, though it may not have been severe enough in all four to merit the term *amnesia* as I am using it in this volume (in this volume, the term *amnesia* is reserved for patients (a) who have severe deficits acquiring new information that extend across modalities and affect everyday functioning and (b) who have no or lesser impairments in memory span and general intellectual functioning.) Of the patients with memory impairment, three demonstrated bilateral lesions, and one had a left-sided lesion. When the anatomical findings from three other cases in the literature with significant memory impairment were mapped along with these author's four cases, only one significant area of overlap was found in the more inferior thalamic sections of the CT scans. This area of overlap included the mammillothalamic tract as it passes through the region of the ventral anterior and ventral lateral nuclei and the adjacent portion of the internal medullary lamina. A small portion of the dorsal medial nucleus, the most anterior tip, was also included in the area of overlap. In the slice midway between the most inferior and the most superior thalamic levels, the areas of overlap included a posterior medial portion of the ventral lateral nucleus, an anterior lateral portion of the dorsal medial nucleus, and the portion of the internal medullary lamina between the affected portions of these two nuclei.

For the two cases who did not show significant disturbance of memory, Cramon et al. found more posteriorly situated lesions. At the more inferior level, the mammillothalamic tract was probably untouched, and the portion of the internal medullary lamina involved was posterior to the portion involved with the cases of memory impairment. At this level, a large portion of the dorsal medial nucleus was involved as well as a portion of the centre median nucleus. At the more superior level, one case involved large portions of the dorsal medial nucleus and a portion of the internal medullary lamina. The other case (unilateral) involved portions of the left ventral lateral, ventral anterior, and dorsal lateral nuclei.

Cramon et al. stated that projections to the dorsal medial nucleus from the amygdala course through the inferior portion of the internal medullary lamina affected in their memory-impairment cases. It was their contention that both these fibers from the ventral amygdalofugal pathway and the mammillothalamic tract (a part of Papez' circuit) had to be affected in order to cause significant memory disturbance after medial thalamic lesion. This was consistent with Mishkin's (1982) contention that diencephalic structures related to both the hippocampal formation and the amygdala had to be affected before severe memory disturbance was seen in monkeys.

The same authors (Cramon, Hebel, & Schuri, 1986) explored the similarity between memory deficits in these same six patients to five other patients with circumscribed vascular lesions of the thalamus. The lesions in these additional five patients were situated unilaterally or bilaterally in the ventral lateral nucleus. None demonstrated significant chronic memory problems, suggesting that the ventral lateral thalamus is not important for memory.

Three case studies published just before or at about the same time as the study of Cramon et al. (1985) have a bearing on the conclusion about the involvement of both the mammillothalamic tract and the internal medullary lamina. Goldenberg, Wimmer, and Maly (1983) reported a case of moderately severe verbal-memory deficit after left thalamic infarction. A CT scan at 2 months postonset demonstrated the lesion to occupy a portion of the ventral anterior nucleus, a portion of the ventral lateral nucleus, a portion of the dorsal medial nucleus, and portions of the internal medullary lamina and the mammillothalamic tract. Winocur, Oxbury, Roberts, Agnetti, and Davis (1984) had described a case of bilateral paramedian thalamic infarction prior to the publication of Cramon et al. (1985). This case had significant persistent memory deficit with intellectual functioning at estimated premorbid levels. The bilaterally symmetric lesions included parts of the dorsal medial nuclei, ventral lateral nuclei, and internal medullary lamina. The authors noted that the mammillothalamic tract was just anterior to the lesion sites and indicated that these structures may have been involved. Swanson and Schmidley (1985) described bilateral infarctions including parts of the dorsal medial nuclei in a case of severe acute amnesia. They also noted involvement of the mammillothalamic tract, and suggested interruption of limbic input to the dorsal medial nuclei similar to the findings of Cramon et al. (1985). However, their localization was less well defined, and their case was reported to have largely recovered by 3 months postonset. No formal testing was reported. The cases of Cramon et al. were chronic cases of memory deficit. Thus, these three cases (Goldenberg et al., 1983; Swanson & Schmidley, 1985; Winocur et al., 1984) could be consistent with the interpretation of Cramon et al. (1985) regarding involvement of the mammillothalamic tract and the internal medullary lamina, but the localization in the latter two cases was not as careful as that of Cramon et al. The transient nature of the memory deficit in the case of Swanson and Schmidley (1985) raises a question as to what percentage of cases with similar lesions would show permanent memory deficits. The answer to this question and its relationship to anatomy have not been well explored.

Several cases have also appeared in the literature since Cramon and colleagues' (1985) study that have confirmed the anterior location of paramedian thalamic infarcts causing significant memory disturbance and/or the involvement of the mammillothalamic tract. Mori et al. (1986) described a case of left thalamic infarction with acute disturbance of language and verbal memory. By 6 to 8 weeks postonset, the language deficit had subsided with only very mild symptoms evident, but significant verbal-memory deficit was still evident. The lesion involved large portions of the ventral lateral nucleus, perhaps portions of the ventral anterior nucleus, the centre median-parafascicularis complex, the mammillothalamic tract, and portions of the internal medullary lamina. Thus, this study seems to confirm Cramon and colleagues' (1985) contention concerning the involvement of the mammillothalamic tract and the internal medullary lamina in thalamic lesions causing significant memory problems.

Kritchevsky, Graff-Radford, and Damasio (1987) studied one case of right medial thalamic infarction and one case of bilateral medial thalamic infarction. The first case involved 15% of the right dorsal medial nucleus as well as parts of the midline and parafascicular nuclei. The second involved about 15% of the dorsal medial nucleus on the left and about 5% on the right; smaller portions of the anterior, parafascicular, ventral posterior, and lateral posterior nuclei were involved on the left, and a small portion of the parafascicular nucleus was involved on the right. In neither case was the mammillothalamic tract involved, and neither case showed severe memory disturbance. The authors concluded that either the amount of the dorsal medial nucleus involved was insufficient to cause memory impairment or the mammillothalamic tract must also be involved to cause serious memory impairment.

Gentilini et al. (1987) found the mammillothalamic tract to be involved in all eight of their cases of paramedian thalamic infarction. However, it was only unilaterally involved in the one case with no memory impairment and also unilaterally involved in one case where memory disorder was detectable only on testing. Five of the other six patients survived long enough for memory assessment. In four of these cases, memory impairment was clinically detectable, and in the other case memory impairment was only evidenced on formal testing. The absence of involvement of the internal medullary lamina in the most severe case of memory impairment cast some doubt on Cramon and colleagues' contention that this structure must be damaged in combination with the mammillothalamic tract to produce severe memory disturbance. All but one case showed relatively good recoveries.

Nichelli, Bahmanian-Behbahani, Gentilini, and Vecchi (1988) provided an interesting twist on Cramon and colleagues' observations. Their patient had a profound amnesia after bilateral thalamic infarction in the territory of the paramedian thalamic artery. This profound amnesia included severe impairment on tests of explicit verbal memory. On the right side, the mammillothalamic tract and the internal medullary lamina, as well as the midline nuclei, portions of the ventral anterior nucleus, and a small portion of the dorsal medial nucleus were damaged. On the left side, at more ventral levels, the authors emphasized that the lesion was more posterior, involving a portion of the dorsal medial nucleus, part of the parafascicular nucleus, and part of the midline nucleus. The coronal section of the MR scan revealed a fact not emphasized by the authors: a portion of the anterior nuclei was involved. Although the authors themselves emphasized that bilateral lesions of the dorsal medial nucleus might hamper communication between the amygdala and frontal lobes, another interpretation seems more likely: damage to both the dorsal medial nucleus and the anterior nuclei is the same as damage to the mammillothalamic tract and the ventral amygdalofugal pathway. Memory deficit will result. The anterior nuclei and the dorsal medial nucleus, of course, are the targets of the mammillothalamic tract and the thalamic continuation of the ventral amygdalofugal pathway, respectively.

Brown, Kieran, and Patel (1989) explored a hemorrhagic lesion which leads to conclusions similar to those just described for the case of Nichelli et al. (1988). Their patient had a left medial thalamic hematoma. Although verbal memory was more affected than visual memory, there was some impairment of both. It is worth noting that even on acute CT scan, there was little mass effect. However, some edema of surrounding white matter was noted. An MR scan 2 months postonset indicated the lesion to be in the dorsal medial nucleus with some extension into the anterior nucleus. Thus, this case is another instance of memory deficit after lesion to both the dorsal medial and anterior nuclei.

Stuss, Guberman, Nelson, and Larochell (1988) reported three cases of paramedian thalamic infarction with memory deficit. Lesions were bilateral in one case, primarily right thalamic in one case, and unilateral left thalamic in one case. The most severe and global memory impairment occurred in the case of bilateral infarction with involvement of the ventral anterior nucleus and mammillothalamic tract bilaterally and the dorsal medial nucleus primarily on the left side. The second case had bilateral dorsal medial nucleus involvement, but damage to the mammillothalamic tract only on the right side. The third case demonstrated involvement of the left mammillothalamic tract, the left ventral anterior nucleus, and a small portion of the dorsal medial nucleus. Portions of the ventral lateral nucleus were involved in all three cases. Thus, the data of Stuss et al. confirm the anterior location and involvement of the mammillothalamic tract suggested by Cramon et al. (1985).

Graff-Radford et al. (1990) performed a study of diencephalic amnesia that has implications both for anatomy and for memory processes. Regarding the anatomical aspects, these authors not only carefully delineated the boundaries of two bilateral medial thalamic lesions that produced amnesias and two such lesions that did not, they also endeavored to more precisely define the anatomical proximity of the mammillothalamic tract and the ventral amygdalofugal pathway as these tracts pass through the thalamus. They accomplished the latter task by using autoradiography in two monkeys. With respect to the path of the ventral amygdalofugal pathway, Graff-Radford and his colleagues noted that this pathway is immediately lateral to the mammillothalamic tract as both pathways proceed superiorly within the ventral anterior nucleus. Fibers of the ventral amygdalofugal pathway continue superiorly to terminate in the dorsal medial nucleus. It should be noted that Cramon et al. (1985) assumed the fibers from the ventral amygdalofugal pathway to be incorporated within the internal medullary lamina, which is medial to the mammillothalamic tract at the level of the ventral anterior nucleus, contrary to the anatomic findings of Graff-Radford and colleagues.

Graff-Radford et al. related their findings in two monkeys to their cases of infarctions in the territory of the paramedian thalamic artery. In two cases the bilateral infarctions demonstrated a relatively anterior location within the thalamus, interrupting both the mammillothalamic tract and the thalamic portion of the ventral amygdalofugal pathway. Both cases were amnesic. A third case had more posterior lesions involving both dorsal medial nuclei, but the mammillothalamic tract and the ventral amygdalofugal pathway were spared. The fourth case had smaller bilateral lesions nicking the ventral amygdalofugal pathway but leaving the mammillothalamic tract untouched. Both of the latter two cases demonstrated less severe memory difficulties, detectable only on delayed-recall tasks. Thus, Graff-Radford et al. confirmed Cramon and colleagues' (1985) finding that more anteriorly placed lesions of the dorsal medial nucleus and surrounding structures cause more severe memory deficits. The anatomical importance of this study is that the authors defined the location of the ventral amygdalofugal pathway within the thalamus, thereby making it a greater certainty that both pathways must be interrupted to cause amnesic syndromes with dorsal medial thalamic lesions.

In summary: A number of recent studies suggest that severe memory problems are produced after thalamic lesions only if either the dorsal medial nucleus or the ventral amygdalofugal pathway *and* either the anterior nuclei or the mammillothalamic tract are both involved. These findings are consistent with the work of Mishkin (1982) in monkeys and can be considered to represent the most current thought regarding medial thalamic structures and memory. What is not clear, however, is how common are cases in which both structures are involved and memory deficits are not severe? And, what does the recovery look like in samples of these cases unselected for chronic memory impairment? For example, Swanson and Schmidley (1985) described good recovery with involvement of the critical structures. It is apparent that continuing description of these cases could continue to lead to valuable insights.

Attentional Mechanisms Related to Memory

Watson et al. (1981) suggested that the thalamic intralaminar nuclei were involved in preparing an aroused organism to respond to a meaningful environmental event. It is unclear how such preparation might relate to the concepts of attention frequently addressed in cognitive models of memory (e.g., see Baddeley, 1990) since Watson et al. did not include the intralaminar nuclei in sensory processing. However, it seems plausible that responding to a meaningful environmental event could involve directing resources for actively processing incoming information. This direction of resources for actively processing incoming information could be referred to as "attention." Attention could impact memory in that the allocation of greater processing resources to specific information would increase the probability that this information would be placed in long-term storage.

Mennemeier and colleagues (Mennemeier, Fennell, & Valenstein, 1990; Mennemeier, Fennell, Valenstein, & Heilman, 1990) studied a case of infarction that primarily involved the posterior left intralaminar nuclei (i.e., centre median and parafasicular nuclei). Portions of the midline nuclei, the dorsal medial, and the ventral lateral nuclei were also involved; however, the mammillothalamic tract and the thalamic extension of the ventral amygdalofugal pathway were untouched. Although left-handed, the patient showed mild verbal-memory deficits. Her pattern of performance on a series of verbal-memory tasks suggested her deficit was primarily attentional in nature. The authors concluded that damage to the centre median-parafascicular complex accounted for this problem.

Jurko and Andy (1973) had earlier studied the effect of stereotaxic lesions on the centre median nucleus. In general, less cognitive deficits appeared to result from lesion of centre median than other thalamic structures. However, the cognitive effects of centre median lesion did include errors in drawing geometric designs, changes in response to an optical illusion, and decreased response to color on the Rorschach Inkblot Test. It is difficult to tell if some of these effects could have been attentional in nature, but patients with centre median lesions did not show effects from lesion on a memory task. The relationship of verbal- and visual-memory performance to side of lesion was not specified.

However, Jurko and Andy (1977) also studied the effects of centre median lesion on patients who had previously undergone unilateral or bilateral amygdalectomies for seizures. Three patients who had thalamectomies in the left centre median nucleus showed decreased memory for verbal paired associates which persisted as long as several months. No consistent effect was seen for patients receiving stereotaxic lesions of the right centre median nucleus. The authors pointed out that the deficits in the left centre median lesions might be due to alerting mechanisms that contribute to mental functions. These data would be consistent with those of Mennemeier et al. (1990).

Attentional processes have been invoked to explain memory phenomena related to thalamic nuclei other than the centre median. Ojemann and his colleagues (Ojemann, 1974, 1977; Ojemann et al., 1971; Ojemann & Fedio, 1968) have studied the effects of verbal object recall during ventral lateral and pulvinar stimulation. Ojemann's 1977 article most clearly explained this research. He showed subjects pictures that they were required to name; subsequently, they counted backward for 6 seconds. Then, they were required to give the name of the object that had just been shown to them. Finally, 4 seconds later, a word-recognition trial was given. Electrical stimulation of the ventral lateral nucleus occurred during object naming only, at recall only, during backward counting only, during both object naming and recall, or not at all for baseline trials.

For ventral lateral stimulation, results affected recall errors in the opposite direction depending upon whether stimulation was done at original presentation or during recall. Error rates during stimulation trials were subtracted from baseline (no stimulation) error rates. Compared to patients with right ventral lateral stimulation, patients with left ventral lateral stimulation showed a significant decrease in recall errors when stimulation was done at the time of initial presentation. However, the left ventral lateral stimulation produced a significant increase in recall errors when it occurred during recall. The author hypothesized a specific alerting response that directs attention to verbal information present in the external environment. Such an alerting response was thought to facilitate short-term memory storage when it occurred during presentation, but to interfere with retrieval if it occurred during recall.

Ojemann (1977) also tested verbal- and nonverbal-recognition paradigms in patients receiving ventral lateral stimulation. In the verbal-recognition task, subjects were required to read aloud one of four words that correctly identified the picture presented on trials as described above. The visual-recognition task involved presentation of irregularly shaped figures. At each presentation, subjects had to answer "Yes" if the shape had been previously presented, and "No" if it had not. A matching-to-sample procedure was also included to ascertain that subjects could discriminate the shape from other shapes. Results for the verbal-recognition task were similar to the recall findings presented above: Compared to right ventral lateral stimulation, left ventral lateral stimulation decreased recognition errors when it occurred at initial presentation, but increased errors when it occurred during the recognition trial. On the other hand, left ventral lateral stimulation tended to increase visual recognition errors no matter when it occurred, though not significantly so. Right ventral lateral stimulation significantly decreased visual recognition errors when it occured during initial presentation, but tended to increase errors when it occured during the recognition trial. On the basis of the recognition data, Ojemann (1977) hypothesized a visual alerting response for right ventral lateral stimulation. This was similar to the specific verbal alerting response discussed above. The effects of left ventral lateral stimulation on visual recognition were explained by the specific verbal alerting response overriding visual processing.

Recall performance of patients stimulated in the pulvinar was examined under different conditions. The task involved subjects naming a series of pictures. After naming the picture presented on a particular trial, subjects were also asked to name the picture from the previous trial. Errors were most dramatically increased when stimulation occurred during recall (i.e., naming the picture on the previous trial). However, errors also increased to a lesser extent if stimulation occurred during initial presentation or during both presentation and recall. This is different from ventral lateral stimulation where recall errors were reduced if stimulation occurred during initial presentation.

Crosson (1984) pointed out that the "verbal"-recall paradigm from these studies of Ojemann and colleagues had an alternate interpretation. Since initial presentation involved showing a picture, recall trials might actually amount to calling up the visual image of the picture from memory, then naming the picture. This explanation could account for increased errors during recall trials for both ventral lateral and pulvinar stimulation; in other words, stimulation could interfere with naming the recalled visual image. However, this explanation does not account for the decreased errors at recall when the stimulation occurred during initial presentation.

Further, a later study by Ojemann (1985) has some bearing on this issue. Patients heard four pairs of dichotic words; each pair differed by only one letter. There was 0.5 seconds between words. After each set of four pairs, subjects reported all words they heard. Left ventral lateral stimulation increased the number of words recalled, and right ventral lateral stimulation had no effect. There was a trend (not statistically significant) for ventral lateral stimulation to increase the number of correctly recalled words in the ear contralateral to stimulation.

One point about the anatomy of ventral lateral stimulation should also be made. This nucleus has some proximity to both the anterior intralaminar nuclei and to the pathways from the intralaminar nuclei to the anterior language cortex which pass through the ventral anterior nuclei. Although spread of stimulation to other nuclei was controlled in the Ojemann studies by keeping it below levels required to evoke sensory phenomena, it is not entirely certain that the intralaminar nuclei or their projections were unaffected by ventral lateral stimulation. Thus, some of the effects noted from ventral lateral stimulation could be due to excitation of efferent intralaminar fibers.

In summary: Studies have implicated thalamic nuclei in the attentional mechanisms necessary to support memory. These nuclei are the intralaminar nuclei and the ventral lateral nucleus. Further study of these phenomena is required. Impairment of underlying attentional processes may create only milder memory deficits such as those seen by Mennemeier et al. (1990). For this reason, study of attentional processes and memory in thalamic lesions will require the close examination of patients with mild to moderate impairment of memory.

Memory Process: Definition of Terms

The memory literature is sometimes inconsistent in usage of various terms, which can cause confusion in the interpretation of findings.

Before discussing research considering diencephalic amnesia and memory processes, I think that logic dictates that I should define terms in several areas. I realize that terms may be used here in a somewhat different way than in many previous works, and that my slightly different usage of terms may be confusing to readers. Nonetheless, a failure to make conceptual distinctions will lead to an even worse confusion regarding memory processes. In order to understand the following discussion, it is important for the reader to have an understanding of how terms referring to memory will be used. This is particularly true for the terms *consolidation, encoding,* and *retrieval.*

Short-Term versus Long-Term Memory

Russell (1981) reviewed the concepts of short-term and long-term memory. Based upon works by Cofer (1976), Norman (1973), Shiffrin (1973), Shiffrin and Schneider (1977), and others, he made several distinctions between short-term and long-term memory. It is of some interest that a distinction similar to the one made herein can be traced to the works of William James. Two properties of short-term memory are of interest. First, it lasts between 20 and 40 seconds, unless it is lengthened by rehearsal. The second property has been called the "limited capacity assumption." According to the limited capicity assumption, short-term memory has a limited capacity of five to ten items. A final point of interest is that short-term memory corresponds to the concept of "conscious awareness" in some models. For such models, it is the stage through which information must pass before it can reach long-term memory, and it is into short-term memory that items in long-term memory are later retrieved. This is a linear model of memory (e.g., Atkinson & Shiffrin, 1968). This type of model has been challenged, for example, by Cowan (1988), who sees short-term memory only as a subset of items within long-term memory.

According to Russell (1981), long-term memory represents a permanent record of events and information learned by the person. Long-term memory may begin as early as 0.5 seconds after an item is attended to. If this is true, there is a period of time during which short-term and long-term memory overlap. Since short-term memory has a limited capacity, information that must be remembered has to be transferred to long-term memory as it is displaced by new information entering short-term memory. This latter concept will be important for interpreting studies of short-term memory.

Remote memory refers to long-term memory stores that are in the more distant past. Operationally in the literature on amnesias, the term *remote memory* is most often used to refer to memories prior to the onset of the amnesic condition.

Episodic versus Semantic Memory

Russell (1981) discussed the distinction made by Tulving (1972) between "episodic" and "semantic" compartments in long-term memory. Episodic memory is characterized by temporal and spatial tags that provide a personal context for specific memories. For example, memory for events would fall under episodic memory because the temporal and spatial context of events are important components of these memories. In semantic memory, temporal and spatial contexts are irrelevant. For example, the ability to remember that a foot consists of 12 inches does not require persons to also remember when and where they learned this fact. Vocabulary could be considered a major component in semantic memory. Cermak (1984) proposed that much information shifts from episodic memory to semantic memory as temporal and spatial contexts become less relevant across the course of years.

Encoding, Consolidation, and Retrieval

I believe that the use of *encoding, consolidation,* and *retrieval* as the primary concepts for memory processes is flawed. One significant problem is that this model does not account for the initial registration of material into long-term memory. Some authors seem to associate initial registration with consolidation whereas others seem to associate it with encoding. In the terminology to be used in this volume, registration of information will be separated from both encoding and consolidation. This separation is justified both conceptually and by the results of studies I will review. All terms discussed in the following paragraph apply to the long-term memory compartment.

For the purposes of this volume, I shall distinguish the following five processes: *Encoding* is the process of transforming information into a format that is eventually used in long-term storage. Encoding involves using the salient aspects of stimuli to relate incoming information to other incoming information or material already in long-term storage. However, it implies neither the registration of that information into long-term storage, nor the maintenance of the information once it has entered long-term storage. *Registration* involves the initial entry of information into long-term memory. This concept assumes that information may fail to reach long-term storage even if it is organized. However, even after registration, information must be maintained in long-term storage. In this volume, the process of maintaining information in long-term storage will be called *consolidation*. However, it should be remembered that initial registration and consolidation are separable processes. *Retrieval* is the process of taking information out of long-term storage for usage at some time after the information was originally acquired. This later usage of information is the purpose of long-term storage and can be triggered by a variety of internal and external circumstances. In addition to retrieval, the process of remembering complex events or information requires the process of *reconstruction*. In other words, the recollection of a complex event or information requires reconstructing individual bits of information stored in long-term memory into a whole. The ability to perform such reconstructions depends, in part, upon how these bits are organized within long-term memory.

Implicit versus Explicit Memory

Roediger (1990) traced the concepts of implicit and explicit memory back to the 19th-century work of Ebbinghaus, though Schacter (1987) has traced concepts similar to implicit memory back to the 17th-century work of Descartes. Ebbinghaus used the terms involuntary and voluntary recollection, which have many parallels between implicit and explicit memory, respectively. Gardner, Boller, Moreines, and Butters (1973) were one of the first groups to apply the term explicit to memory. They used this term to refer to a memory for the task in which material was learned. They indicated that reference to the earlier task may be an important cue in recall and might be selectively impaired for some amnesic patients. In later usage of the term (e.g., Graf, Squire, & Mandler, 1984), explicit memory is operationally defined as memory in which instructions are given to remember the material during initial exposure and/or in which instructions to recall or recognize a specific set of information are given during the recall or recognition exercise. In a little more conceptual rendition (e.g., Butters & Stuss, 1989; Graf & Schacte, 1985; Roediger, 1990; Schacter, 1987), others emphasize that explicit measures of memory reflect conscious recollection of the past. In other words, explicit memory involves conscious attempts to recall or recognize specific happenings or information.

By contrast, Graf and Schacter (1985), Roediger (1990), and Schacter (1987) have emphasized that implicit tests of retention do not require conscious recollection of recent events for their performance. Butters and Stuss (1989) suggested that prior experiences unconsciously facilitate performance in implicit memory. According to some (e.g., Graf et al., 1984; Shimamura & Squire, 1984), implicit memory would involve circumstances during which a preexisting element of semantic memory is activated in a task not explicitly defined as involving memory and after which the probability of a given response is tested in a task not explicitly requesting recollection of an earlier event. For example, a subject might be presented with a pair of words and asked to rate their degree of relatedness, but no mention of remembering the words is made. Later, subjects may be asked to free-associate to the first word in the pair to ascertain if the probability of giving the second word has increased. (Note that no reference to the earlier task has been made.) However, this activation explanation for implicit memory does not fit all the data since amnesic patients sometimes show priming for new information as well as information already in semantic memory (see Schacter [1987] for further discussion).

In some circles, it has been common to categorize some implicit-memory tasks as belonging to procedural memory (e.g., Squire, 1987). However, in at least some experimental paradigms, important distinctions can be drawn between implicit and procedural memory (e.g., Graf et al., 1984; Shimamura & Squire, 1984). For example, some priming experiments depend upon the use of existing semantic-memory stores to increase the probability that an item in semantic memory will be given in response to other situations. Procedural memory does not depend on preexisting semantic stores. Procedural memory, on the other hand, involves the tuning and sequencing of elements into a specific procedure, but priming paradigms do not depend upon such turning and sequencing. In some priming paradigms, the effects are temporary, while procedural memory endures over periods up to months (e.g., Cohen & Squire, 1980). Thus, Schacter (1987) questioned the inclusion of all forms of implicit memory under the rubric of procedural memory. In keeping with this observation, it seems prudent for the time to consider implicit versus explicit and declarative versus procedural as potentially separate dimensions of memory.

Procedural versus Declarative Memory

Cohen and Squire (1980) were among the first to emphasize the distinction between declarative and procedural memory. The terminology was borrowed from artificial intelligence, and its application was based in part on their own data and in part on previous observations that amnesic patients could demonstrate normal learning of motor tasks (e.g., Brooks & Baddeley, 1976; Corkin, 1968; Milner, 1962). According to Squire and Cohen, declarative memory was data-based memory, whereas procedural memory was the encoding of operations or procedures. Procedural memory is rule-based. Another way of thinking about this distinction is that procedural memory involves knowing how to do some task, but declarative memory requires knowing some fact (i.e., familiarity with some piece of data). Thus, a motor skill like performance with a pursuit rotor or a cognitive skill like mirror reading would be classified as procedural learning. Learning factual information would be an example of declarative memory.

Diencephalic Dysfunction and Memory Processes

Ultimate understanding of diencephalic participation in memory demands not only knowledge of which diencephalic structures are involved in memory, but also of how they participate. Studies of various memory processes after diencephalic damage have provided the best window into its memory functions. Two primary bodies of literature are relevant to this area: the study of memory processes in alcoholic Korsakoff's syndrome and the study of memory processes after other acquired diencephalic damage. I will cover the literature on alcoholic Korsakoff's syndrome first.

Memory Processes in Alcoholic Korsakoff's Syndrome

Alcoholic Korsakoff's syndrome is a condition of some chronic alcoholics in which there is a profound incapacity to enter information into long-term memory storage in spite of relatively intact intellectual functioning. Acute onset is most frequently marked cognitively by the confusional state of Wernicke's encephalopathy, though onset is sometimes insidious. As noted above, patients with alcoholic Korsakoff's syndrome show damage in the midline diencephalon, notably the dorsal medial thalamus and mammillary bodies (Victor et al., 1971). Although damage may also be present in other structures (see discussion below), alcoholic Korsakoff's syndrome has been taken as a model for diencephalic amnesia. As such, some understanding of the involvement of the diencephalon in memory may be gained by examining research into the memory deficits of patients with this disorder. Because alcoholic Korsakoff's syndrome has been studied for so long, the number of cognitive studies in the area dwarfs the number of cognitive studies done in other areas. Since the alcoholic Korsakoff's research acts as a departure point for other cognitive investigations of the subcortical amnesias, it seems appropriate to cover it first. This does not mean that the information regarding the cognitive aspects of other diencephalic amnesias, of basal forebrain amnesias, or of basal ganglia disorders should be treated as an afterthought. There is simply less data available in these areas.

As just noted, the literature on alcoholic Korsakoff's syndrome is vast; indeed, it could easily be the subject of a separate volume. It would be impossible to cover the entire literature on the topic in depth; therefore, I have made some choices regarding which studies to review in the current volume. Studies relevant to the main controversies concerning this syndrome will be addressed. But many studies of amnesic syndromes (e.g., Baddeley & Warrington, 1973; Squire, Shimamura, & Graff, 1987; Warrington & Weiskrantz, 1970; Weiskrantz & Warrington, 1970) have mixed alcoholic Korsakoff's patients with patients who have amnesic syndromes of a different origin. Since such a mixture of etiologies may obscure characteristics of the disorder, which is primarily diencephalic in nature, I will not review studies in which the performance of alcoholic Korsakoff's subjects cannot be separated from that of other types of amnesic patients.

Further, in the way of introduction, I should note that this literature is riddled with problems. Many major findings have been challenged in significant ways. One difficulty is that the same subject pools have been tested repeatedly, so it is not always clear how much a subject sample in one study overlaps with samples of previous studies from the same laboratory. This fact was clearly stated in Squire and Shimamura's (1986) discussion of characteristics of their "standing" sample of amnesic patients. This problem can limit generalization of findings to other samples. A related problem is differences between laboratories in inclusion and exclusion criteria, which can lead to differences in findings. For example, Baddeley (1990) has noted careful attempts to exclude amnesic subjects who have other cognitive deficits in his laboratory, while other laboratories have relied only upon basic intelligence and memory tests to define their samples. Further, memory paradigms used in studies have been incompletely understood, and concepts of memory functions sometimes have varied implicitly between studies.

One further problem with using alcoholic Korsakoff's syndrome as a model for diencephalic amnesia is that damage is not limited to the diencephalon. Victor et al. (1971) described extension of the lesions into the brain stem. Arendt, Bigl, Arendt, and Tennstedt (1983) described loss of cholinergic neurons in the basal forebrain (nucleus basalis, nucleus of the diagonal band, medial septal nucleus) in alcoholic Korsakoff's syndrome. Shimamura, Jernigan, and Squire (1988) demonstrated that Korsakoff's patients, like nonamnesic alcoholics, have significant cortical atrophy in the frontal and peri-Sylvian cortices on CT scan. Roche, Lane, and Wade (1988) studied the CT scan of an acute Wernicke's encephalopathy patient who evolved into a state of chronic severe memory loss. In addition to diencephalic lesion, the authors identified the anterior columns of the fornix and the interventricular septum as involved in the patchy hemorrhagic damage. This finding indicated that the latter structures are involved in at least some cases of alcoholic Korsakoff's syndrome.

Finally, before reviewing the memory-process data for alcoholic Korsakoff's syndrome, the status of other cognitive functions in this disorder should be explored briefly. Many such functions are intact. For example, Talland (1965) found digit span to be within normal limits for this population, and this finding has rarely been disputed before or since. But supraspan tests of memory (i.e., tests that include more bits of information than can be stored in short-term memory) did show impairment for his Korsakoff's syndrome patients. Talland also found his alcoholic Korsakoff's patients to perform within normal limits on standardized, composite measures of intelligence. Indeed, subsequent studies have sometimes used the discrepancy between standardized intelligence tests and memory tests as an inclusion criterion for studies of this population. Nonetheless, patients with alcoholic Korsakoff's syndrome do show impairment on some tests of problem solving (e.g., Oscar-Berman, 1973; Talland, 1965). For example, these patients demonstrate difficulty in shifting conceptual sets on tests of problem solving.

Thus, the following facts should be recognized: (1) Alcoholic Korsakoff's patients may not be perfect models of diencephalic amnesias because other structures including the frontal lobes, the anterior columns of the fornix, and the basal forebrain may be damaged. (2) Alcoholic Korsakoff's patients show deficits in reasoning that could be related to changes in these other structures. (3) Experimental paradigms and interpretation of results may reflect an incomplete understanding of memory processes. (4) Because of repeated testing from the same pools of subjects, generalization of findings within laboratories cannot always be assumed to apply to other subject pools. These statements should be considered caveats applicable to the following review.

As noted above, major themes do run through the memory literature on alcoholic Korsakoff's syndrome. The discussion that follows will be organized by these major themes. In order of coverage, these themes include retention in short- and long-term memory, proactive interference, depth-of-processing and related paradigms, implicit memory, procedural memory, and temporal gradient in retrograde amnesia.

Retention in Short-Term and Long-Term Memory

Retention of items in short-term and long-term memory has been explored in several studies. Regarding the simple retention of information in short-term memory, studies attempting to establish whether a deficit exists for alcoholic Korsakoff's patients will be explored below. An inability to maintain information in short-term memory could have implications for how much information is registered in long-term memory. Other studies that explore the nature of such a short-term memory deficit (e.g., proactive interference or semantic organization) will be explored in separate sections. It should be noted that many of the studies interpreted as involving retention in short-term memory have used the Peterson and Peterson (1959) paradigm. Difficulties in using this task solely as an indicator of short-term retention will be discussed at the end of this section. As it turns out, results of the Peterson and Peterson paradigm may reflect the influence of long-term as well as short-term retention.

Although long-term registration of information in alcoholic Korsakoff's syndrome is defective, other studies discussed below indicate that some information can reach long-term stores. It is of interest to ascertain if there is an abnormal loss of that information that reaches long-term memory in this patient population. Studies that address this question will also be covered toward the end of this section.

Talland (1965) had alcoholic Korsakoff's patients and controls learn supraspan lists of nonsense syllables and words and tested recall at varying lengths of time up to 12 minutes after learning. For Korsakoff's subjects, the largest drop-off in performance occurred between recalls at zero and 90 seconds, suggesting that the loss of information may have occurred between short-term and long-term memory. Some further drop-off occurred between 90 and 180 seconds, but performance began to level off after that.

One commonly used method for assessing stability of short-term memory is the Peterson and Peterson (1959) paradigm. In this procedure, subjects are provided with bits of information that are within the limited capacity of short-term memory. For example, a single word or triads of consonants, numbers, or words might be used. In some trials, an immediate recall is requested, but in other trials a delay of varying length is interposed. The delay is usually less than the maximum length of normal short-term memory, as described above.

One commonly used set of intervals is 3, 9, and 18 seconds. During the delay, subjects are given a task (e.g., counting backward by 3's or naming colors). The purpose of the task is to prevent the subject from rehearsing the information, relying upon the strength of the "trace" created only by initial presentation. This method was used in many of the early studies of alcoholic Korsakoff's syndrome to investigate several aspects of short-term memory.

Butters, Lewis, Cermak, and Goodglass (1973) gave alcoholic Korsakoff's subjects and controls verbal (consonant trigrams) and nonverbal (spatial patterns) stimuli in visual, tactile, and auditory modalities. The Peterson and Peterson paradigm was used with no delay and with 9- and 18-second, distraction-filled intervals. The distraction was counting backward. At the end of the interval, subjects were exposed to a second trigram or pattern and had to tell if the second stimulus was the same as the first. In general, Korsakoff's patients showed impairments relative to normals for verbal material with both delay intervals; however, no such impairments were shown for nonverbal materials. The authors interpreted their findings to demonstrate a material-specific (verbal) memory impairment for Korsakoff's patients in short-term memory. They further speculated that a failure to employ semantic strategies could underlie the material-specific deficit. However, an alternate conclusion offered by the authors is more plausible: since the interpolated distraction task was verbal in nature, it probably generated a greater amount of interference for verbal than for nonverbal materials. It should also be noted that the earlier results of Samuels, Butters, Goodglass, and Brody (1971) were not so clear that alcoholic Korsakoff's patients were unimpaired relative to controls on a visual-memory task presented in the Peterson and Peterson paradigm.

Cermack, Butters, and Goodglass (1971) presented consonant trigrams, single words, and word triads to alcoholic Korsakoff's patients. The Peterson and Peterson method was used with distraction intervals of 3, 9, and 18 seconds. With consonant triads and single words, the Korsakoff's subjects recalled significantly fewer items than alcoholic and normal controls at the 9- and 18-second delays. For word triads, Korsakoff's subjects recalled significantly fewer items than alcoholic and normal controls at the 3-, 9-, and 18-second delays. Thus, results indicated that short-term retention was worse for alcoholic Korsakoff's patients than for controls. When a recognition as opposed to a recall paradigm was used with word triads, Korsakoff's patients still performed significantly below alcoholic controls at the 3-, 9-, and 18-second delays. However, they were able to recognize more information than they could recall, indicating that the recall method did not allow them to retrieve all the information available. Finally, Cermak et al. presented a list of six paired associates 16 times or until the list was learned over each of 4 consecutive days. It took the Korsakoff's subjects significantly more trials to perform the list without errors on every day but the 4th, when there were no significant differences with alcoholic controls. On each consecutive day, it took the Korsakoff's patients less trials to achieve one perfect performance than on the previous day. According to the authors, these data indicated that some information was able to enter the long-term memory of the Korsakoff's subjects, though less efficiently and more slowly than for controls.

The Peterson and Peterson (1959) paradigm has not always yielded inferior performance for patients with alcoholic Korsakoff's syndrome. Mair et al. (1979) used this method with two alcoholic Korsakoff's patients and controls. Three 3-letter words were presented with distraction-filled intervals of zero, 5, 10, 15, 30, and 60 seconds. Both patients showed equal or superior performance to controls. Kopelman (1985) presented word triads with counting backward as a distraction. Recall was tested at 0, 2.5, 5, 10, and 20 seconds. Performance of Korsakoff's patients did not differ from that of controls, even though the performance of Alzheimer's disease subjects was significantly below that of both Korsakoff's and normal subjects once the distraction was introduced.

Turning our attention to long-term memory, investigators have determined that memories decay over time after they have been registered into long-term memory. Consolidation, as defined above, is the maintenance of information in long-term memory. To the degree that decay is prevented, memories are consolidated in long-term memory. Figure 6-1 illustrates different rates of forgetting (i.e., rates of decay) for hypothetical groups. In this figure, a "yes-no" recognition task with a random response rate of 50% has been used, similar to many of the studies discussed below. Group N shows the percentage of correct responses for the hypothetical normal group. Group A demonstrates a normal rate of response soon after initial presentation of the stimuli, but the abnormally rapid rate of forgetting leads to a lower performance at 24 hours and 1 week later. Group B began at a lower rate of performance but demonstrates what appears to be a normal rate of forgetting at first glance. However, Group B's performance approaches random levels by 1 week after presentation, and it is not expected that their performance would go below a random level. Since Group B is close to the worst performance level expected, it is difficult to estimate their true rate of forgetting.

Before rates of forgetting in alcoholic Korsakoff's syndrome could be compared to that of normals, however, some way of equating their

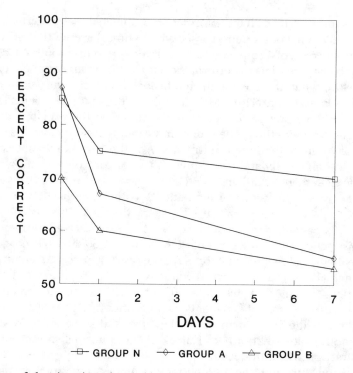

Figure 6-1. A hypothetical rate-of-forgetting experiment. A "yes–no" response paradigm for recognition memory is used; therefore, the 50% performance level represents random chance responding. Group N shows a normal rate of forgetting. Group A starts at a normal level of performance but demonstrates an accelerated rate of forgetting. Group B's performance starts below normal levels. Because Group B's performance level approaches random chance after 7 days, it is difficult to tell if their rate of forgetting is parallel to the normal curve of Group N.

performance to that of normals would be desirable. In this way the effects of initial rate on later levels of performance could be controlled. A study by Huppert and Piercy (1977) seemed to provide a way for equating performance. They exposed pictures to alcoholic Korsakoff's subjects and controls for three different durations (0.5, 1, 2-seconds) at three different frequencies (1, 2, 4 times). Recognition memory was tested using a "yes-no" response format at 20 minutes after exposure. For each exposure duration by frequency of exposure cell, controls performed significantly better than patients. However, both groups improved when duration of exposure, frequency of exposure, or both were increased. When the total exposure time was 4 to 8 times greater for the amnesic patients than for the controls, performance was equivalent. The authors concluded that Korsakoff's patients demonstrated an initial registration deficit that could be overcome by increasing the total exposure time. The ability to equate performances between amnesic and nonamnesic groups was used by the authors in subsequent experiments.

Huppert and Piercy (1978) provided a more clear demonstration that alcoholic Korsakoff's patients could retain information in long-term memory. They showed normal controls and Korsakoff's subjects magazine pictures and equated their recognition memory performance after a 10-minute delay. The authors accomplished the latter by exposing pictures for either 4 or 8 seconds to Korsakoff's patients while using only a 1 second exposure for controls. Subsequently, the recognition memory performance of controls and amnesic patients also was equivalent after 1 day or 7 days. Huppert and Piercy concluded that alcoholic Korsakoff's patients had difficulty in the initial learning of the information. However, when amnesic performance is equated for initial learning, they show a normal rate of forgetting and are capable of maintaining information in long-term storage.

Huppert and Piercy (1979) repeated the same procedures with patient H. M., who had amnesic syndrome after bilateral removal of mesial temporal lobe structures. Pictures were exposed to H. M. for either 10 or 15 seconds. After both exposure intervals, H. M. demonstrated an accelerated rate of forgetting compared to controls and/or alcoholic Korsakoff's patients. The authors concluded that amnesia associated with diencephalic lesion was due to initial registration deficits, while amnesia associated with bilateral temporal lobe dysfunction was a deficit in consolidation. Similarly, Butters, Miliotis, Albert, and Sax (1984) demonstrated a faster rate of forgetting in a postencephalitic patient with extensive bilateral mesial temporal damage than in normal controls or diencephalic amnesia.

In comparison to patients with presumed temporal lobe memory deficits (i.e., patients receiving electroconvulsive therapy), Squire (1981) also demonstrated that patients with alcoholic Korsakoff's syndrome did not show an abnormally high rate of forgetting up to 32 hours after exposure. Moss, Albert, Butters, and Payne (1986) similarly found that patients with alcoholic Korsakoff's syndrome did not show an abnormal rate of forgetting like patients with senile dementia of the Alzheimer's type. The intervals were much shorter for the Moss et al. study than the Squire study (i.e., rate of forgetting was assessed by comparing 15-second recall versus 2-minute recall). Memory also was being assessed by a more difficult recall paradigm in the Moss et al.

study, whereas Squire used a recognition-memory task. Recall as opposed to recognition introduces greater retrieval demands. Thus, some caution must be exercised in interpreting these latter results.

Martone, Butters, and Trauner (1986) verified normal rates of forgetting for pictures in alcoholic Korsakoff's patients as well as in Huntington's disease patients. In a second experiment, subjects were asked to recognize a previously presented picture versus a foil stimulus either by presentation of the whole picture, a main object, or a peripheral object. Performance was equated by exposing pictures 2 seconds for controls, 8 seconds for Huntington's patients, and 12 seconds for alcoholic Korsakoff's patients. There were no group differences in performance for whole picture, main object, or peripheral object. Thus, when given enough time, amnesic patients are able to register similar visual information to controls.

When Kopelman (1985) compared picture-recognition memory at 10 minutes, 24 hours, and 7 days after presentation, normal subjects gave more correct responses than alcoholic Korsakoff's or Alzheimer's disease patients in spite of the fact that the latter groups were given greater exposure times in an attempt to equate learning. Nonetheless, there were no differences in rates of forgetting between groups. Alzheimer's disease patients showed more false recognitions. The author interpreted his findings to mean that memory problems were caused by initial registration deficits for both patient groups. It should be noted that his Alzheimer's disease patients were very close to a random performance level on the task, making it less likely for them to show a greater rate of forgetting as predicted.

One caution should be noted regarding equating initial performance by varying length of exposure between groups. Martone et al. (1986) exposed pictures to older normals for 1 second and to younger normals for 0.5 second. Although performance level was equal between groups after 10 minutes, the younger group with the shorter exposure showed inferior recognition memory after 1 week. The authors noted that equal performance between subject groups after 10 minutes does not necessarily equate the groups with respect to the amount learned. Therefore, some caution must be used when interpreting studies that attempt to equate initial performance by using longer exposure for groups with memory problems.

Further, one should note that the rate of forgetting explanation for temporal lobe amnesic syndrome in general, and for patient H. M. in particular, has been questioned. Freed, Corkin, and Cohen (1987) tested H. M.'s recognition memory over varing intervals (10 minutes, 24 hours, 72 hours, 1 week) with two recognition memory paradigms. H. M. was given two 10-second exposures to pictures that controls saw once for 1 second. (Note the increased exposure over the previous study with H. M.) When he was required to say "Yes" for pictures that had been exposed during the learning phase or "No" for pictures that had not, H. M.'s performance was equivalent to controls after 10 minutes, but performance dropped significantly below controls after 24 hours. H. M.'s performance level did not appear to change from 24 to 72 hours or from 24 hours to 1 week. Control's performance, on the other hand, continued to fall such that there was no significant difference between H. M. and controls after 72 hours and 1 week. The authors interpreted the findings to show that H. M. showed "a normal rate of forgetting over a 1 week delay interval." An alternative interpretation is that H. M.'s lowest level of performance for this 1-week interval had been raised above previous levels (Huppert & Piercy, 1979) by additional exposure. The fact that he approached this lowest level of performance more rapidly than controls may indeed mean that his rate of forgetting was more rapid.

More troublesome for the rate-of-forgetting explanation of temporal lobe amnesia were Freed and colleagues' (1987) findings on picture recognition when the authors tested H. M.'s recognition memory by asking him to choose which of two pictures he had seen during the learning phase of the experiment. Exposure durations were the same as for the "yes-no" recognition task. There were no significant differences between H. M.'s and controls' performance at any delay (10 minutes, 24 hours, 72 hours, 1 week). In fact, H. M.'s performance was actually insignificantly above that of controls at the 72-hour and 1-week intervals.

These data do not spell the doom of rate-of-forgetting explanations for temporal lobe amnesia as suggested by the authors; they do, however, call attention to the complexities of interpreting data from rate-of-forgetting experiments. Not only must one consider equating performance at an initial delay, one must consider where subject's performance levels off, and how quickly performance approaches that leveling-off point. It is also important to consider the potential interaction between strength of initial registration and the ability to consolidate material into long-term memory, as opposed to considering registration and consolidation as entirely separate processes (e.g., see Martone et al., 1986).

In spite of the controversy about rate of forgetting in patients with bilateral mesial temporal damage, there is some converging evidence regarding the ability of alcoholic Korsakoff's patients to retain information in long-term memory once the initial registration phase has been accomplished. For example, Lhermitte and Signorette (1976) compared visual memory performance of a patient with alcoholic

Korsakoff's syndrome to the performance of a patient with bilateral mesial temporal lesions, the performance of a patient with bilateral cingulate lesions, and the performance of controls. In their task, the subjects had to learn where in a 3 X 3 grid each of nine pictures went. Once the subjects had learned the positions to criterion (three consecutive perfect trials), they were required to describe each picture and where it went (free recall) and to point to the square where a picture went when the picture was presented (cued recall). These recall trials were done at 3 minutes, 1 hour, 24 hours, and 4 days. Normal controls required between one and four trials to learn the task. The patient with bilateral mesial temporal lesions took 16 trials to learn the task and had very little or no recall on either free or cued recall as soon as 3 minutes after reaching criterion. The authors concluded that the information failed to be transferred from short-term to long-term memory. The patient with bilateral cingulate lesion learned the task in one trial, but showed little memory for the pictures and positions on free recall. However, performance was perfect on cued recall. Since the patient was able to perform well with cues, the authors reasoned that a retrieval deficit was the cause for poor performance on free recall. The patient with Korsakoff's syndrome took 12 trials to learn the task, had no recollection during free recall, but showed performance within normal limits on delayed cued recall. Since the patient took a long time to learn the task, the authors reasoned that there was difficulty transferring the information from short-term to long-term memory. Based on performance in their task and previous literature, they reasoned that the Korsakoff's patient also had a retrieval and information-processing deficit since performance was adequate only on cued as opposed to free recall. The performance of the Korsakoff's patient confirms that information can be retained once it is placed into long-term storage as evidenced by cued-recall performance, but it also suggests that a retrieval deficit is active in alcoholic Korsakoff's syndrome.

Based on the above data, a few conclusions now will be drawn regarding the retention of information in short- and long-term memory. The Peterson and Peterson paradigm has been interpreted as tapping short-term memory. If one uses an Atkinson and Shiffrin (1968) approach, one might surmise that this paradigm depends only upon short-term memory because material is kept from long-term memory by preventing rehearsal. Studies finding impairment in alcoholic Korsakoff's syndrome using this technique might be interpreted as demonstrating a deficient ability to maintain information in short-term memory, in accordance with this view. However, there is a second possible interpretation *if* short- and long-term memory are considered to be overlapping: information is lost from short-term memory, especially at longer delays, perhaps because of decay or maybe even due to displacement of information by the distraction task. As short-term memory thereby becomes less effective in retaining the information, normal subjects become more dependent upon the rudimentary (i.e., without elaboration) registration of the material in long-term memory. Korsakoff's patients become deficient at the longer intervals because of deficient registration of the material in long-term memory. The lack of differences between Korsakoff's patients and normals in some studies (Koppleman, 1985; Mair et al., 1979) may be due to the longer exposure times used in these studies (i.e., 2 or 3 seconds vs. 1 second)

Although rate-of-forgetting studies in some ways have been controversial, they have provided quite consistent evidence vis-à-vis patients with alcoholic Korsakoff's syndrome: given enough time, these amnesic patients can register information into long-term memory and can show normal rates of forgetting as measured by recognition-memory tasks. The controversy is more whether alcoholic Korsakoff's patients differ from temporal lobe amnesics because the existence of abnormally high rates of forgetting has been questioned in the latter population. Regarding rates of forgetting, it may be that there is an interaction between strength of initial registration and consolidation such that extremely brief periods of registration produce higher rates of forgetting (e.g., Martone et al., 1986) or extremely long exposure periods will produce lower rates of forgetting (possibly Freed et al., 1987). Thus, the question with temporal lobe amnesics becomes: do they show simply quantitative differences in strength of registration of material into long-term memory, or do they show a different kind of deficit with abnormally high rates of forgetting?

Proactive Interference

The term *proactive interference* refers to the tendency of previously learned information to interfere with the recall of more recently learned information. For example, a group of subjects is required to learn and recall List A; then, they are required to learn and recall List B. If recall on List B is less than recall on List A, then proactive interference may be active. Certain factors are known to increase proactive interference, such as the semantic similarity of items on List A and List B or massed as opposed to distributed practice. *Retroactive interference* occurs when recently learned information interferes with the recall of previously learned information. Data indicate that alcoholic Korsakoff's patients may be abnormally sensitive to proactive interference. As explained below, proactive-interference tasks (i.e., failure to release from proactive interference with taxonomic category shifts) also have been used to argue that these patients have difficulty attending to semantic information. The possible causes of proactive-interference effects in alcoholic Korsakoff's syndrome will be discussed at the end of the section.

Talland (1965) included tests of proactive and retroactive interference among the numerous other tests he performed on his sample of patients with alcoholic Korsakoff's syndrome. He looked at both types of interference with both nonsense syllables and words. With both stimuli, controls were significantly affected by retroactive interference but not by proactive interference compared to noninterference trials. Amnesic patients showed no differential effects of interference over noninterference trials for words and nonsense syllables. But Korsakoff's patients did show greater retroactive-interference effects than controls when the task was to learn a ten-word sentence. It is likely that the former tasks (i.e., learning of nonsense syllables and words) involved a "floor" effect for the Korsakoff's patients that obscured the effects of interference, whereas the latter task (sentence learning) did not involve such an effect. The intertest intervals make it likely that Talland's procedures tapped long-term as opposed to short-term memory effects.

In another early study, Cermak and Butters (1972) explored the sensitivity of alcoholic Korsakoff's patients to interference from previous lists. They employed the Peterson and Peterson (1959) technique with distraction-filled intervals of various length. Their first list consisted either of three consonants or three short words. Their second list consisted of three short words. Compared to alcoholic controls, alcoholic Korsakoff's subjects showed a relatively greater loss of information under high proactive-interference conditions (words followed by words) than under low proactive-interference conditions (consonants followed by words). The authors concluded that the amnesic patients' memories were more sensitive to disruption by proactive interference. The authors seemed to confirm the sensitivity to proactive interference by using trials spaced by a 6-second interval (massed practice) versus trials with a 1-minute intertrial interval (distributed practice). Distributed practice gives proactive interference a chance to dissipate. When compared to controls, the Korsakoff's subjects demonstrated a relatively worse performance on the massed-practice than on the distributed-practice trials.

The ability of patients with alcoholic Korsakoff's syndrome to use semantic information in verbal memory has been tested using several paradigms. The dominant idea has been that these patients may be unable to encode information in the most efficient format. Use of meaning, as opposed to use of other strategies (e.g., acoustic similarities), has been assumed to be the most efficient means of organizing verbal information for memory (e.g., Cermack, Butters, & Gerrein, 1973).

Buildup of proactive interference has been used to study the sensitivity of alcoholic Korsakoff's patients to semantic information. In the release-from-proactive-interference paradigm, subjects are given a number of short lists with a free recall requested after each presentation. Until the final trial, all words in the successive lists are from the same semantic category. Across trials a proactive interference (i.e., an interference of items of previous lists in the recall of the present list) builds up. Thus, recall declines on each successive trial. On the final trial, words are presented either from the same semantic category as other trials or from a different category. If the same category is continued, proactive interference remains in effect, and performance continues to decline. If a different semantic category is used, there is a release from proactive interference, and performance of normal subjects increases after the shift of semantic category. Sometimes, alcoholic Korsakoff's patients fail to demonstrate a release from proactive interference, and their performance remains low after semantic-category changes. This has been taken as an indication that they are insensitive to the information contained in semantic categories. Figure 6-2 shows how results from a hypothetical release-from-proactive-interference experiment might look.

For example, Cermak, Butters, and Moreines (1974) explored several aspects of proactive interference. They provided alcoholic Korsakoff's patients and alcoholic controls with five learning trials, with either a category shift or no category shift on the fifth trial. In one paradigm, either letter or number triads were used on the first four trials. In the shift condition, the fifth trial consisted of a number triad instead of the letter triads used on the first four trials, or vice versa. In a second paradigm, triads consisted of words from set semantic categories. The semantic category was the same for the first four trials. In the shift condition, the category changed on the fifth trial, whereas there was no category change in the no-shift condition. A distraction-filled interval of 15 seconds was used between presentation and recall for each trial. Compared to controls, alcoholic Korsakoff's subjects showed a normal release from proactive interference in the letter-number task, but failed to show a release from proactive interference when the shift was from words of one semantic category to words of another category. As noted above, the authors interpreted this finding to reveal an insensitivity to semantic properties of the stimuli in the

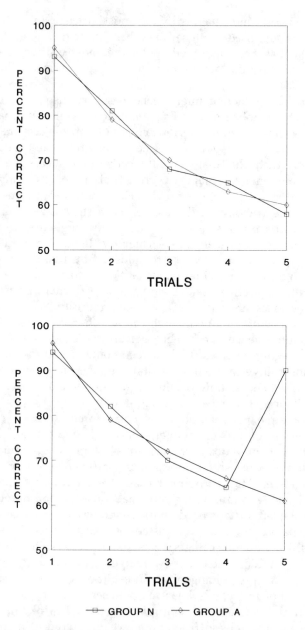

Figure 6-2. A hypothetical release-from-proactive-interference experiment. *Top:* The buildup of proactive interference across all five lists occurs for both Group N and Group A when items from each of the five lists come from the same category. *Bottom:* However, when there is a category shift for list words in Trial 5, Group N demonstrates a normal release from proactive interference, but Group A does not.

category-shift task. The study also demonstrated that Korsakoff's patients could show a release from proactive inteference under some conditions. Finally, the authors noted that amnesic subjects showed a significantly greater decrement by Trial 4 in both the letter-number and word tasks, confirming Cermak and Butters's (1972) contention that alcoholic Korsakoff's patients were more sensitive to proactive interference.

Squire (1982) confirmed the failure to release from proactive interference in patients with alcoholic Korsakoff's syndrome. In addition, these patients demonstrated an inability to make judgments about temporal order. However, this group of amnesic patients did show some ability to use semantic information in recognition memory, though their ability was not as great as that of alcoholic controls. The failure to release from proactive inteference along with deficits in temporal-order judgments correlated with performance on frontal lobe tasks. Squire noted that previous studies had shown frontal lobe patients to demonstrate failure to release from proactive inhibition (Moscovitch, 1982) and deficits in temporal-order judgments (Milner, 1971). Further, a patient with verbal-memory deficit after left diencephalic injury from a stab wound did not show either of these problems. Thus, Squire concluded that failure to release from proactive interference and deficits in temporal-order judgments were due to frontal lobe changes frequently seen with alcoholic Korsakoff's syndrome.

In this context, it is worth noting that Speedie and Heilman (1983) and Crosson (1985) suggested that frontal lobe deficits after dorsal medial thalamic lesions might be due to the prolific connections of this diencephalic structure with the frontal lobes. This observation is relevant, of course, because of the dorsal medial thalamic pathology in alcoholic Korsakoff's syndrome (Victor et al., 1971). However, the above-mentioned patient with dorsal medial thalamic lesion after stab wound did not show deficits typical of frontal lobe damage, suggesting that deficits in frontal lobe tasks in alcoholic Korsakoff's syndrome may not be attributable solely to the connections of the dorsal medial nucleus with the frontal lobe.

Glass and Butters (1985), on the other hand, attempted to explain the greater buildup of proactive interference in patients with alcoholic Korsakoff's syndrome that was found in the Cermak and Butters (1972) and the Cermak et al. (1974) studies. Their experiment involved measuring the reaction time necessary to distinguish words from nonwords given different primes appearing 700 milliseconds prior to the stimuli. Half of the primes signaled that a word from a set category (e.g., body parts) would follow 75% of the time, and half of the primes were neutral with respect to the word that ensued. In one set of trials 3 X's were used as the prime, and 3 O's were the neutral cue. In a second set of trials, the prime was a semantic category (e.g., bird) and the word that followed was an exemplar of a different category (e.g., body parts). As shown in previous studies using the 700-millisecond interval, normal and alcoholic controls responded more quickly to items from the expected category with both types of primes (i.e., X's or category) than in the neutral condition. Alcoholic Korsakoff's subjects responded more quickly to words from the expected category when X's were the prime, but they demonstrated no difference between words from the expected-category and the neutral-cue condition when a conflicting category was the prime. The authors considered the results evidence that Korsakoff's patients were unable to inhibit normal associations to the conflicting prime. They further suggested that proactive interference may not be the product of poor encoding as previously suggested (e.g., Butters and Cermak, 1980). Rather, proactive interference may be the cause of poor encoding through interference with succeeding items.

The concept of proactive interference is relevant to intrusion errors when such intrusions come from prior items in a series. For example, Samuels et al. (1971) presented a number of auditory and visual stimuli using the Peterson and Peterson paradigm to alcoholic Korsakoff's subjects and subjects with cortical lesions. Korsakoff's patients repeated more responses from prior items than did patients with cortical lesions. Butters and colleagues (Butters et al., 1987; Butters et al., 1986) presented series of stories to alcoholic Korsakoff's patients, Huntington's disease patients, Alzheimer's dementia patients, and controls. Korsakoff's patients tended to show more intrusions from prior stories than did controls or Huntington's disease subjects, but Alzheimer's dementia patients also committed prior story intrusions. The authors related prior story intrusions to abnormal susceptibility to proactive interference. It should be noted that alcoholic Korsakoff's patients also show other types of extra-story-intrusion errors.

Huppert and Peircy (1976) performed an experiment that may shed light on proactive interference in some situations. When they found that alcoholic Korsakoff's patients performed better on recognition memory for low-frequency than high-frequency words, they wondered if this result was due to an inability to recognize the context in which the more familiar words had been presented. On Day 1 of their second experiment, Korsakoff's subjects and controls were shown 80 magazine pictures on three occasions for a total of 22 seconds. On Day 2, they were shown 80 magazine pictures, half of which had been presented on Day 1. After 10 minutes, subjects were presented with four classes of pictures: those that had been seen on Day 1 only, those that had been seen on Day 2 only, those that had been seen on both Day 1 and Day 2, and those that had not been seen previously. For each picture, subjects were asked, "Did you see this picture *today*?" If subjects said "No," they were then asked if they had seen the picture before. Replies to the first question determined whether subjects were able to make a judgment as to the temporal context in which they might have seen the picture. Replies to the second question, when combined with replies to the first, provided an estimate of how well subjects could determine if the picture had been seen before without respect to context. For pictures presented on Day 1, both Korsakoff's patients and controls recognized those pictures presented on both Day 1 and Day 2 as having been presented on Day 2. However, the Korsakoff's subjects incorrectly recognized significantly more pictures presented on Day 1 as having been presented on Day 2 than did controls. Thus, they had difficulty making judgments about temporal context. Both groups were able to accurately discriminate pictures that had not been presented before from other categories, indicating that Korsakoff's patients could make judgments about familiarity of pictures if context was not a factor. If one applies these data to prior-list- and prior-story-intrusion errors made by Korsakoff's patients, then one can hypothesize that prior-list- and prior-story-intrusion errors occur because alcoholic Korsakoff's patients are unable to discriminate the temporal contexts in which items or ideas have been presented.

Winocur and Kinsbourne (1978) also demonstrated that alcoholic Korsakoff's patients could not overcome the tendency to give prior list intrusions on a paired associates task. They had subjects learn a list of highly associated pairs and then changed only the second item of the pairs for a new set of learning trials. Although the Korsakoff's subjects could not overcome the proactive interference, controls could. The authors went on to demonstrate that manipulating the environmental contextual cues associated between the two lists could lower the interference.

In summary: Alcoholic Korsakoff's subjects are abnormally sensitive to the buildup of proactive interference. A failure to demonstrate normal release from proactive interference after shifts of semantic categories probably indicates that alcoholic Korsakoff's patients do not process semantic cues normally. However, Squire (1982) presented convincing evidence that this phenomenon may be a product of frontal lobe as opposed to diencephalic dysfunction. Greater proactive interference may be related to prior list and prior story intrusions found in many studies. Both may be caused by an inability to make use of contextual information in memory processes. It follows that the inability to use contextual information could result from frontal lobe impairment and is consistent with deficits in temporal-order judgments shown by Korsakoff's and frontal patients. Finally, greater buildup of proactive interference with alcoholic Korsakoff's patients is an indication that they have some memory representation of items from prior trials. Since the buildup of proactive interference typically occurs over intervals too long to encompass short-term memory, and since explicit long-term storage can be assumed defective with these patients, a different type of memory storage must be present. Thus, abnormal buildup of proactive interference may be an indication of implicit memory representation of prior items and an interference of such implicit representations with explicit recall.

Depth-of-Processing and Related Paradigms

Other experimental paradigms have been used to study the ability of alcoholic Korsakoff patients to respond to semantic characteristics of stimuli to be remembered. However, the concept of semantic process-ing is somewhat restrictive because it only applies to verbal paradigms. In a more general sense, the argument has been made that patients with alcoholic Korsakoff's syndrome might fail to use efficient strategies for processing nonverbal as well as verbal material. Thus, a more general way of stating this tendency is that the amnesic patients may process information with superficial but not deep strategies. In verbal memory paradigms, results of the studies discussed below generally have been interpreted to indicate that alcoholic Korsakoff's patients do not spontaneously use semantic information under normal learning conditions. However, they can benefit from semantic cues, and they use semantic information if given more exposure time to verbal stimuli.

Weiskrantz and Warrington (1970) found that giving recall cues 1 minute after lists were presented improved the performance of amnesic patients, just as it does in normals. However, Cermak and Butters (1972) found that alcoholic Korsakoff's subjects performed worse on cued than free recall when recall was required immediately after presentation. Cermak, Butters, and Gerrein (1973) clarified the discrepancy by demonstrating that it was the 1-minute delay that produced the improvement for Korsakoff syndrome patients upon cued recall; cued-recall performance was still worse than free recall if there was no delay. In all three studies the cues were semantic. This indicated that these amnesic patients can respond to the semantic characteristics of stimuli when they are used as cues during recall.

However, Cermak et al. (1973) went on to explore this issue further. They found that when instructed to do so, alcoholic Korsakoff's patients could use semantic, associative, or acoustic cues. However, they also presented a recognition task in which semantic, associative, or acoustic errors could be made. In a long list of words, subjects had to state when a word had appeared previously in the list. In addition to repeated words, there were homonyms, synonyms, and associates of other list words. Compared to alcoholic controls, the Korsakoff's subjects made a greater number of false recognitions on homonyms and associates than on synonyms. The authors interpreted this finding to mean that the amnesic patients use less efficient organization strategies (acoustic or associative) when not instructed to what aspects of the stimuli to attend. Further, they suggested that these patients were deficient in their utilization of semantic information.

Gardner et al. (1973) explored the effectiveness of three types of cueing on the word-list memory of alcoholic Korsakoff's patients. In the reference-to-task condition, subjects were told, "A few moments ago I asked you to remember some words. Do you remember what they were?" In the categorical-cue condition the category to which the to-be-remembered word belongs was given both at presentation of each word and following a delay. Only after the delay, subjects had to provide the first word from the category that came to their mind and five other exemplars. In the third condition, both reference-to-task and the category cue were used. It took both the task and category cues to improve the memory of Korsakoff's subjects, while alcoholic controls increased performance under both the reference-to-task and the reference-to-task + category-cue conditions. The authors suggested that the amnesic patients could not spontaneously draw upon their semantic knowledge of the list words during the reference-to-task condition, but they could respond to semantic cues when they were provided. The merits of storage versus retrieval explanations were discussed. It is also of interest that the category cue only condition did demonstrate some increase over baseline responses to the category for the Korsakoff's patients. This is actually an early example of an implicit-memory task, and the authors did distinguish this task from "explicit" memory. They suggested that repetition of an item might alter its probability in the hierarchy of responses to a category even in patients with explicit-memory deficits.

Jaffe and Katz (1975) examined the effects of providing semantic cues at initial presentation and at recall on the recall performance of a single patient with alcoholic Korsakoff's syndrome. In addition to the recall condition, a recognition condition was used. The patient's recall approached the same level as recognition performance when the semantic cues (i.e., category of item) were provided at both initial presentation and at recall. Cueing only at initial presentation or only at recall was not sufficient to increase recall performance. Although recognition performance was superior to recall performance (except when cues were given at both times), recognition performance was still noticeably less than might be expected. The authors felt that the below-par recognition performance was an indication that some items were not registered in long-term memory. However, the discrepancy between recognition and recall under most conditions indicates that the patient also could not adequately retrieve information that was registered into long-term memory. This study again indicates that Korsakoff's patients can improve recall with semantic cueing, though this patient required the structure of the cue for both initial encoding and retrieval in order to improve performance.

Cermak and Reale (1978) required subjects to process words either by physical features (upper- or lowercase), phonemic analysis (rhyme), or semantic analyses (three different tasks). When alcoholic Korsakoff's patients and alcoholic controls were given 60 words in succession and required to process them by one of these methods, controls performed best at recognizing those words that they had to process semantically. Korsakoff's patients did not show greater recognition performance under the semantic as opposed to the phonemic or physical features conditions. Only when the task was broken down into 12-word, as opposed to 60-word, lists did the Korsakoff's subjects demonstrate significantly better recognition for semantically processed words as opposed to words processed by physical features. Speed of processing was generally similar for the two groups for the different types of processing. The authors reasoned that the latter finding (amnesics' memory for semantically processed words is better under some conditions) supported the assumption that decreased depth of processing is at least partially responsible for their memory deficit. In other words, since their memory does improve when forced to semantically process words, their normal propensity not to process words in this fashion leads to memory problems. However, the authors also pointed out that since semantic processing did not improve recognition performance in all cases, other factors must also be considered as responsible for the memory deficits in amnesic patients. The authors were unable to elaborate on such other factors.

Using a recognition-memory paradigm, Wetzel and Squire (1980) compared depth of processing in alcoholic Korsakoff's patients, patient N.A. with a stab wound affecting the dorsal medial thalamus, and patients receiving electroconvulsive therapy. Stimulus words were presented, and subjects were asked to state whether words were printed in upper- or lowercase letters, whether words rhymed with a word provided by the experimenter, or whether a word belonged to a semantic category provided by the experimenter. Different words were used for each type of question. The answer to each type of question was affirmative for half of the words and negative for half of the words. Korsakoff's patients, N.A., and electroconvulsive therapy patients all performed lower than their respective controls. However, N.A. and electroconvulsive therapy patients demonstrated increased recognition performance when they were asked to pay attention to the category and the answer was affirmative. This was the same pattern demonstrated by controls. The Korsakoff's patients did not demonstrate improved recognition under this latter condition. The authors concluded that the relatively widespread neuropathology in the Korsakoff's patients caused them to be unable to benefit from semantic encoding compared to patient N.A. Squire's (1982) later interpretation is more specific and applicable to this earlier study. He thought the difference between alcoholic Korsakoff's patients' and N.A.'s ability to perform semantic encoding was due to frontal lobe involvement in the former but not in the latter.

Wetzel and Squire (1980) also ran normal subjects with fast and slow presentations and with 1-minute and 3-day delays before recognition. The rationale was that these conditions might reduce the recognition of normals, causing them to be unable to use semantic information. Although the increased delay did cause reduced recognition performance, the pattern was the same in all conditions: normals demonstrated increased performance for words presented under the category condition with an affirmative answer. These results suggest that it was not the level of recognition performance determining the lack of benefit from the semantic information in alcoholic Korsakoff's patients, but the inability to perform semantic encoding.

Mayes, Meudell, and Neary (1980) assessed the ability to process nonverbal stimuli in patients with alcoholic Korsakoff's syndrome. Patients and controls viewed nonsense shapes and faces in a recognition-memory study. With each type of stimulus (faces, shapes), patients were given a superficial processing strategy and a deep processing strategy. For faces, the deep strategy was to rate the friendliness of the face, and the superficial strategy was to rate the straightness of the hair. For shapes, the deep strategy was to provide a name for the figure, and the superficial strategy was to count the sides. The authors equated performance in amnesics and controls by providing unusually long exposures to the stimuli, and by doing the recognition testing of controls at longer intervals after exposure to stimuli and/or after exposure to a greater number of stimuli. The authors reasoned that if Korsakoff's patients processed stimuli less deeply, they would benefit more from the deep-processing strategies than controls. Their findings indicated that deep-processing strategies resulted in better recognition performance than no strategy for both groups. Superficial-processing strategies resulted in worse recognition performance than no strategy for both groups. However, there were no differences between groups with any strategy or stimulus type. Mayes et al. reasoned that a deficit in deep processing by Korsakoff's patients would lead to greater benefit when they were required to use a deep-processing strategy. Since such a finding did not occur, they concluded that Korsakoff's subjects' tendency to ignore meaningful aspects of stimuli does not contribute to their memory problem. There are other potential reasons for these findings. One is that the experimental task was constructed so as to maximize the performance of the Korsakoff's patients. Perhaps depth-of-processing deficits are overcome with greater processing time, and therefore not shown when performance has been maximized for Korsakoff's patients.

Some studies have shown that story content can affect the ability of alcoholic Korsakoff's patients to remember stories. Davidoff et al. (1984) presented stories with neutral, sexual, and aggressive themes to Korsakoff's patients, alcoholic patients, and neurologically normal controls. Korsakoff's patients recalled more ideas from the sexual stories both at immediate recall and after a 30-second, distraction-filled delay, but the other groups did not. The amnesic patients also lost information from immediate to delayed recall regardless of theme, whereas the other groups did not lose significant information. Granholm, Wolfe, and Butters (1985) confirmed the superior memory in alcoholic Korsakoff's subjects for stories with sexual content versus happy, sad, or neutral content. Huntington's disease patients and controls did not show this tendency.

To summarize: Under "normal" learning conditions, alcoholic Korsakoff's patients may fail to respond to semantic information in verbal-memory tasks. However, if they are instructed to process information by its semantic attributes and/or if they are given semantic cues at recall, performance improves. In other words, if given the same brief exposure adequate for normal learning, these amnesic patients do not spontaneously use semantic information in memory tasks, even though they are otherwise capable of responding to such information. Increasing processing time, however, may enable alcoholic Korsakoff's patients to respond spontaneously with greater depth of processing. It is uncertain if deficient depth of processing applies to visual information.

Implicit Memory

According to Schacter (1987), *repetition priming* is the facilitation of the processing of a particular stimulus because of a recent exposure to that stimulus. Since priming experiments usually do not explicitly request subjects to remember the primed stimuli, they belong to the realm of implicit memory. Word priming is one type of methodology used to explore implicit memory. One type of word priming is word-stem completion. In this paradigm, subjects are exposed to a list of words in some sort of nonmemory task. Perhaps subjects are asked to rate how much they like or dislike words (e.g., Shimamura et al., 1987). Subsequently, subjects are given a word stem consisting of the first few letters of the words to which they were exposed. There are several possibilities for each stem. Subjects are requested to complete the stems with the first words that come to mind. The experimenter counts the number of times a word from the "nonmemory" task is given for its stem. Baseline guessing rates are taken into account by having subjects complete stems for words to which they were not exposed and measuring the number of times they give a specific predetermined response. When words are used in priming experiments, it is usually assumed that subjects have had prior exposure to the words and therefore have knowledge of their meaning. To put it another way, words have preexisting representations in semantic memory. In general, the studies reviewed below have revealed that alcoholic Korsakoff's patients have shown positive effects for priming when words have been used as stimuli. Priming experiments involving nonwords, without preexisting representations in semantic memory, have not shown such consistent results (see Schacter, 1987).

Graf et al. (1984) presented a word-stem-completion task to patients with alcoholic Korsakoff's syndrome, other amnesic patients, and controls. The word-stem completion was presented within the context of two different initial tasks, and under two different completion procedures. Regarding initial task presentation, subjects had to state whether consecutive words contained the same vowels or had to rate how much they liked the words. In one word-stem-completion condition (priming) subjects had to write the first word that came to mind, but in the other condition (cued recall), they were told to use the stem as a cue to recall the list words. Free-recall and recognition conditions were also used. (Statistical analyses did not separate Korsakoff's subjects from other amnesics, but individual group graphs of results make it possible to verify which results apply to Korsakoff's subjects.) Relative to controls, Korsakoff's patients were impaired on free recall for both the vowel and liking conditions. For the recognition and cued recall,

Korsakoff's subjects were comparatively impaired in the liking but not the vowel condition. Priming was comparable between groups in both the liking and vowel conditions. It is apparent that the liking condition required initial semantic processing of the word, whereas the vowel condition did not. This feature probably accounts for the group difference in the liking condition while no group difference existed in the vowel condition for recognition and cued recall. Under the condition requiring semantic processing with stem-completion priming, the authors concluded that both alcoholic Korsakoff's subjects and controls demonstrated activation of words in preexisting semantic memory. When elaboration (or active processing) is required for the explicit memory tasks, Korsakoff's patients show impairment.

Shimamura et al. (1987) confirmed that patients with alcoholic Korsakoff's syndrome and patients with Huntington's disease demonstrated normal word-stem-priming effects, whereas patients with senile dementia of the Alzheimer's type were deficient in word-stem-completion priming. The authors suggested that the priming failure in Alzheimer's disease reflected an inability to activate representations in lexical (word) memory. Such an interpretation would not only account for word-finding and semantic-memory deficits in Alzheimer's disease, it would imply that the ability to activate such representations is intact in Korsakoff's syndrome and that exposure to stimuli can alter the probability of response for these patients.

Shimamura and Squire (1984) studied the relationship between paired-associates learning and priming in alcoholic Korsakoff's subjects. These authors cited previous literature noting that Korsakoff's patients could demonstrate normal learning for related associate pairs. One purpose of their study was to ascertain if patients' learning for related paired associates might be possible through priming effects. In their first experiment, the authors demonstrated that Korsakoff's patients had impaired learning on unrelated paired associates, even though they had normal priming for the first words in the associate pairs. In the second experiment, subjects were given explicit instructions to learn paired associates during their presentation. The Korsakoff's patients showed an ability to learn related paired associates, though they performed below alcoholic controls on this task. However, amnesics' performance fell to a chance level by 2 hours after learning while performance of normals remained significantly above chance levels. The forgetting of associate pairs by amnesics followed the same time course as stem-completion priming, indicating that recall of related associates might indeed be dependent upon the type of memory used in priming tasks (i.e., implicit memory or activation). In a third experiment, subjects were asked to rate how highly related paired associates were. The associates had been chosen because of their high relatedness. Korsakoff's patients produced as many associates as controls when asked to free associate to the first word of the pair. In a fourth and final experiment, the subjects were asked to rate words in accordance with how much they liked the words. They were then asked to free associate to words that were related to words from the original list. Korsakoff's patients showed a performance roughly equal to that of controls immediately after presentation, and they showed a drop to chance levels of performance 2 hours later. As expected, when asked to recall the word list, amnesic performance was inferior to that of controls. The latter two experiments indicate that semantic priming for alcoholic Korsakoff's subjects was not limited to the stem-completion paradigm. Results also indicated that superiority of controls' performance on the paired associates task was dependent on explicit-memory instructions.

Cermak, Talbot, Chandler, and Wolbarst (1985) explored the proposition that perceptual priming in patients with alcoholic Korsakoff's syndrome is dependent upon a preexisting representation in semantic memory. They presented subjects with 10-word lists, then performed recognition-memory or perceptual-identification tasks. The perceptual-identification task involved presenting words that were on the lists and words that were not on the lists for 35 milliseconds. Each time the subject failed to identify a word, it was presented again for 10 milliseconds longer until correct identification occurred. When there was no delay before recognition memory, the Korsakoff's patients showed an equivalent performance to alcoholic controls. But, when the perceptual identification was interposed between list exposure and the recognition trial, the Korsakoff's subjects performed significantly more poorly than alcoholic controls. Both immediately and after a delay, Korsakoff's patients and controls took less time to identify list as opposed to nonlist words. When nonwords were used for the perceptual-identification task in a second experiment, alcoholic controls demonstrated facilitation for previously presented nonwords as opposed to nonwords that had not been presented. Korsakoff's patients did not show such a facilitation effect for nonwords. For this latter task, the authors concluded that perceptual identification could be primed in controls based upon their episodic memory for nonwords, but Korsakoff's patients could not rely upon their defective episodic memory for priming with nonwords. On the other hand, a preexisting representation of actual words in semantic memory was enough to produce priming of perceptual identification.

To summarize: Alcoholic Korsakoff's patients demonstrate priming equal to that of controls for both word-stem-completion and paired-associates tasks. It is of some interest that Roediger (1990) distinguished between perceptually driven and semantically driven tasks. He noted that most priming experiments have involved perceptual similarities; for example, word-stem completion involves visual and phonological characteristics of the primed words but does not depend upon the semantic aspects. On the other hand, the type of priming task using free association and paired associates depends more on semantic properties of the words to be primed. According to Roediger, results of priming tasks may depend on whether they are perceptually or semantically driven, and may not need to invoke the explanation of separate explicit and implicit memory systems. In other words, since most priming experiments have been perceptually driven, the characteristics of perceptually driven memory tasks versus semantically driven tasks may account for differences in priming versus recall or recognition experiments without resorting to implicit- versus explicit-memory systems. If this were true, and if one takes into account difficulties in semantic processing for alcoholic Korsakoff's syndrome patients, one might predict that Korsakoff's subjects would have difficulty with a semantically driven task involving free association and paired associates in priming. Thus, the results of Shimamura and Squire (1984) are important because they indicate that semantically driven and perceptually driven priming not only produce similar results for this population, but also produce similar patterns of temporal decay. This would indicate that some forms of implicit memory are independent of the memory system that is so severely damaged in alcoholic Korsakoff's syndrome.

Procedural Memory

Attempts have also been made to explore procedural memory after the onset of alcoholic Korsakoff's syndrome. For the procedural-memory studies discussed below, results have been most consistent on tasks involving motor skills, where patients with alcoholic Korsakoff's syndrome generally demonstrate relatively intact learning. For example, Talland (1965) included several examples of skill learning in his studies of alcoholic Korsakoff's syndrome. In a task where subjects were required to move beads with a plunger apparatus, both Korsakoff's subjects and controls showed improvement across trials, though the Korsakoff's subjects were slower than controls. On a task in which the beads had to be moved with crossed forceps, neither group showed consistent improvement across trials. On tests of procedural learning that do not involve a motor-skill component (map puzzle, maze), the Korsakoff's patients had greater difficulty learning the task and showed less retention of the skill than normals. These results raise the question whether retained procedural learning in Korsakoff's patients can be applied to all procedural-learning tasks, or only to motor skills. Yet, it should be remembered that on the map and maze learning, Talland made no attempt to equate groups for initial performance or task difficulty. Further, it was not clear to what extent subjects may have depended upon explicit verbal learning of task demands for performance. Talland concluded that his amnesic patients showed motor-skill learning, but they had difficulty on tasks where they had to retain maps or plans of action.

This latter point was also made by Cermak, Lewis, Butters, and Goodglass (1973). They gave a pursuit-rotor and a finger-maze task to patients with alcoholic Korsakoff's syndrome, alcoholics, and normal controls. The pursuit-rotor task required subjects to keep a stylus on a small metal target on a turntable that rotated at 45 rpm. The finger mazes had 4- and 6-choice points where subjects had to make either a right or a left turn. All groups made equal improvement on the pursuit-rotor task, indicating equivalent motor-skill learning. However, the Korsakoff's patients performed significantly worse than the other two groups on the finger mazes. The authors concluded that the comparatively poor performance on the finger mazes by the amnesic patients was probably the product of covert verbal learning on the task by nonamnesic subjects.

Cohen and Squire (1980) had Korsakoff's patients learn to read triads of words presented as a mirror image. Five blocks of trials were given on each of 4 days; within each block of trials, half of the triads were new, and half of the triads were repeated. The amnesic subjects acquired the mirror-reading skill at the same rate as normal controls, as measured by their performance on the new triads. However, the amnesics were inferior at reading the repeated-word triads, suggesting that they benefited less from memory of the repeated words. The authors implied that the difference in pattern of performance on the new words and the repeated words reflected that alcoholic Korsakoff's patients had normal procedural learning since they learned to mirror read, but impaired declarative learning since they did not profit to a normal degree from repeated triads.

Martone et al. (1984) replicated Cohen and Squire's findings that alcoholic Korsakoff's patients learned mirror reading at a normal rate, but failed to benefit from repetition as much as normals. Further, the patients with Korsakoff's syndrome were inferior in identifying words that had been used in the mirror-reading task in a recognition-memory paradigm. In contrast, patients with Huntington's disease did not acquire the mirror-reading skill at a normal rate, though they did demonstrate improvement in reading repeated words and recognition memory comparable to that of normal controls. The authors cited this as proof that the procedural and declarative learning could be dissociated in the two patient populations.

In summary: Patients with alcoholic Korsakoff's syndrome do demonstrate an ability to learn motor skills and mirror reading. Thus, learning of these skills represents a preserved type of memory in alcoholic Korsakoff's syndrome in addition to priming. On procedural learning tasks that may be mediated by explicit memory, however, these amnesic patients were impaired relative to controls. There is some evidence that patients with Huntington's disease do show impaired motor skill and procedural learning. This fact will be discussed further in Chapter 7.

Temporal Gradient in Retrograde Amnesia

Another important facet in the memory disturbance of patients with alcoholic Korsakoff's syndrome is patterns of remote-memory impairment, that is, impairment of memories from times prior to the onset of the amnesic disorder. In general, such memory disorders are referred to as "retrograde amnesia." This phenomenon can be noted in other neurological disorders, such as head injury, in addition to Korsakoff's syndrome. Clinical experience has indicated that patients with alcoholic amnesic disorders have greater difficulty in remote memory the closer it gets to the onset of the disorder (Selzer & Benson, 1974). Some investigators have sought to empirically validate this clinical observation by testing remote memories common to the entire subject pool across decades. Examples of such remote memories would be famous faces, public events, or famous voices. Figure 6-3 shows a temporal gradient on a hypothetical task for three fictional groups. The task has been equated for difficulty across decades. Group N shows normal memory across decades; Group A shows a temporal gradient with more severe loss for recent memories; and Group C shows equal losses across decades.

Selzer and Benson (1974) were among the first to formally assess temporal gradient in retrograde amnesia for alcoholic Korsakoff's syndrome. They administered a multiple-choice, remote-memory questionnaire to patients with alcoholic Korsakoff's syndrome and controls. Patients had their onset within 4 years of the study. Compared to controls, amnesic patients indeed demonstrated greater difficulty on the more recent items. There were significantly fewer correct responses to questions about events in the most recent 15 years than to questions about events in the 15 years after age 10 for

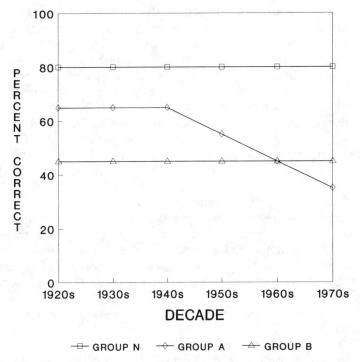

Figure 6-3. A hypothetical retrograde-amnesia experiment. Difficulty of items has been equated across decades. Group N demonstrates a normal performance across decades. Group A never shows a normal performance but does particularly poorly on material from more recent decades. In other words, Group A's performance demonstrates a temporal gradient. Group B performs at uniformly low levels across decades.

Korsakoff's subjects. Controls showed a roughly equal number of correct responses for the two periods.

Albert, Butters, and Levin (1979) devised tasks to ensure that the temporal gradient exhibited by patients with alcoholic Korsakoff's syndrome was not a function of varying difficulty of items across decades. Within each decade, they had easy and difficult items (as verified by a pilot study) for each of three tasks. The first task was recalling names for pictures of famous faces; the second was recall of public events; the third was recognition of public events. When compared to neurologically intact subjects, patients with Korsakoff's syndrome demonstrated a greater difficulty with recent than more remote information for easy faces, difficult faces, easy-event recall, difficult-event recall, and difficult-event recognition. They only failed to demonstrate a temporal gradient for easy-event recognition.

Additionally, Albert et al. found that Korsakoff's patients had significantly greater difficulty recognizing older versus younger pictures of famous persons when compared to controls. The authors concluded that temporal gradients were genuine and not a function of greater difficulty on more recent items. Finally, unlike anterograde-memory problems, phonemic versus semantic cues did not differentially affect the recall of Korsakoff's versus control subjects. Based on the latter finding, the authors concluded that difficulties in recall from remote memory did not parallel difficulties in recall for the anterograde compartment, since Korsakoff's patients had been shown to favor phonemic over semantic cues in anterograde-memory tasks (e.g., Cermak et al., 1974).

Meudell, Northen, Snowden, and Neary (1980) extended findings of retrograde amnesia for famous faces to retrograde amnesia for famous voices. Alcoholic Korsakoff's subjects were significantly worse at identifying famous voices, and the deficit was worse in comparison to controls for more recent decades. Since the Korsakoff's subjects did not differentially improve in comparison to controls when cues were given or when a recognition format was used, the authors reasoned that the retrograde defect for amnesic subjects was not simply a retrieval deficit.

Albert, Butters, and Brandt (1981) found that Huntington's disease patients and alcoholic Korsakoff's patients both demonstrated significant retrograde amnesia for events and faces. However, only patients with alcoholic Korsakoff's syndrome had a temporal gradient in retrograde amnesia for the faces and events. This study showed that the temporal gradient demonstrated by patients with alcoholic Korsakoff's syndrome is not demonstrated by all patients with retrograde memory losses.

Zola-Morgan, Cohen, and Squire (1983) asked alcoholic Korsakoff's patients and alcoholic controls to recall personal episodes related to specific words given them by the examiner. Without being prompted, Korsakoff's subjects were able to recall fewer episodes than controls. However, if subjects were given examples or prompted to be more specific when difficulty responding arose, there was no difference between groups. Korsakoff's patients drew significantly more experiences from more remote time periods, similar to their responses on famous faces or famous events tasks. Thus, there may be some temporal gradient for remote memory of personal episodes.

Shimamura and Squire (1986) studied the relationship between performance on nine anterograde memory measures and three remote-memory measures in a pool of alcoholic Korsakoff's patients tested over the years. Anterograde-memory deficit was correlated with remote-memory deficit only for the most recent decades. The authors concluded that a single explanation for remote- and anterograde-memory deficits could not be applied in these patients. A common deficit (e.g., retrieval difficulty) would demand equal correlations between anterograde and remote memories for all decades.

Butters and Stuss (1989) gave two possible explanations for the temporal gradient in remote memory for alcoholic Korsakoff's syndrome. The first is that chronic alcoholism prior to the onset of amnesic disturbance causes memories to be stored in a partial or degraded fashion. These degraded "engrams" are then more subject to disruption by the subsequent brain damage that causes the amnesic syndrome. The second explanation was originally put forth by Cermak (1984). He noted that newly acquired knowledge may be episodic in nature, that is, it maintains its temporal and spatial contexts. As time passes and the knowledge is rehearsed and connected to other new and old information, the knowledge becomes independent of temporal and spatial contexts. In other words, it becomes a part of semantic (as opposed to episodic) memory. According to this viewpoint, the more attached knowledge is to a temporal and spatial context, the more vulnerable it is to disruption in amnesic syndromes.

Butters and Stuss (1989) reviewed evidence that alcoholics without amnesic syndromes do demonstrate some decrement in more recent memories, but only for the most difficult items (Albert et al., 1980; Cohen & Squire, 1981). However, they felt that such deficits alone were not enough to account for the more severe temporal gradients seen in the remote memories of patients with alcoholic Korsakoff's syndrome. Ultimately, Butters and Stuss considered the episodic versus semantic explanation of Cermak (1984) to be the most probable cause of temporal gradients in amnesic syndromes. Squire, Haist, and Shimamura (1989) showed that patients with amnesic syndrome of presumed temporal lobe origin show temporal gradients in remote memory similar to those shown by patients with alcoholic Korsakoff's syndrome. These data also favor the hypothesis that memories make a transition from episodic to semantic storage, and that episodic storage is more prone to disruption. On the other hand, according to the data of Zola-Morgan et al. (1983), remote memory for personal episodes are also better remembered by Korsakoff's patients in the more distant past. It would be hard to argue that memory for personal episodes eventually falls into semantic memory.

In summary: Temporal gradient in the remote memory of patients with alcoholic Korsakoff's syndrome is a robust finding. Alcoholics also may show some temporal gradient in retrograde memory, but it does not appear great enough to account for the magnitude of deficit seen in alcoholic Korsakoff's syndrome. Although temporal gradients are not found in Huntington's disease, there is some evidence that bitemporal amnesics also show a temporal gradient. Some believe that more recent memories are more disrupted in Korsakoff's syndrome because they are episodic, and episodic memories are more susceptible to disruption. The fact that alcoholic Korsakoff's patients demonstrate temporal gradients in personal episodic memories suggests that this episodic-memory explanation cannot account for temporal gradients.

Conclusions Regarding Alcoholic Korsakoff's Syndrome

Taking this literature review into account, several conclusions can be drawn about memory dysfunction in alcoholic Korsakoff's syndrome: (1) Retention difficulties at longer intervals in Peterson and Peterson paradigms most likely reflect long-term not short-term memory deficits. (2) If longer exposure intervals are used, patients with alcoholic Korsakoff's syndrome can retain at least some types of information as long-term memories. It is unclear just how true this might be for patients with bitemporal amnesias. (3) Patients with alcoholic Korsakoff's syndrome are susceptible to proactive interference. (4) If given·exposure intervals adequate for normal memory, these subjects tend spontaneously not to use semantic information as much as normal controls. If given proper instructions, however, Korsakoff's subjects sometimes can make use of semantic information. (5) Implicit memory, as measured by some types of priming tasks, is intact in alcoholic Korsakoff's syndrome. (6) In these patients, remote memory is worse in the few years just prior to onset of the syndrome; that is, they show a temporal gradient for retrograde-memory loss. This pattern applies to personal episodic as well as to more generic memories. (7) Several cautions must be taken into account in applying alcoholic Korsakoff's data to diencephalic memory functions. For example, difficulty processing semantic information may be more related to frontal than to diencephalic dysfunction. Or the repeated testing of the same subject pools leads to questions about the generalizability of data. Thus, it would be desirable to confirm patterns of deficit from alcoholic Korsakoff's studies in investigations involving other types of diencephalic amnesia.

Memory Processes after Medial Thalamic Infarction and Other Lesions

Research regarding memory processes after diencephalic lesions from infarcts, hemorrhages, or stab wound cannot be as easily grouped by issues as research with alcoholic Korsakoff's syndrome. Although memory-process research with such Korsakoff's patients has provided a starting point for studies of discrete thalamic lesion, the experimental paradigms from the Korsakoff's literature have just begun to be applied to studies of these other lesions. These latter studies have involved single cases, or, at most, a handful of subjects, and different studies have chosen to focus on different aspects of memory. For these reasons, the best way to present the data is to review details of the individual studies separately, with the exception of a couple of general issues. Thus, I will briefly cover the general issues of lateralization and confabulation, and then proceed to discuss individual cases.

In spite of the fact that paramedian thalamic infarctions are often bilateral, unilateral infarcts are not uncommon. The existence of unilateral paramedian thalamic infarcts offers us an opportunity not available in the study of alcoholic Korsakoff's syndrome: to observe whether lateralization of cerebral functions extends to memory at the level of the diencephalon. Speedie and Heilman (1982) noted greater verbal- than nonverbal-memory deficits in their case of left dorsal medial thalamic infarction. Further, these authors (Speedie & Heilman, 1983) later found a case of right medial thalamic infarction in which visual memory showed greater impairment than verbal memory. The case of Goldenberg et al. (1983) was a relatively small left thalamic lesion occupying portions of several structures. Like the case of Speedie and Heilman (1982), verbal memory was affected in the presence of a relatively intact visual memory. The case of N.A. (e.g., Cohen & Squire, 1980; Squire, 1981; Squire et al., 1989; Squire & Moore, 1979) also confirms that greater left than right diencephalic damage can cause more impairment of verbal than nonverbal memory. In the more chronic stages, the case of Mori et al. (1986), with left thalamic infarction, showed only minimal language deficits, but significant verbal-memory deficits continued. Visuospatial memory was unimpaired in Mori's case, similar to the case of Speedie and Heilman (1982). It should be noted that Stuss et al. (1988) confirmed greater visual-memory deficits with right paramedian thalamic infarction and greater verbal-memory deficits in left paramedian thalamic infarction. The case of Brown et al. (1989) had a hemorrhagic lesion in the left dorsal medial and anterior nuclei. Verbal memory was severely affected, but there was also a lesser impairment of visual memory. To summarize, lateralization of verbal- versus visual-memory functions extends in most cases to the level of the medial thalamus. This fact would indicate that it is the ipsilateral influences of the medial thalamus that are important in memory.

Regarding the issue of confabulation, a few studies of vascular lesion of the medial thalamus have contributed observations. Choi et al. (1983) found confabulation acutely in one of three cases of thalamic hemorrhage. Gentilini et al. (1987) found confabulation acutely in three of six patients with memory impairment resulting from paramedian thalamic infarction. Stuss et al. (1988) noted acute confabulation in all three of their cases of paramedian thalamic infarction. However, a milder form of the confabulation persisted only in the case of bilateral paramedian infarction with the most severe memory impairment. By way of comparison, it is of interest that confabulation was once considered a hallmark of alcoholic Korsakoff's syndrome. However, Talland (1965) covered this topic at some length. In the more acute phases of Wernicke's encephalopathy, most, if not all, patients confabulate. When Wernicke's encephalopathy evolves into the more chronic Korsakoff's syndrome, confabulation disappears in many patients and becomes more circumscribed in most others. Confabulation during the more acute phase in Wernicke's encephalopathy may be related to factors other than diencephalic dysfunction. On the other hand, data of Choi et al. (1983) and especially the infarct cases of Gentilini et al. (1987) and Stuss et al. (1988) indicate that there may be a relationship between confabulation and diencephalic dysfunction in some patients. Talland (1965) indicated that acute confabulation in Wernicke's encephalopathy drew upon patients' recollection of actual experience, but they reconstructed and recombined the content of actual experience in such a way as to produce distorted memory. To the extent confabulation reflects such a process, it may be reflective of impairment in reconstruction of memories.

Turning to the individual studies, as noted above, many of the paradigms used in alcoholic Korsakoff's syndrome have recently been applied to cases of vascular lesion. This includes tasks normally conceptualized as reflecting frontal lobe functioning. However, there has been a great deal of inconsistency regarding which of the many paradigms have been used. The most consistent findings indicate that patients with vascular lesions in the medial thalamus do not demonstrate procedural-learning difficulty and frequently do show failure to release from proactive interference.

Speedie and Heilman (1982) found greater verbal- than nonverbal-memory deficits in their case of left dorsal medial thalamic infarction. They also noted impairment of frontal lobe functions on the Wisconsin Card Sorting Test, serial hand positions, and arrangement of words into sentences. Although the sudden onset of memory problems ties them to the infarction, the same cannot be said of the frontal lobe deficits. Frontal lobe dysfunction on similar tasks is not only common to patients with alcoholic Korsakoff's syndrome (e.g., Oscar-Berman, 1973), it is also common in schizophrenia (Weinberger, Berman, & Zec, 1986) of which the patient had a history. However, Speedie and Heilman (1983) found a case of right medial thalamic infarction in which visual memory showed greater impairment than verbal memory. This case, too, showed significant frontal lobe impairments on a number of tasks. Although a stronger case can be made for infarction accounting for frontal lobe impairment in this second case of Speedie and Heilman, it must be noted that this patient had a mild depression which predated the memory dysfunction and thalamic infarction.

The case of Goldenberg et al. (1983) was a relatively small left thalamic lesion occupying portions of several structures. His verbal memory was affected in the presence of a relatively intact visual memory. Because there were defects in acquiring new verbal memories, in naming, and in remote verbal knowledge, the authors concluded that a retrieval deficit was the only explanation that could account for all the dysfunctions.

The case of N.A. (e.g., Cohen & Squire, 1980; Squire, 1981; Squire et al., 1989; Squire & Moore, 1979) also had greater verbal- than nonverbal-memory impairment. With respect to verbal memory, there were some similarities between N.A. and patients with alcoholic Korsakoff's syndrome. Neither N.A. nor patients with alcoholic Korsakoff's syndrome demonstrated an abnormal rate of forgetting like patients with presumed temporal lobe dysfunction (Squire, 1981). Also like patients with alcoholic Korsakoff's syndrome, N.A. could learn a mirror-reading task at a normal rate, but he failed to demonstrate a normal benefit from repeated word triads (Cohen & Squire, 1980). Thus, there are indications of preserved procedural learning for patient N.A. in spite of deficits in verbal memory.

The performance of N.A. has also differed from patients with alcoholic Korsakoff's syndrome in some important aspects. In spite of the fact that failure to release from proactive interference and deficits in judgment of temporal order were shown in alcoholic Korsakoff's syndrome, N.A. has demonstrated neither of these problems (Squire, 1982). Further, N.A. did not demonstrate an inability to profit from imposed semantic processing like alcoholic Korsakoff's patients (Wetzel & Squire, 1980). It is worth noting that frontal lobe functions (e.g., card sorting and word fluency) and intellectual functions were also normal to excellent for N.A. Although intellectual functioning is within normal limits for alcoholic Korsakoff's patients, performance on frontal lobe tests is not (e.g., Oscar-Berman, 1973). On the basis of this data, Squire (1982) concluded that failure to release from proactive interference and deficits in temporal-order judgment were not essential components of diencephalic amnesia, but a reflection of frontal dysfunction in patients with alcoholic Korsakoff's syndrome. Since N.A. did not demonstrate frontal dysfunction, he did not have a failure to release from proactive interference or defects in temporal-order judgment.

Another difference between N.A. and alcoholic Korsakoff's patients involves remote memory. On tests of remote memory, N.A. exhibited no retrograde amnesia on six of eight tests, though he did show some evidence of retrograde memory deficit on recall of public events and a test of autobiographical memory (Squire et al., 1989). Thus, the degree to which retrograde amnesia is a function of diencephalic lesion may also be called into question. It could be related to additional frontal damage in alcoholic Korsakoff's syndrome, or perhaps bilaterally symmetric diencephalic damage may be required to produce severe retrograde memory deficits. Swanson and Schmidley (1985) noted a variable retrograde amnesia in their case of anterograde amnesia accompanying bilateral medial thalamic infarction. The patient had grossly recovered by 3 months postonset.

It should be stated at this point that Butters and Stuss (1989), Speedie and Heilman (1983), and Crosson (1986) have noted with respect to alcoholic Korsakoff's syndrome that damage to the dorsal medial thalamus may impact frontal functioning because of the extensive interconnection of the frontal lobes and the dorsal medial thalamus. Indeed, some of the frontal lobe atrophy noted in alcoholic Korsakoff's syndrome (Shimamura et al., 1988) could even reflect transneuronal retrograde degeneration secondary to damage to the dorsal medial thalamus. To the extent these factors are related, Butters and Stuss maintained that "frontal" symptoms should be considered as integral to diencephalic amnesia, not as ancillary.

Cramon et al. (1986) found normal digit span and short-term retention of verbal stimuli in their cases of memory deficit after thalamic infarction. One of their four patients was said to have experienced an increased rate of forgetting. All four patients were noted to be impaired in "verbal-learning" tasks.

In the more chronic phase, Mori and colleagues' (1986) case of left thalamic infarction showed minimal language deficits but significant problems in verbal memory. As noted above, visuospatial memory was unimpaired. Concerning verbal memory, immediate recall was impaired, but there was a significant loss of information to delayed recall. Further, recognition memory was quite impaired. Given the impaired problem solving in cases of alcoholic Korsakoff's syndrome, it is of interest that this patient's performance on the Wisconsin Card Sorting Test was apparently unimpaired.

The case of Winocur et al. (1984) was notable for its extensive testing of certain aspects of the patient's anterograde-memory deficits. On memory for consonant trigrams (Peterson & Peterson, 1959) with distraction-filled intervals of various length (0, 3, 6, 9, 18 seconds), the patient's (B.Y.) performance depended upon the length of exposure of the stimulus. With a 2-second exposure, B.Y. showed increasing deficits compared to controls with increasing length of delay. However, with a 4-second exposure, he showed significant impairment only after the 18-second delay. The authors suggested that B.Y.'s initial processing of information had been negatively affected, and that longer exposure time allowed him to compensate to some degree for this encoding deficit.

Tests of long-term memory confirmed that B.Y.'s memory for verbal and nonverbal information was more impaired compared to controls after a delay than after immediate recall; however, one should note that delayed recall in the case of verbal memory took place after a 30-second, distraction-filled interval, while delayed recall of visual material took place after 40 minutes. B.Y.'s immediate verbal-recall performance showed primacy and recency effects like controls, but unlike controls, his delayed recall performance did not demonstrate such effects.

Compared to controls, B.Y.'s performance on forced-choice recognition of words and faces was impaired, but probably better than that of patients with amnesic syndrome or alcoholic Korsakoff's syndrome. Nonetheless, on recall tasks where partial cueing was provided, B.Y.'s performance was worse than that of previously tested alcoholic Korsakoff's syndrome and other amnesic patients.

Regarding interference, B.Y. did show a failure to release from proactive interference, similar to previously reported studies of alcoholic Korsakoff's syndrome (e.g., Squire, 1982). Yet he did not show the high degree of prior list intrusions characteristic of patients with alcoholic Korsakoff's syndrome on a task (negative transfer) that should have elicited such errors. The authors offered two possible explanations for the latter difference between B.Y. and previously tested Korsakoff's syndrome patients. The first is that B.Y. experienced a lesser degree of brain damage; the second is that he did not have damage to significant structures that may have been affected in the Korsakoff's subjects.

Winocur et al. (1984) concluded that B.Y.'s deficit most likely reflected incomplete representations of experienced events during initial processing. As evidence, they cited his improvement with increased length of presentation, his drop in performance after a delay, and the fact that his less-impaired immediate recall of lists was primarily due to a recency effect. It appears that these results do represent what is called in this text an incomplete registration of material in long-term memory. The authors themselves had difficulty excluding deficits in consolidation. This confusion arises from interpretation of the Peterson-Peterson paradigm as possibly reflecting problems in consolidation and a failure to measure loss of information at an interval longer than 24 hours. Thus, as consolidation is understood in this volume, the authors cannot make any inferences about it based upon their data.

Nichelli et al. (1988) performed an extensive neuropsychological evaluation of their patient with thalamic amnesia. They found profound impairment of long-term verbal memory on several tests and severe impairment of visual supraspan memory. This was consistent with the clinical amnesia. Included in their explicit verbal memory tests were the findings that there was a loss of primacy effects in list recall and impaired verbal recognition, suggesting that initial storage of verbal material was limited. Regarding implicit and procedural memory, several results were of interest. The patient learned a mirror-tracing task, but the learning seemed to be specific to the figure on which he was trained. He was able to learn and apply a simple mathematical rule, even though he had no idea he had learned it. The patient also was able to learn a mirror-reading task. Unlike the findings of Cohen and Squire (1980) and Martone et al. (1984); however, Nichelli and colleagues found that their patient showed normal improvement with repeated words. Results with nonrepeated words were more difficult to interpret. The authors attributed the discrepancy between their patient and Korsakoff's subjects' inability to improve on repeated word triads to the fact that they only used one word in mirror reading while previous studies had used triads. The authors believed that in the latter technique the first word gave normal subjects cues to the second and third words, allowing them to improve their times on repeated triads more than the amnesic patients. Thus, the authors confirmed evidence of intact implicit and procedural memory with their case of thalamic amnesia; however, they challenged the idea that intact procedural memory could be applied to thalamic amnesia in a blanket fashion. They suggested that some effects might be task-specific. It is unfortunate that methodological differences prevent strict comparisons to previous studies of alcoholic Korsakoff's syndrome.

Stuss et al. (1988) also performed a number of memory tests on their three cases of paramedian thalamic infarction. In one task, they gave patients 12-word lists in which words were drawn from three different semantic categories. Recall was done either in an unconstrained free recall or using category cues. Semantic categories were called to the patients' attention on some trials but not on others. In general, patients' performance deteriorated with category cues at recall, but calling attention to the semantic categories during initial learning aided later recall for the two patients with left thalamic lesions. These data would support an encoding-deficit hypothesis of diencephalic amnesia. Retrograde amnesia was tested and confirmed in the most severe case of memory deficit, but there was no indication of temporal gradient.

The case of Brown et al. (1989) had a hemorrhagic lesion in the left dorsal medial and anterior nuclei. Verbal memory was severely affected, but there was some impairment of visual memory as well. The patient did quite well on a card-sorting test thought to measure frontal functions. Results of the Selective Reminding Test showed the patient to have a tendency to overrely on short-term memory. His recall of consonant trigrams in a Peterson and Peterson task was actually better than that of controls, and he showed no buildup of proactive interference. The authors concluded that short-term memory was intact in spite of the significant impairment in acquiring new long-term memory.

In addition to making a contribution to the anatomy of diencephalic amnesias, Graff-Radford et al. (1990) have contributed to our understanding of diencephalic lesions and memory processes. It will be recalled that two of their four patients with infarctions in the territory of the paramedian thalamic artery had amnesic syndromes. Those two patients had lesions that probably included both the mammillothalamic tract and the ventral amygdalofugal pathway. Both patients scored in the extremely impaired range on a number of standard memory tests including the Rey Auditory Verbal Learning Test, Wechsler Memory Scale paragraphs and verbal paired associates, the Benton Visual Retention Test, and the Rey-Osterreith Complex Figure (30-minute delay). There were some similarities to patients with alcoholic Korsakoff's syndrome. Both of Graff-Radford and colleagues' patients demonstrated a failure to release from proactive interference. It has been argued that this latter problem is a sign that patients are failing to process the semantic characteristics of the stimuli (Cermak et al., 1974). It has been further argued that this problem is due to frontal lobe damage in patients with alcoholic Korsakoff's syndrome (Squire, 1982), but neither of Graff-Radford and colleagues' patients demonstrated structural changes in the frontal lobes. On the other hand, both patients showed some impairment on card-sorting and verbal-fluency tasks thought to tap frontal lobe functions. These latter findings are similar to those of Speedie and Heilman (1982, 1983) and would be consistent with their suggestion that the prolific connections of the dorsal medial thalamus with frontal lobe structures accounts for frontal lobe dysfunction in cases of medial thalamic lesion. Also like alcoholic Korsakoff's patients, one patient showed a temporal gradient in her ability to identify famous events. But she showed the temporal gradient on only one of five tasks. The second amnesic was too young for the usual tests of remote memory to be valuable, but he did well on a personal-history questionnaire.

Some similarities to patients with basal forebrain lesions were also noted. The first case had difficulty in temporal orientation and temporal sequencing of remote events. Her recall was greatly aided by cueing in remote-memory tasks. The second patient whose memory was less impaired did well on a personal-history questionnaire, and was too young for standard remote-memory tests to be of use. These potential similarities between basal forebrain and thalamic amnesic syndromes require further investigation. In light of the anatomic pathways running through both the basal forebrain and the thalamus, the similarities and differences between cases with these types of amnesic syndromes is an important issue. It will be discussed further in the next chapter.

Mennemeier et al. (1990) have made an important contribution to the study of diencephalic functions. They studied memory processes in a case, B.E., whose lesion involved primarily the centre median-parafascicular complex. On standardized tests of verbal memory, B.E. demonstrated mild memory impairment. The uniqueness of this case is the attempt to unravel the nature of memory impairment in a case of less-than-severely-disturbed memory. Others (e.g., Cramon et al., 1985; Graff-Radford et al., 1990) have not considered such cases worthy of extended discussion, but Mennemeier and colleagues have demonstrated that there is much to be learned from examination of these cases.

Before discussing the formal memory studies in B.E., it is worth noting that she complained of memory and concentration problems. She had difficulty remembering conversations, material she read, and dates. Perhaps more importantly, she complained of an inability to perform simultaneous activities which she described herself as previously able to accomplish. This problem was one factor in her inability to work.

Her performance on two tasks led the authors to conclude that B.E. had retained her ability to process semantic information. First, B.E. demonstrated a normal release from proactive interference, and second, she showed superior memory for semantically processed words over words processed for physical or phonological characteristics. In fact, although the patient showed performance equal to that of controls for semantically processed words, her performance was inferior to controls for words processed by orthographic characteristics. Further, her performance on the longer distraction-filled delays of a Peterson and Peterson task was also significantly below that of normals. On the Selective Reminding Test (Buschke, 1973), the patient demonstrated an overreliance on short-term memory, reduced long-term storage, and a lack of consistency in retrieval from long-term memory. It is also worth noting that the authors described the patient as showing a normal rate of forgetting.

B.E.'s greater difficulty with orthographically processed material may have indicated difficulty with processing strategies more typically associated with short-term memory, while she could process information in a way (semantically) more frequently associated with long-term memory (see Baddeley, 1990). Another way of saying this, according to Mennemeier et al., is that the patient's ability to store information in long-term memory was impaired when she was required to use a less robust method for encoding information into long-term memory. The authors pointed out that difficulty on the Peterson and Peterson paradigm is probably due to interference from stimuli presented on previous trials. Therefore, B.E.'s deficit on this task indicated susceptibility when multiple stimuli compete for processing resources. (This interpretation was also consistent with her self-reported difficulties.) Finally, her performance on the Selective Reminding Test suggested difficulty transferring information into long-term storage. The authors concluded that the pattern of deficit when stimuli compete for processing resources and of impairment when required to use a less robust means of encoding were consistent with an attentional deficit. It should be pointed out that their inferences were based primarily on memory tasks at this point, though attempts are being made to independently confirm an attentional deficit.

In summary: Cases of vascular lesion and stab wound of the medial thalamus have contributed to our knowledge of how the diencephalon participates in memory processes. Lateralization of verbal- versus visual-memory functions at the level of the medial thalamus suggests that the anterior and dorsal medial thalamic nuclei are part of a specialized intrahemispheric memory system. Like the data from alcoholic Korsakoff's syndrome, studies of vascular lesion and stab wound indicate that the diencephalon plays a role in initial registration of material into long-term memory (Brown et al., 1989; Nichelli et al., 1988; Squire, 1982; Winocur et al., 1984). Stuss et al. (1988) provided some data that medial thalamic lesions also cause problems with encoding information into long-term memory. However, certain indicators of impaired semantic processing, such as failure to release from proactive interference, may be related to frontal lobe dysfunction (Graff-Radford et al., 1990; Squire, 1982). Carrying the inference one step further, these results suggest that semantic processing deficits may not be a necessary component of diencephalic memory disturbance (Squire, 1982). Since impairment on "frontal lobe" tasks can be found in some cases of dorsal medial thalamic lesion without frontal lobe damage (Graff-Radford et al., 1990; Speedie & Heilman, 1983), it may be concluded that the deficits in "frontal lobe" tasks in such cases are related to the connections of the dorsal medial thalamus with the frontal lobes. Continued careful application of paradigms developed in alcoholic Korsakoff's syndrome research to cases of vascular lesion in the diencephalon should help us to refine our understanding of how diencephalic structures participate in memory.

Conclusions

Several conclusions can be drawn about the role of diencephalic structures in memory. Regarding the structures involved, the mammillary bodies, the dorsal medial thalamus, and the anterior thalamic nuclei are the primary diencephalic candidates for involvement. There is some possibility that the midline thalamic nuclei are important as well. There are virtually no studies showing that exclusive involvement of one of these structures leads to the profound memory disturbance found in amnesic syndromes. Even animal analog studies that purport to demonstrate the exclusive importance of one of these structures for memory have shown damage to other structures. There is some evidence that the ventral lateral nucleus (Ojemann, 1977) and intralaminar nuclei (Mennemeier et al., 1990) may be important for attentional processes supporting memory.

Cramon (1989) has emphasized that one must not only consider these nuclei, but the white matter pathways leading into and away from them. Thus, the connections from the hippocampus to the anterior thalamic nuclei and the mammillary bodies are probably important for the communication between the hippocampus and these structures in memory processes. The mammillothalamic tract links the mammillary bodies to the anterior thalamic nuclei. The ventral amygdalofugal pathway supplies fibers from the amygdala to the dorsal medial thalamus and may also play a role in memory.

Thus, in agreement with Mishkin's (1982) model, there are two systems originating in the temporal lobes that play a role in memory. The first corresponds to Papez circuit. It originates with the hippocampal formation and includes the fornix, the mammillary bodies, the mammillothalamic tract, and the anterior thalamic nuclei. The second system originates with the amygdala and includes the ventral amygdalofugal pathway and the dorsal medial thalamus. Profound memory impairment (amnesic syndrome) is most likely to occur when both of these systems have been involved on a bilateral basis. This statement can be considered to be the prevailing thought concerning the neuroanatomy of diencephalic memory deficit. However, it is likely that this view, too, will be refined as research progresses.

It is also important to consider how diencephalic structures participate in memory. Studies of memory process in alcoholic Korsakoff's syndrome and after other diencephalic lesion provide our main window concerning these processes. Table 6-1 compares disturbances of memory processes in patients with alcoholic Korsakoff's syndrome, patients with other medial thalamic lesions, and patient N.A. A comparison of findings provides some insights regarding diencephalic participation in memory.

Perhaps the most telling finding is that patients with alcoholic Korsakoff's syndrome rarely, if ever, have shown an abnormal rate of forgetting when their initial learning was equated to that of controls. Patient N.A. also has shown a normal rate of forgetting. In other cases

Table 6-1. Impairments for Alcoholic Korsakoff's Syndrome, Medial Thalamic Lesion, and Patient N.A.

	Subject sample		
Kind of impairment	Alcoholic Korsakoff's	Medial thalamic lesion	Patient N.A.
1. Abnormal rate of Forgetting	Never	—	No
2. Failure to release from proactive interference	Usually	Frequently	No
3. Presence of retrograde amnesia	Always	Sometimes	Minimal
4. Temporal gradient in retrograde amnesia	Usually	Rarely	No
5. Confabulation	Sometimes	Sometimes	—
6. Impaired procedural learning[a]	No	No	No
7. Impairment on frontal lobe tasks	Usually	Sometimes	No

[a]Referring only to procedural learning tasks that cannot be mediated by explicit memory.

of diencephalic lesion, rate of forgetting generally has not been tested. Cramon et al. (1986) did describe one of their patients as having an abnormal rate of forgetting, but this was not well documented. This phenomenon is important because it does indicate that patients with diencephalic amnesia do have a deficit in the initial registration of information into long-term memory. If given long enough exposure, this registration deficit can be overcome, at least for some recognition-memory paradigms. It also indicates that the problem in alcoholic Korsakoff's syndrome does not appear to be consolidation of material once it is registered into long-term memory. If consolidation was a problem, we would expect to see an accelerated rate of forgetting in alcoholic Korsakoff's syndrome.

Recognition-memory paradigms minimize retrieval demands, which may either reduce difficulty accessing information or allow for the use of weaker memory traces. Since most rate-of-forgetting experiments have been done with recognition memory as opposed to recall, it is impossible to surmise from these studies whether a deficit in retrieval exists with longer exposure times. To the extent that cueing and recognition versus recall have been shown to improve the memory performance of patients with diencephalic amnesia (e.g., Cermak et al., 1973; Jaffe & Katz, 1975), then it can be conjectured that retrieval deficits are a part of their memory problems. Of course, poor retrieval may be due to poor encoding since the ability to retrieve information depends upon the way in which it is encoded. When memory performance is equated to that of controls, alcoholic Korsakoff's patients do appear capable of responding with more extensive processing of information (e.g., Cermak & Reale, 1978; Mayes et al., 1980). If recall were still abnormal under such circumstances, a retrieval deficit in the absence of an encoding deficit could be presumed. Such an experiment has yet to be performed.

Patients with temporal lobe lesions have demonstrated abnormal rates of forgetting in some cases when initial memory has been equated (e.g., Butters et al., 1984; Hupert & Piercy, 1978; Squire, 1981), but Freed and colleagues (1987) indicated there were circumstances under which patients with amnesia after mesial temporal lesion did not show an abnormal rate of forgetting. Some resolution of this problem for mesial temporal amnesias would contribute to our understanding of diencephalic amnesia. A key question to be explored is do cases of diencephalic amnesia show the same type of initial registration deficit as patients with mesial temporal lesions, only a little less severe? Or, do patients with diencephalic amnesia show only initial registration deficits, while patients with mesial temporal lesions show both initial registration and consolidation deficits?

Failure to release from proactive interference most likely does indicate an encoding problem for patients with alcoholic Korsakoff's syndrome. However, the centrality of this symptom for diencephalic memory deficit can be questioned. First, the fact that patient N.A. does not demonstrate such a failure (Squire, 1982) indicates that semantic-processing deficits may not be a necessary component of a severe diencephalic memory deficit. Squire (1982) had suggested this pattern of processing might be related to frontal lobe dysfunction. Nonetheless, some patients with medial thalamic infarct do demonstrate this difficulty (e.g., Graff-Radford et al., 1990; Winocur et al., 1984). However, a second line of evidence indicates some problems with the encoding interpretation. This is the evidence cited above that depth-of-processing deficits may disappear when performance is equated to that of normals. This would indicate that semantic-processing deficits are a by-product of deficient registration of material into long-term memory. Since long-term memory is more likely to operate on a semantic basis than short-term memory (Baddeley, 1990), it may be assumed that semantic-processing difficulties result from the inability to engage long-term memory processes.

Whether a temporal gradient in retrograde amnesia is a necessary component of diencephalic amnesia also can be questioned. When tested, some patients with medial thalamic infarction have shown retrograde memory deficits, but they infrequently demonstrate the temporal gradient of alcoholic Korsakoff's syndrome (Graff-Radford et al., 1990; Stuss et al., 1988; Swanson & Schmidley, 1983).

As long as procedural-learning tasks are not mediated easily by explicit memory, patients with alcoholic Korsakoff's syndrome (Cermak et al., 1973; Cohen & Squire, 1980; Martone et al., 1984; Talland, 1965), patients with medial thalamic infarction (Nichelli et al., 1988), and patient N.A. (Squire, 1981) all seem to demonstrate intact procedural learning. Priming experiments demonstrating intact priming in alcoholic Korsakoff's patients have not been adequately tested in patients with other diencephalic lesions.

The contribution of frontal lobe dysfunction to the pattern of memory deficits in diencephalic amnesia is also of some interest. Squire (1982) maintained that failure to release from proactive interference was due to frontal lobe deficits in patients with alcoholic Korsakoff's syndrome. Indeed, frontal processing deficits are often seen in these patients (e.g., Oscar-Berman, 1973; Squire, 1982). It is uncertain in these cases if the frontal lobe impairment is a direct result of frontal lobe damage, or an indirect result of damage to the dorsal medial nucleus which is intimately connected to the frontal lobes. It is of interest that cases of dorsal medial infarction without frontal damage sometimes demonstrate frontal lobe dysfunction (Graff-Radford et al., 1990; Speedie & Heilman, 1983). But other cases of medial thalamic infarction (Mori et al., 1986), hemorrhage (Brown et al., 1989), or stab wound (Squire, 1982) have not shown frontal lobe deficits. Ultimately, this may depend upon location of lesion within the dorsal medial nucleus. Areas specifically connected to the dorsal lateral frontal lobes might be particularly vulnerable in this respect. The resolution of this issue will require better localization within the dorsal medial nucleus.

Finally, it is clear that the hemispheric specialization for processing verbal and visual information applies to memory functions at the level of the diencephalon (Brown et al., 1989; Mori et al. 1986; Speedie & Heilman, 1982, 1983; Squire & Moore, 1979; Squire et al., 1989; Stuss et al., 1988). The integrity of this specialization for memory at the diencephalic level is consistent with the specialization for language discussed in Chapter 3. It is a further indication that diencephalic structures interact as a part of hemispheric systems, along with cortical structures, for processing language and storing memories.

Many of these issues will be discussed further in Chapter 8 when theoretical implications are explored in greater detail. Before doing so, however, it is necessary to turn our attention to the role of the basal ganglia and the basal forebrain in memory processes. Once these aspects have been addressed, we will be in a better position to explore the question of how diencephalic structures participate in a memory system.

7

The Basal Forebrain and the Basal Ganglia in Memory

Since the early 1980s, increasing attention has focused on two additional sets of structures and their role in memory. The first set of structures is collectively called the basal forebrain. More specifically, as noted in Chapter 5, the cholinergic cells of the basal forebrain appear to participate in memory. These cells can be found in the nucleus basalis of Meynert, the nucleus of the diagonal band of Broca, and the medial septal nucleus. These cells are the source of cholinergic innervation to the neocortex (nucleus basalis), hippocampus (nucleus of the diagonal band and medial septal nucleus), and amygdala (nucleus basalis) (Mesulam, Mufson, Wainer, & Levey, 1983). Although interest in these structures arose partly because of evidence of cholinergic deficit in Alzheimer's disease (e.g., Arendt et al., 1983; Bird, Stranahan, Sumi, & Raskind, 1983; Coyle, Price, & DeLong, 1983; Perry et al., 1978; Terry & Katzman, 1983; Whitehouse, Price, Clark, Coyle, & DeLong, 1981; Whitehouse et al., 1982), many complications cloud interpretation of the memory deficits of Alzheimer's patients as due primarily to cholinergic deficit. For this reason, I will not exhaustively explore memory in Alzheimer's-type dementia in this work. Such an exploration simply cannot lead to clear statements regarding the role of the basal forebrain in memory. However, other evidence implicating the basal forebrain cholinergic cells in memory can be found in what has become an extensive animal literature and in human studies of patients with vascular lesions.

The second set of structures, the basal ganglia, consists of the caudate nucleus, the putamen, the ventral striatum (nucleus accumbens, olfactory tubercle, ventral caudate, and ventral putamen), and the globus pallidus. As I noted in Chapter 1, the basal ganglia are key parts of parallel loops starting and ending in the cortex (Alexander et al., 1986). Multiple cortical structures project into the caudate, putamen, and ventral striatum. These striatal structures, in turn, project into the globus pallidus, where large disc-shaped dendritic fields are in a position to integrate striatal inputs (Percheron, Yelnik, & Francois, 1984). The globus pallidus then projects to various thalamic nuclei, including the ventral anterior nucleus, the ventral lateral nucleus, the dorsal medial nucleus, and the intralaminar nuclei. Thalamic fibers finally partially close the loop by projecting back to the anterior cortical area which is one of the structures projecting into the striatal portion of the loop. Several loops, anatomically distinct at all levels, exist. Although there are other anatomic considerations concerning the basal ganglia, any role in memory for these structures probably is mediated through these loops.

The most extensive evidence concerning the basal ganglia in memory has come from the study of Huntington's disease patients and to a lesser extent from the study of Parkinson's disease patients. Many of the studies on Huntington's disease patients have used models and concepts that were found useful in the study of alcoholic Korsakoff's syndrome. Studies of vascular lesion cases and other disease entities have also made some contribution. Studies of Huntington's and Parkinson's disease patients are not free from difficulties in reflecting the role of the basal ganglia in memory. Effects on the cerebral cortex can be found in both entities, and even the basal forebrain has been implicated to some degree in Parkinson's disease (Arendt et al., 1983). Thus, any results relying upon these disease entities to establish a role for the basal ganglia in memory can be considered controversial.

In the current chapter I will focus first on the evidence concerning the basal forebrain in memory. I will discuss human vascular lesion studies implicating the basal forebrain in memory, and consider anatomical complications in interpreting these studies and the role of animal lesion studies in resolving anatomical issues. Subsequently, I will review evidence regarding the basal ganglia in memory. I will place some emphasis on process studies that address a specific role for the basal ganglia in memory. Finally, I will make a few concluding remarks.

The Basal Forebrain and Memory

As I mentioned in Chapter 5, cholinergic neurons in the basal forebrain are the main suppliers of acetylcholine to the neocortex and hippocampal formation. These cholinergic neurons reside mainly within the nucleus basalis of Meynert in the substantia innominata, within the nucleus of the diagonal band of Broca, and within the medial septal nuclei. One impetus for consideration of the basal forebrain in memory has been findings in the 1970s and 1980s that cortical cholinergic activity is reduced in senile dementia of the Alzheimer's type. Memory loss is one of the earliest and most debilitating symptoms in this type of dementia.

For example, Perry et al. (1978) showed significant reduction in cortical choline acetyltransferase activity for Alzheimer's patients compared to normals, patients with depression, and patients with multi-infarct dementia. By contrast, alterations in the gamma amino butyric acid (GABA) system were found in all nonnormal groups. Further, the authors found a correlation between cholinergic activity and numbers of senile plaques in these populations, but found no significant correlation between GABA activity and numbers of senile plaques. Finally, reduced cholinergic activity also correlated with decreases in cognitive functions, whereas no such correlation existed for GABA activity. In another example of such findings, Bird et al. (1983) found reduced cholinergic activity in the frontal cortex, temporal cortex, hippocampus, and cerebellum for early onset Alzheimer's patients. Late onset Alzheimer's patients demonstrated decreased cholinergic activity only in the hippocampus. Decreased cholinergic activity was also measured in the nucleus basalis of Meynert in Alzheimer's disease patients.

These latter findings have led to studies of morphologic changes in the basal forebrain. For example, Whitehouse, Price, Clark, Coyle, and DeLong (1981) demonstrated significant cell loss in the nucleus basalis of Meynert for an Alzheimer's disease patient compared to a control patient. Whitehouse et al. (1982) followed up by showing similar changes in the nucleus basalis of Meynert in a sample of five Alzheimer's patients as compared to controls. Cell loss was also shown in the nucleus of the diagonal band for these patients. Arendt et al. (1983) demonstrated such findings in a larger sample of Alzheimer's disease patients (n = 14). While the average neuron loss was greater in the neurons imbedded within the substantia innominata, neuron loss was also shown in the nucleus of the diagonal band and the medial septal nucleus. It is of some interest that this pattern of cell loss was not unique to the Alzheimer's patients: patients with idiopathic Parkinson's disease and with alcoholic Korsakoff's syndrome also demonstrated loss of large cholinergic cells in these areas. The authors considered this pattern of cell loss in Alzheimer's disease the morphologic correlate of cortical cholinergic deficiency. Reviews of the cholinergic system dysfunction in Alzheimer's disease have found loss of cholinergic neurons in the nucleus basalis to be consistent with evidence of decreased cholinergic activity in the cortex since the basal forebrain is the main source of acetylcholine for the cerebral cortex (Coyle, Price, & DeLong, 1983; Terry & Katzman, 1983).

Although findings of decreased cholinergic activity and basal forebrain cell loss in Alzheimer's-type dementia have been relatively consistent in these and other studies, some care must be exercised when drawing conclusions. The coexistence of memory loss and basal forebrain cholinergic cell loss in Alzheimer's disease does not imply that the cholinergic cell loss causes the memory dysfunction; for example both phenomena could be caused by some other factor. Structural changes in the cortex of Alzheimer's patients, including the hippocampal formation, are so pervasive that they must be considered as the probable direct cause of much of the dysfunction manifested in Alzheimer's disease. In other words, other evidence for participation of basal forebrain structures in memory must be sought.

Vascular Lesion of the Basal Forebrain

Cases of lesion to the basal forebrain have been one important source of such evidence. Most of these cases involve vascular lesion and/or aneurysm surgery around the anterior communicating artery. In general, studies of anterior communicating artery aneurysm hemorrhage support a role for the basal forebrain in memory. However, it is uncertain if certain characteristics demonstrated by patients with these lesions are caused by damage to the structures or by combined damage to the basal forebrain plus other structures, such as the frontal lobes. The characteristics in question include confabulation and difficulty in temporal sequencing.

Some of the earlier studies resulting from anterior communicating artery anomalies predated widespread use of the CT scan, and therefore do not include detailed analysis of the anatomy of lesions. For example, Lindqvist and Norlen (1966) studied memory and cognitive functions in 33 patients on whom surgery for ruptured anterior communicating artery aneurysm was performed. In 17 of 33 cases, symptoms similar to those of alcoholic Korsakoff's syndrome were present acutely. In 11 of these 17 cases, the memory disorder disappeared mostly or entirely within 6 months after operation. Five cases had significant persisting memory disturbance, and one case had only a mild memory disturbance and could not be followed over time.

The description of memory disturbance in Lindqvist and Norlen's (1966) cases is of some interest. Since they tested cognitive functions other than memory, they were able to exclude attentional disorders or more extensive cognitive dysfunction as a cause of the memory symptoms. Confabulation was often present; sometimes confabulated details were repeated across time. Retrograde amnesia was present acutely and often disappeared later. In both cases described in detail, patients were noted to have greater difficulty recalling material happening closer to the operations, suggesting some temporal gradient. At times, patients were unable to recall particular items of information, but at other times they were able to recall the same items, especially with cues. This pattern indicates some difficulty accessing information that is held in long-term memory. In fact, one patient was described as able to remember details close to the time of the operation, but had difficulty putting them into the proper chronological order. Performance on recognition and recall tests of memory was impaired. Patients had difficulty recognizing their memory deficits and seemed to be unconcerned about the future.

In an earlier analysis of some of these cases, Norlen and Lindqvist (1964) had suggested that the memory deficit was due to cortical (gyrus rectus) involvement as opposed to subcortical damage. However, this analysis is not entirely consistent with the subsequent analysis of other authors (see Damasio et al., 1985; Gade, 1982; Phillips et al., 1987, below), though orbitofrontal damage may be related to some symptoms.

Talland had applied his knowledge of alcoholic Korsakoff's syndrome to the examination of amnesia after anterior communicating artery aneurysm rupture and repair (Talland, Sweet, & Ballantine, 1967). In two cases, these authors found fabrications and disorientation in the acute postoperative phase. Errors in temporal or situational placement were common and led to confabulation thereafter. Memory for consonant trigrams after brief periods of counting backward was normal for the first patient and only slightly impaired for the second. Neither patient could learn lists of nonsense syllables; memory for paragraphs was impaired, especially after a delay. Picture recognition was impaired initially in the first patient but recovered; the second patient demonstrated a lower-than-normal number of correct recognitions in the acute phase, but showed numerous false-positive recognitions in the chronic phase. Some evidence indicated that cueing aided recall for recent public events. Both patients showed average IQ's during intellectual assessment. Acutely, both patients showed a lack of concern for their condition, though this was apparent chronically only in the second patient. It is of some interest that Talland and colleagues saw these patients as quite similar to alcoholic Korsakoff's patients with whom Talland had extensive experience. The reader may recall that Graff-Radford et al. (1990) saw similarities between the amnesias in paramedian thalamic infarctions and basal forebrain lesions. Talland et al. hypothesized that damage extended into structures related to Papez' circuit.

Logue, Durward, Pratt, Piercy, and Nixon (1968) analyzed sequelae of anterior cerebral artery and anterior communicating artery rupture. Unfortunately, the authors did not separate the two territories. In their 79 patients, memory was more often impaired than intellect. Acute confabulation appeared to predict later memory deficit on testing, as 16 of 18 patients with acute confabulation later demonstrated memory deficit. In 26 cases of anterior communicating artery aneurysm treated by surgery, Sengupta, Chiu, and Brierley (1975) found memory deficit to be common, but, contrary to Logue et al. (1968), no more common than intellectual deficit. In comparing their study with that of Logue et al., Sengupta et al. noted that the Logue study had excluded surgically treated patients, while their own study included only patients who had received surgical treatment.

Okawa, Maeda, Nukui, and Kawafuchi (1980) found amnesic syndromes of varying severity in 40 of their 85 cases with anterior communicating artery aneurysm presurgically. The number increased to 53 postsurgically, but only 19 of 73 patients receiving long-term follow-up demonstrated memory deficits of varying degree. Confabulation was also relatively common acutely: 14 of 85 patients presurgically, and 28 of 85 postsurgically. However, only 3 of 73 patients showed chronic confabulation.

Volpe and Hirst (1983) studied two patients who developed amnesia after surgery for anterior communicating artery aneurysm repair but who showed no evidence of infarction on CT scan. Neither patient confabulated on a chronic basis, and both showed high average IQ's on intellectual testing. Memory testing revealed severe impairment of free recall. Relative to the mean and standard deviation of controls, however, their performance improved on cued-recall and recognition tasks, suggesting a retrieval deficit. Compared to normal controls, patients demonstrated increased prior-list intrusions, similar to patients with alcoholic Korsakoff's syndrome (e.g., Butters et al., 1987; Butters et al., 1986).

Vilkki (1985) compared the performance of five patients who had surgery for aneurysm of the anterior communicating artery to the performance of normal controls. As a group, the surgery patients showed normal performance on selected subtests of the Wechsler Adult Intelligence Scale, and normal short-term memory (repetition of digits forward and backward). Their performance was within normal limits for remembering word triads when repetition of a different triad was interpolated as interference. However, they demonstrated impairment of memory for geometric designs. Their incidental recall of a word list was severely impaired, but improved with cueing. Their incidental visual recognition was impaired relative to controls. Only two patients showed confabulation, and both of these patients demonstrated orbitofrontal lesion on CT scan. One of the other three patients showed frontal lesion. The author suggested that frontal lesion was a prerequisite for confabulation in these patients. He noted variability in the presence of confabulation, the presence of other frontal symptoms, and the degree to which cueing aided recall.

Gade (1982) was among the first to detail anatomic considerations in amnesic syndromes after anterior communicating artery aneurysm repair. He noted that between 3 and 13 perforating arteries depart from the anterior communicating artery. When surgical procedures compromise the distribution of these perforating arteries (trapping of aneurysm), the incidence of amnesic syndrome is high, with 9 of 11 cases in his series. However, when the distribution of these perforating arteries is less disturbed (ligation of aneurysm neck), then the incidence of amnesic syndrome dropped dramatically, with 6 of 37 cases in the author's series. When the latter type of operative procedure was used, Du Cros and Lhermitte (1984) reported a somewhat higher incidence of memory disturbance than Gade (1982), but Hori and Suzuki (1979) had reported an even lower long-term incidence of memory dysfunction than Gade. Gade reported the distribution of the perforating arteries from the anterior communicating artery to include the septal region, the subcallosal area (including the diagonal band), the columns of the fornix, the anterior hypothalamus, the optic chiasm, the mesial part of the anterior commissure, the lamina terminalis, and perhaps portions of the corpus callosum and anterior cingulate. He surmised that memory deficit and other postoperative symptoms might be due to damage in these areas. It should be noted that Gade did not include the nucleus basalis among the involved structures; it appears to be lateral to the region of involvement described.

Alexander and Freedman (1983) also reported amnesic syndromes after anterior communicating artery rupture in 11 patients. Initially, the patients exhibited a confusional state with confabulation and an inability to recognize the deficit. After some weeks, the disorder evolved into an amnesic state with dense anterograde-memory deficit and variable retrograde amnesia. Infarction was common, but the amnesic state could be seen when there was no accompanying infarction, when there was unilateral infarction, or when there was bilateral infarction. Patients were described as often demonstrating apathy or unconcern, similar to those of Lindqvist and Norlen (1966).

Alexander and Freedman suggested that damage to the septal region or the anterior hypothalamus was responsible for the memory deficits. Attempts to pharmacologically compensate for potential acetylcholine loss or dopamine loss (through damage to medial forebrain bundle) were unsuccessful.

Damasio et al. (1985b) studied five cases of basal forebrain lesion; four had lesions secondary to rupture of anterior communicating artery aneurysms, and one had lesions secondary to resection of an arteriovenous malformation. Basal forebrain involvement included the septal nuclei, the nucleus accumbens, the nuclei of the diagonal band, and medial portions of the substantia innominata. The amnesic syndrome involved the retrograde and anterograde compartments, with mild impairment in three cases and severe impairment in two cases. All cases showed impairment of verbal and nonverbal memory on formal testing.

Four symptoms characterized the memory disorder: (1) Patients were able to learn information in separate modalities, but they were unable to match information across modalities. For example, the patients were able to learn the names of their doctors, their faces, and other characteristics, but they were not able to match faces or other characteristics with the doctors' names. (2) Patients were unable to apply time-tags to new and old information, and therefore had difficulty with temporal ordering of events. (3) Patients confabulated freely. Fabrications included elements of current realities as gleaned from the news and other sources. (4) Cueing strongly benefited both recall and recognition.

All cases included unilateral damage of the orbitofrontal lobes, as well as damage of mesial temporal structures. Damasio et al. (1985b) concluded that orbitofrontal damage could not be responsible for symptoms since orbitofrontal damage sparing the basal forebrain does not cause memory deficit. However, ventral medial frontal damage can produce amnesic symptoms. The authors concluded that basal forebrain connections with mesial temporal lobe structures were responsible for the memory deficit. Since cueing improved memory and patients performed better on recognition memory than recall, the authors concluded that their patients suffered from a retrieval deficit.

Actually, the suggestion that basal forebrain connections with the mesial temporal lobes may be important in memory symptoms was consistent with the findings of Volpe, Herscovitch, and Raichle (1984). These authors found decreased oxygen metabolism in the mesial temporal lobes of two patients with chronic amnesic syndrome after anterior communicating artery aneurysm rupture and repair. Orbitofrontal and thalamic metabolism were not decreased in these patients.

When herpes encephalitis caused bilateral mesial temporal and anterior lateral temporal lobe damage in addition to bilateral basal forebrain damage, Damasio et al. (1985a) found a profound amnesic syndrome. This patient demonstrated a dense anterograde-memory deficit, but the episodic-memory deficit extended not only into the anterograde compartment, but also into the retrograde compartment. The patient's remote memory was almost completely devoid of autobiographical, contextual memories. Confabulation and some evidence of loss of temporal tagging were consistent with other basal forebrain cases reported by the same group (see above). Memory tests demonstrated intact short-term memory with profound loss of the ability to establish new memories in both the verbal and nonverbal modalities. Episodic-memory loss extended to famous faces. The authors surmised that the hippocampus determined the relationship between stimuli in different modalities and the relationship between new incoming information and established memories. Thus, damage to the hippocampus would interfere with establishing new episodic memories. They also concluded that there must be a separate register for cross-indexing multiple stimuli to support episodic memory, and that this register might be located in the anterior lateral temporal lobes. Destruction of this register might lead to the loss of remote episodic memory.

Phillips et al. (1987) were able to do a postmortem study of a patient with an anterior communicating artery aneurysm rupture who developed an amnesic syndrome after surgical treatment. In addition to the hemosederin staining of the right gyrus rectus and the para-olfactory areas from hemorrhage, there was bilateral necrosis in the septal region, the nucleus of the diagonal band, a small portion of the anterior inferior globus pallidus, the inferior portion of the anterior limb of the internal capsule, and the paraventricular hypothalamus. The lesion was almost symmetrical but slightly more extensive on the right, and the presumed cause was inadvertent sacrifice of the perforating branches of the proximal anterior and anterior communicating arteries. It is worth noting that nucleus basalis was spared, consistent with Gade's analysis.

The amnesic syndrome of Phillips and colleagues' patient was characterized by intact short-term memory, but a severe inability to establish new long-term memories. After the operation, the patient was described as having a "tendency to confabulate." It is unclear if the patient confabulated spontaneously after his acute postsurgical "global-confusional state" cleared, but confabulation was provoked by prompting during delayed-recall tests of memory 6 months postonset. There was a variable retrograde amnesia. Neuropsychological assessment at 6 months postsurgery indicated the memory deficit to be relatively isolated, that is, other cognitive functions were grossly intact. Personality changes included apathy and a loss of spontaneity. Thus, descriptions of amnesic syndrome are consistent with those of Damasio et al. (1985b). It is of interest that the often mentioned nucleus basalis of Meynert may not have to be involved to produce amnesic syndrome. Memory loss may be specific to the neurons in the septal region and the nucleus of the diagonal band, which are the cholinergic supply for the hippocampus.

DeLuca and Cicerone (in press) examined confabulation in patients with hemorrhage as a result of anterior communicating artery aneurysm (n = 9) and a second group consisting of patients with hemorrhages elsewhere in the brain (n = 17). These authors reported that confabulation was observed in both groups when patients were not oriented to person, place, month, and year. However, with the return of orientation, all of the patients with hemorrhage secondary to anterior communicating artery aneurysm hemorrhage continued to confabulate, whereas confabulation persisted in only 1 of 17 subjects in the other hemorrhage group. This latter subject was the only patient in the other hemorrhage group with clear frontal lobe involvement. DeLuca (personal communication) reported that all patients with anterior communicating artery aneurysm hemorrhages in the DeLuca and Cicerone study displayed a significant anterograde amnesia, structural changes in the frontal lobes (CT scan), and psychometric evidence of frontal lobe dysfunction (Wisconsin Card Sorting Test) in addition to confabulation. This finding is significant because those cases of Damasio et al. (1985b) and Vilkki (1985) who confabulated all had at least some frontal lobe damage. DeLuca and Cicerone's conclusion that frontal lobe deficit must be present in addition to memory disturbance before confabulation was found was consistent with the findings of Vilkki (1985) as well as those of Damasio et al. (1985b). It is of further interest that DeLuca (1990) reported an anterior communicating artery aneurysm patient with clear frontal lobe lesions on CT and clear psychometric evidence of frontal lobe dysfunction (2 categories and 96 perseverative errors on Wisconsin Card Sorting Test). This patient was not amnesic and did not confabulate. Thus, while frontal lobe dysfunction may be necessary for confabulation following anterior communicating artery aneurysm hemorrhage, it is clearly not sufficient. DeLuca (personal communication) hypothesizes that both frontal dysfunction and amnesia (i.e., basal forebrain lesion) are necessary for confabulation to be expressed.

In summary: Memory disturbance is a common sequela of rupture of anterior communicating artery aneurysms or surgery to repair anterior communicating artery aneurysms. (It should be noted that the incidence of postsurgical memory deficit has decreased as surgical techniques have improved.) In some cases, memory symptoms improve, but in others it is a more-or-less permanent dysfunction. The amnesic syndrome is characterized by variable retrograde amnesia but consistent inability to establish new memories. Frequently, cueing has been noted to improve recall (Damasio et al., 1985b; Vilkki, 1985; Volpe & Hirst, 1983), and recognition memory performance may improve relative to recall (Volpe & Hirst, 1983). The classical interpretation of this pattern of deficits suggests that patients with basal forebrain lesions, in part, are having difficulty accessing information that does exist in long-term stores. It should be noted, however, that most amnesics show some improvement from free recall to recognition.

It has also been found that this group of patients has trouble with the temporal ordering of events in new and remote memories (Damasio et al., 1985b; Talland et al., 1967). Damasio et al. (1985b) have suggested that temporal tagging of memories was deficient after basal forebrain lesion. A related issue is confabulation, which is frequent in these cases. It has been suggested that frontal lobe damage in addition to basal forebrain damage may be necessary for the appearance of confabulation (DeLuca & Cicerone, 1989; Vilkki, 1985). Since the cases of Damasio et al. (1985b) all had frontal damage, it is possible that the temporal-tagging deficit may also be related to frontal dysfunction.

Relatively early in the documentation of memory deficit after anterior communicating artery aneurysm rupture or repair, Talland et al. (1967) noted similarities between these patients and patients with lesions of the dorsal medial thalamus and mammillary bodies (i.e., alcoholic Korsakoff's syndrome patients). Some parallels have since been drawn by Graff-Radford et al. (1990) in reference to patients with medial thalamic infarctions. Indeed, if the examination of tracts as well as nuclei is relevant to medial thalamic lesion, it is just as important for basal forebrain lesions. Gade (1982) noted that the columns of the fornix, supplying the mammillary bodies with input from the hippocampal formation as a part of Papez' circuit, are in the distribution of the perforating arteries originating from the anterior communicating artery. If Gade's analysis is correct, however, ischemic lesions involving arteries branching from the anterior communicating artery are unlikely to extend laterally enough into the substantia innominata to damage the portion of the ventral amygdalofugal pathway destined for the dorsal medial thalamus. On the other hand, there may be damage to the medial septal nucleus, which receives input from the amygdala. Thus, one of the output pathways of the hippocampus and a nucleus connected to the amygdala are both damaged in the type of basal forebrain lesion examined above. This circumstance may be similar to dorsal medial thalamic lesions where amnesic disorders are produced only if the mammillothalamic tract and the ventral amygdalofugal pathway are both damaged.

Given these anatomical complexities regarding the basal forebrain, studies of human vascular lesions cannot resolve the question of how important the cholinergic neurons of the basal forebrain are for memory. Exploration of other approaches to this problem is necessary. Therefore, a brief (but not exhaustive) exploration of the animal literature and studies of cholinergic functions in normal humans will help to resolve some of this ambiguity.

Animal and Pharmacological Studies

Given the small number of studies regarding human basal forebrain lesions and the anatomical ambiguity they leave, the examination of animal analog studies has particular importance in this area. In general, animal studies across species have suggested that basal forebrain structures play a role in memory and that this role is dependent upon cholinergic activity.

The nucleus basalis magnocellularis of the rat is thought to be analogous to the human nucleus basalis of Meynert. Numerous investigations of memory after lesion to this structure have been performed in the rat. Bilateral lesion of the nucleus basalis magnocellularis has led to impaired acquisition of new learning (Flicker, Dean, Watkins, Fisher, & Bartus, 1983; Murray & Fibiger, 1985, 1986). Performance deficits have also been noted on tasks that require memory from trial to trial after bilateral lesion (Bartus et al., 1985; Dunnett, 1985; Helper, Olton, Wenk, & Coyle, 1985; Tilson et al., 1988) and unilateral lesion (Beninger, Jhamandas, Boegman, & El-Defrawy, 1986a) to the nucleus basalis magnocellularis. Nucleus basalis lesions usually create decreases in cholinergic activity of the neocortex, but not the hippocampus. This is consistent with evidence that the nucleus basalis supplies the neocortex but not the hippocampus (Mesulam et al., 1983). Cholinergic input to the hippocampus is supplied from the medial septal region and the nucleus of the diagonal band. Occasionally, performance deficits in tasks learned before lesioning have occurred with bilateral lesion (Murray & Fibiger, 1986) and unilateral lesion (Beninger, Jhamandas, Boegman, & El-Defrawy, 1986b) to the nucleus basalis. Impaired performance on tasks requiring trial-to-trial memory has also been noted after bilateral lesion to the medial septal area (Helper et al., 1985), bilateral lesion to the medial septal area plus the nucleus of the diagonal band (Kessler, Markowitsch, & Sigg, 1986), and bilateral lesion to the medial septal area plus the nucleus basalis (Helper et al., 1985; Knowlton, Wenk, Olton, & Coyle, 1985).

Two facts regarding these animal studies are perhaps more germane to this discussion of the human basal forebrain. First, many of the lesions causing memory deficit in these studies were created with ibotenic acid (Bartus et al., 1986; Dunnett, 1985; Flicker et al., 1983; Helper et al., 1985; Kessler et al., 1986; Knowlton et al., 1985; Murray & Fibiger, 1985, 1986). Ibotenic acid has an affinity for selectively damaging cholinergic cells. Thus, while it may be difficult to separate vascular lesion of the nucleus basalis from vascular lesion to the ventral amygdalofugal pathway in humans, it is possible to selectively lesion these cholinergic neurons in rats, and memory impairment does indeed result. Second, the administration of cholinergic agonists or cholinest-erase inhibitors in the right dosages almost invariably leads to some improvement of memory performance in rats with basal forebrain lesions (e.g., Casamenti, Bracco, Bartolini, & Pepeu, 1985; Kwo-On-Yuen, Mandel, Chen, & Thal, 1990; Murray & Fibiger, 1985, 1986; Tilson et al., 1988). Memory deficit with selective lesion of cholinergic basal forebrain neurons and memory improvement after the administration of cholinergic agonists in rats with basal forebrain lesion do suggest that the cholinergic system itself is of direct importance in memory. In fact, there is some evidence that the frontal cortex may be the site of action for cholinergic agonists in nucleus basalis–lesioned rats. Harountunian, Mantin, and Kanof (1990) found that administration of a cholinergic agonist (physostigmine) enhanced one-trial passive-avoidance learning for rats with and without nucleus basalis lesions. Lesions of the frontal cortex abolished this improvement.

Of course, some care must be taken in applying results in rat studies to humans. First, there is evidence that rats may perform some memory tasks well after nucleus basalis lesion (Murray & Fibiger, 1986). Second, one study (Kessler et al., 1986) noted more severe memory deficits after lesion to midbrain cholinergic centers than after lesion to basal forebrain structures. Third, similar structures may not perform analogous functions between species as divergent as rats and humans. However, with respect to this later criticism, it should be noted that irreversible memory deficits have been produced after bilateral ibotenic acid lesion to the nucleus basalis of Meynert in the monkey (e.g., Irle & Markowitsch, 1987). Wilson and Rolls (1990) have shown that neurons in the basal forebrain of monkeys respond differently to stimuli based upon their current reinforcement value, that these differential responses are maintained across a number of intervening trials, and that rapid adjustments can be made to changes in reinforcement value. The authors concluded that responses of basal forebrain neurons represented encoding of the learned reinforcement value. Thus, animal lesion studies must be seen as generally supportive of the concept that cholinergic neurons of the basal forebrain play some role in memory.

Furthermore, studies have shown that pharmacologic alteration of cholinergic activity can affect memory and cognitive functions in humans. For example, Drachman (1977) found that administration of the cholinergic antagonist scopalamine to normal humans reduced cognitive and memory functioning. Physostigmine, an antagonist of scopalamine, mitigated the effects of scopalamine, whereas amphetamine, a stimulant, did not do so. The author concluded that cholinergic neurons had a direct role in cognitive and memory functions as opposed to an indirect role through arousal mechanisms. Davis and Yamamura (1978) reviewed several similar studies in which scopalamine produced decreases in long-term memory storage. McEvoy (1987) found that standard clinical doses of anticholinergic antiparkinson drugs impaired the acquisition of new memory in healthy young and old adults. Older subjects on anticholinergic medication exhibited significantly more extralist intrusions. Short-term memory was not affected. Thus, the literature has consistently shown decreased ability to acquire new information in normal humans taking anticholinergic drugs. These findings would be consistent with a role in memory for cholinergic systems, probably including the basal forebrain.

Conclusions

In summary: Animal analogue data and experiments with cholinergic medications in normal humans can shed some light on the relationship of basal forebrain lesion to human memory dysfunction. First, studies in rats have consistently shown that lesions in the basal forebrain lead to decreased performance in memory and learning tasks. This decreased performance is accompanied by lowered cholinergic activity in the cortex. Administration of cholinergic agonists or cholinesterase inhibitors mitigates decreased performance on memory tasks. There is even some information suggesting the frontal cortex to be the site of action for improving memory performance with cholinergic agonists after basal forebrain lesion (Harountunian et al., 1990). While some care must be taken in applying this information across species, there is evidence that the basal forebrain is involved in memory for other species. For example, memory deficits have been found in monkeys after nucleus basalis lesions (Irle & Markowitsch, 1987), and basal forebrain neurons may respond differentially to stimuli based upon their learned reinforcement value (Wilson & Rolls, 1990). Finally, humans show decreased memory performance with administration of anticholinergic medications.

When taken together with data regarding patients with anterior communicating artery aneurysm bleeds and/or repairs, it can be concluded that the basal forebrain plays a role in memory and that this role is based upon the basal forebrain's cholinergic efferents. However, many questions remain to be answered. For example, to what degree does damage to pathways coursing through the basal forebrain play a role in memory deficits noted with basal forebrain lesions? Are symptoms such as temporal tagging and confabulation due to basal forebrain damage, frontal lobe damage, or a combination of the two? To what extent do basal forebrain structures play a role in retrieval versus other memory processes? In order to increase our understanding of the role of the basal forebrain in memory, future studies will have to address these issues.

The Basal Ganglia and Memory

Extensive consideration of the basal ganglia in memory processes has been a relatively recent phenomenon. One impetus for the interest was some early comparisons done between alcoholic Korsakoff's syndrome patients and Huntington's disease patients. Recently, Nelson Butters and his colleagues have completed a number of memory studies with Huntington's disease patients, in part using the concepts and experimental paradigms developed in their research with alcoholic amnesic syndromes.

Another impetus for examining memory in Huntington's and Parkinson's disease patients is the concept of "subcortical dementia." An extensive discussion of the problems with this concept is beyond the scope of this chapter. However, one of the most obvious problems with the concept of subcortical dementia is germane: most patient groups with so-called subcortical dementias also have cortical involvement. For example, there is evidence that the frontal cortex is the first part of the cortex to atrophy in Huntington's disease, before atrophy moves to more posterior cortical regions as the disease progresses (Sax et al., 1983). In fact, with the excitotoxic hypothesis of Huntington's disease (e.g., Perry & Hansen, 1990), it is possible that cortical changes may precede changes in the caudate nucleus and actually produce caudate nucleus degeneration by somehow supplying toxic levels of glutamate to the caudate nucleus.[1] It is clear in Parkinson's disease that the degeneration of the substantia nigra, pars compacta, affects mesocortical dopamine projections as well as the nigrostriatal dopaminergic system. Potential effects of mesocortical dopamine projections cannot be discounted. Finally, the so-called cortical dementias also show structural changes in various subcortical sites (e.g., McDuff & Sumi, 1985). Thus, memory studies with Parkinson's and Huntington's diseases must be evaluated with the knowledge that cortical changes may occur and affect memory in these entities. In this section, I will first cover studies with Huntington's disease, then studies with Parkinson's disease, and finally studies with other basal ganglia disorders.

Memory Dysfunction in Huntington's Disease

Since atrophy of the caudate nucleus is among the first structural changes that can be identified on CT scan and appears at the onset of the movement disorder (e.g., Sax et al., 1983), Huntington's disease is considered to provide a means for studying the role of the basal ganglia in cognition. The fact that these patients demonstrate cortical atrophy as the disease progresses was mentioned above as a complicating factor in this interpretation. Many of the more recent studies have used paradigms developed in studies with alcoholic Korsakoff's syndrome, and these design parallels will be reflected in the organization of the next few paragraphs about Huntington's disease. Parts of the first section will cover the ability of Huntington's patients to encode memory for long-term storage. A few more general studies of memory also will be reviewed. Then, the following topics will be covered: studies implicating retrieval, studies of procedural memory, studies of implicit memory, and, finally, studies of remote memory.

Encoding and Other Memory Studies

In general, encoding (as defined in Chapter 6) does not appear to be the problem for Huntington's patients that it is for alcoholic Korsakoff's patients. Butters, Tarlow, Cermak, and Sax (1976) studied the effects of proactive interference in patients with Huntington's disease, patients with alcoholic Korsakoff's syndrome, and alcoholic controls. In

1. It is also possible, of course, that excess glutamate remains in the area of striatal synapses because mechanisms for clearing it in Huntington's disease are dysfunctional (e.g., Perry & Hansen, 1990). This explanation is more consistent with the fact that the caudate nucleus appears to be the most heavily involved site early in the disease process, but it does not explain the eventual cortical involvement.

repeating consonant trigrams or single words after a distraction-filled delay (Peterson & Peterson, 1959), both groups scored significantly below controls at longer delays (9 and 18 seconds). On the proactive-interference task, word or consonant triads were presented in blocks of two trials. Triads were repeated after a distraction-filled delay. In the high-proactive-interference condition, word triads on the first trial were followed by word triads on the second trial. In the low-proactive-interference condition, consonant triads were followed by word triads. Under the high-proactive-interference condition, both Huntington's and Korsakoff's patients performed below controls, but in the low-proactive-interference condition, only the Huntington's patients performed below controls. The authors concluded that Korsakoff's but not Huntington's patients were abnormally susceptible to proactive interference. These findings were essentially replicated in massed presentation (6-second intertrial interval) versus distributed presentation (60-second intertrial interval) of word triads. The massed presentation is thought to carry greater proactive interference because of the greater temporal proximity of trials.

Butters et al. (1976) also studied false-positive errors on a "yes-no" recognition task in these three groups. After the word list was presented in a written format, foil items were interspersed among actual list items in the recognition trial, which was also presented in a written format. Foil items included semantically associated items, homonyms, synonyms, and unrelated items. Replicating Cermak et al. (1973), Korsakoff's patients were found to make more mistakes than controls on homonyms and semantically associated items but not on synonyms. However, the Huntington's patients demonstrated an equal number of errors across types of foils. Thus, memory problems in Huntington's patients could not be attributed to the use of more superficial processing strategies, as has been implied for alcoholic Korsakoff's syndrome. It is also worth noting that Huntington's patients endorsed significantly fewer list items that were repeated during the recognition trial than alcoholic controls, but their total number of false-postitive errors did not differ from that of controls.

Sax et al. (1983) studied memory, cognitive functions, and caudate atrophy in patients in various stages of Huntington's disease. As measured by the Wechsler Memory Scale (Wechsler, 1945), memory dysfunction generally seemed to increase as the disease progresses. Degree of caudate atrophy was correlated with composite scores and some individual subtests on the Wechsler Memory Scale. However, Russell (1975) has criticized this instrument because it does not contain measures of delayed recall; thus, it is difficult to separate short-term from long-term memory deficits using this instrument.

Given previous indications of encoding deficits in Huntington's disease (Butters et al., 1976; Weingartner, Caine, & Ebert, 1979), Beatty and Butters (1986) felt it appropriate to further study encoding capacity with this population. The authors required Huntington's patients and normal controls to learn lists of 14 words including 7 high-imagery words and 7 low-imagery words. Subjects received four learning trials and had a delayed-recall trial after 30 minutes. Although Huntington's patients recalled fewer words than controls, both groups recalled more high-imagery words than low-imagery words, as expected for nonimpaired populations. This effect favoring highly imageable words was noted both on learning trials and on the delayed-recall trial. Imageability did not significantly affect delayed-recognition perform- ance for Huntington's patients; controls' errors were too few to make a meaningful analysis. Huntington's patients did perform significantly below controls on the recognition trial. These results were contrary to those of Weingartner et al. (1979), and the authors suggested the difference might be that there was a greater difference in their high and low imageability words than there was in the Weingartner et al. study.

Beatty and Butters (1986) also tested release from proactive interference with these two groups, and they found that both controls and Huntington's disease patients demonstated a normal release from proactive interference. The authors interpreted the results from both their experimental tasks as indicating that normal encoding can be maintained in the face of the caudate degeneration present in Huntington's disease. These authors made one further observation based upon these data: since patients with frontal lobe damage and memory deficit do demonstrate a failure to release from proactive interference, memory deficit in Huntington's patients does not match that of frontal dysfunction. Thus, memory deficit in Huntington's patients cannot be entirely blamed upon frontal cortical dysfunction.

Martone et al. (1986) used Huppert and Piercy's (1978) task to measure rate of forgetting in Huntington's patients, alcoholic Kor- sakoff's patients, and controls. The durations of exposure for these groups were 4 seconds, 8 seconds, and 1 second, respectively. These exposure durations equated the groups' performance on the two- alternative, forced-choice recognition task at 10 minutes after exposure. The groups did not differ in performance either at 6 hours or at 7 days later. The authors concluded that Huntington's patients could consoli- date information into long-term memory, and that their results could be consistent with a retrieval deficit for these patients. (See discussion below for further evidence regarding retrieval deficit.)

Martone et al. (1986) also tested similar patient groups by exposing them to pictures with one main and one peripheral element. Exposure durations were 2 seconds, 8 seconds, and 12 seconds for the controls, Huntington's patients, and Korsakoff's patients, respectively. Groups performed at similar levels of accuracy on yes-no recognition regardless of whether they saw the whole picture, the main element only, or the peripheral element only. The authors surmised that Huntington's and Korsakoff's patients analyzed the pictures in equal detail when given adequate time. The fact that both patient groups required longer times to process information suggests that either their initial registration or their encoding was less efficient than that of controls.

Memory span, the number of items that can be held in immediate attention at one time, is often taken as an indicator of short-term memory capacity. Orsini et al. (1987) tested spatial and verbal memory span in normal controls, Huntington's disease patients, Parkinson's disease patients, and patients with progressive supranuclear palsy. Spatial memory span was tested with the Corsi Block Test (Lezak, 1983), and verbal memory span was tested with forward digit span. The Corsi Block Test requires subjects to tap blocks on a nine-block board in the same sequence as the examiner. Huntington's disease patients scored significantly lower on spatial span than did controls and Parkinson's patients. On verbal span, Huntington's disease patients scored more poorly than Parkinson's patients, progressive supranuclear palsy patients, and controls. The authors suggested that findings represented a severe attention deficit in Huntington's patients but not the other groups. Since focused attention is a prequisite for memory span, this interpretation is plausible; however, results could also represent a specific deficit in short-term memory processes.

Granholm and Butters (1988) studied the effect of different types of cues at initial presentation and at recall upon the ability of Alzheimer's patients, Huntington's patients, and controls to retrieve words. In their experiment, cue words were given at both initial presentation and at recall in four conditions. In one condition, the same strong cues were given at both presentation and recall. In the second condition, the same weak cues were given at both presentation and recall. In the third experimental condition, strong cues were given at initial presentation, but weak cues were given at recall. In the fourth condition, weak cues were given at presentation and strong cues were given at recall. In a fifth condition, no cues were given either at presentation or at recall. The tendency of cues attended to at encoding to facilitate subsequent recall has been termed "encoding specificity" (Thomson & Tulving, 1970). Huntington's patients were inferior to control subjects in terms of total words recalled. However, similar to intact subjects, Huntington's patients benefited from strong cues at recall if they had also been given during initial presentation of the words, and they performed worse with weak cues at recall when strong cues had been given during presentation. Alzheimer's patients responded to strong cues at recall whether or not these cues had been used at initial presentation. Thus, Huntington's patients and controls demonstrated similar patterns of using semantic relationships of cue words and to-be-remembered words to encode information. The authors attributed Huntington's patients' poorer recall performance to an inability to retrieve information from memory since their encoding pattern appeared normal. However, this reasoning is convincing only if one fails to separate initial-registration and semantic-encoding processes. It could be argued that Huntington's patients may have been influenced by poor initial registration of material into long-term memory as well as by a retrieval deficit. Since the list in this experiment exceeded short-term memory span, it can be assumed that subjects had to use long-term memory for some portion of their recall. Unfortunately, the immediate recall procedure did not allow for the separation of short-term and long-term memory processes.

Although memory dysfunction is one of the first signs of cognitive disturbance in Huntington's disease (Brandt & Butters, 1986; Josiassen, Curry, & Mancall, 1983), Brandt, Folstein, and Folstein (1988) found greater impairment of memory for Alzheimer's disease patients who scored at the same level as Huntington's disease patients on a standardized mental status examination. The Huntington's patients did more poorly than the Alzheimer's patients on serial 7 subtractions; the authors thought this latter deficit was related to deficits in attention and conceptual tracking.

Recently, genetic tests have been developed that can identify patients who will develop Huntington's disease with a fairly high degree of accuracy. Jason et al. (1988) found that Huntington's disease patient family members with a high probability of developing chorea had lower visual-memory scores than Huntington's family members with a low probability of developing choreiform symptoms. No difference between these two groups was found in verbal-memory tasks. The high-probability group also showed some difficulty on a task thought to tap frontal lobe functions (Wisconsin Card Sorting Test). Huntington's patients' difficulty on frontal lobe tasks such as the Wisconsin Card Sorting Test (Grant & Berg, 1948) or the Porteus Maze Test (Porteus, 1959) has been found in other studies as well (e.g., Fisher, Kennedy, Caine, & Shoulson, 1983).

Kramer, Levin, Brandt, and Delis (1989) studied memory in Huntington's, Parkinson's, and Alzheimer's patients, using the California Verbal Learning Test (Delis, Kramer, Kaplan, & Ober, 1987). A discriminant function analysis demonstrated that Parkinson's and Huntington's patients could be statistically separated from each other, as well as from patients with Alzheimer's disease. Huntington's patients repeated items significantly more during recall trials (perseverations) but had a significantly slower rate of forgetting (20-minute delay) than did Parkinson's patients. Alzheimer's disease patients made more intrusions than either Huntington's or Parkinson's patients, had a more rapid rate of forgetting than Huntington's patients, and made more perseverations than the Parkinson's group. The authors concluded that Parkinson's and Huntington's patients demonstrated different patterns of verbal-memory deficit, suggesting that the term "subcortical dementia" is too simplistic to be applied to both groups.

To summarize: Studies have occasionally suggested encoding deficits for Huntington's disease patients, but a number of findings suggest encoding deficits are not prominent with Huntington's disease patients. For example, Huntington's disease patients, unlike alcoholic Korsakoff's patients, show a normal release from proactive interference (Beatty & Butters, 1986). They do not demonstrate evidence of preferentially using more superficial forms of encoding in a recognition-memory paradigm (Butters et al., 1976). In at least some instances, Huntington's patients do demonstrate greater memory for highly imageable words (Butters & Beatty, 1986), and, if given enough time, they process pictures in as much detail as normals (Martone et al., 1986). Their pattern of cue utilization at presentation and recall is similar to that of normals, while Alzheimer's patients demonstrated a different pattern (Granholm & Butters, 1988). Thus, the weight of the evidence is against an encoding explanation for memory deficit in Huntington's disease patients.

As an aside, it is of some interest that Huntington's patients do show normal release from proactive interference (Beatty & Butters, 1986) in spite of the fact that they show frontal deficits (e.g., Brandt et al., 1988; Fisher et al., 1983). These data from different studies demonstrate that frontal impairment and release from proactive interference may be dissociable at least in this population, contrary to the suggestions of Squire (1982). However, this hypothesis should be tested in a single study to explore the relationship between these two functions in Huntington's patients.

Where, then, does the memory deficit lie with Huntington's disease? A normal rate of forgetting (Martone et al., 1986) suggests that Huntington's patients are able to consolidate information into long-term memory. The fact that they must be given longer exposures to stimuli to equal normal performance levels indicates that initial registration of material into long-term stores may be deficient. Further, some studies (e.g., Brandt et al., 1988; Orsini et al., 1987) have suggested that short-term memory and/or attention may be deficient for Huntington's patients. Nonetheless, retrieval processes must also be explored; this is the topic of the ensuing section.

Retrieval Studies

Several studies have focused on the issue of retrieval deficit in Huntington's disease either in design or interpretation. Evidence for retrieval deficits in Huntington's patients is not entirely unequivocal. Even if one accepts the notion of a retrieval deficit, deficient performance in situations where retrieval demands are low suggests that defective registration of material in long-term memory may also be a factor.

Weingartner et al. (1979) presented ten highly imageable words and ten less-imageable words in a list-learning task. Subjects were Huntington's patients and normal controls. The list was presented by the method of Buschke (1973). On the first trial, all 20 words are presented, but on subsequent trials, only words missed on the immediately previous trial are presented again. The subject's goal is to recall as many of the 20 words as possible on each trial. Performance of Huntington's patients was inferior to that of controls across trials. Furthermore, normal controls learned the highly imageable words more quickly than the less-imageable words, but Huntington's patients were insensitive to this difference in their learning performance. Huntington's patients, however, were able to discriminate highly imageable and less-imageable words. Generally, Huntington's patients were less likely to consistently retrieve a word across trials than were controls. The authors concluded that Huntington's patients demonstrated a retrieval deficit due to their inability to adequately encode stimuli, consistent with previous interpretations (Caine, Ebert, & Weingartner, 1977). The failure to show a better performance for highly than less-imageable words was interpreted to indicate an inability to use characteristics of stimuli that could aid encoding. This interpretation is inconsistent with studies indicating that Huntington's patients do not demonstrate the same kind of processing deficits as alcoholic Korsakoff's patients, as discussed above. Further, it is inconsistent with the results of Beatty and Butters (1986); they did find Huntington's patients to perform better with highly imageable words. However, the inconsistency of retrieval across trials is consistent with a retrieval deficit.

Butters et al. (1985) evaluated retrieval by administering two versions of a 15-item word-learning task to Huntington's disease patients, amnesics, and normal controls. The first version consisted of five learning trials with free recall after each trial; a delayed recall was obtained after 20 minutes. The second version consisted of five learning trials with a yes-no recognition trial after each learning trial; a delayed-recognition trial was obtained after 20 minutes. On the recall version, controls recalled more words than both Huntington's and amnesic patients, and the latter two did not differ. When performance on the first trial was subtracted from performance on the fifth trial, controls showed greater learning than both patient groups, but the Huntington's patients demonstrated greater learning than amnesics. Similarly, when delayed-recall performance was subtracted from the fifth learning trial, controls showed less forgetting than both patient groups, but the Huntington's patients showed less forgetting than the amnesic patients. A different pattern arose on the recognition version. On a composite measure of accuracy (d'), controls again scored better than both patient groups; however, the Huntington's patients scored better than amnesics on the five learning trials, unlike the recall version. Huntington's disease patients correctly recognized more list items than amnesic patients but less than controls. However, Huntington's patients made as many false recognitions as amnesics but more than controls. The fact that Huntington's subjects performed better than amnesics on recognition memory but not on recall and the fact that Huntington's patients correctly recognized more items than amnesics was taken as an indication that information had been stored, but that the Huntington's patients could not access the information as easily by recall as by recognition. In other words, a retrieval deficit was a part of their problem on recall performance. On the other hand, the fact that Huntington's patients still scored lower on recognition memory than normals indicates that more than a retrieval deficit was operating in their case.

Butters et al. (1986) replicated the results of Butters et al. (1985) using early and advanced Huntington's patients and an amnesic group consisting only of alcoholic Korsakoff's patients. The results were precisely the same as the earlier Butters et al. study, with the following exceptions: Although early Huntington's patients again showed greater learning than amnesics from the first to the fifth learning trial in the recall task, the advanced Huntington's patients were equal to amnesics in this respect. Also on the recall task, neither Huntington's group differed in rate of forgetting from the controls, though all three of these groups forgot less than the Korsakoff's group. In the latter study, word-list generation also was performed. Controls performed better than all patient groups, and alcoholic Korsakoff's patients were superior to advanced Huntington's patients. Korsakoff's patients repeated more words within trials than did other groups. Finally, the authors also tested recall and recognition memory for stories. On the recall task, controls were superior to alcoholic Korsakoff's and to Huntington's patients. The patient groups did not differ in recall. Multiple stories were used in the story recall, and Korsakoff's patients gave more prior-story-intrusion errors than did controls or Huntington's patients. For story recognition, controls were superior to both patient groups, but as in list recall, the Huntington's patients recognized significantly more ideas than did Korsakoff's patients. Thus, Huntington's patients showed improved performance on recognition tasks relative to alcoholic Korsakoff's patients for both list and story recall. On the other hand, Huntington's patients were inferior to Korsakoff's patients on word-list generation. The authors' interpretation of this latter finding was that the Huntington's patients were not able to meet the retrieval demands of word-list generation as well as the controls and the amnesic patients, consistent with other evidence of a retrieval dysfunction.

Although Huntington's, alcoholic Korsakoff's, and Alzheimer's patients did not differ in the number of story units recalled, Butters et al. (1987) again found Huntington's patients did not emit numerous prior-story-intrusion errors like Korsakoff's and Alzheimer's patients. On word-list generation by initial letter, both Huntington's and Korsakoff's patients demonstrated fewer correct responses than their respective control groups, but Alzheimer's patients did not differ from their control group. Huntington's disease patients repeated fewer words (i.e., made fewer perseverations) than either the Alzheimer's or Korsakoff's patients. All three patient groups demonstrated impaired word-list generation by semantic category. Thus, the Huntington's patients were distinguished from Alzheimer's and Korsakoff's patients in that they did not show prior-story-intrusion errors and in that they showed fewer perseverations on word-list generation by initial letter. The authors concluded that the Huntington's patients had a qualitatively different memory disturbance than either the Korsakoff's or Alzheimer's patients. Further, the authors felt that decreased word-list-generation scores were consistent with a retrieval deficit for Huntington's patients, though results did not strongly corroborate such a hypothesis.

Moss et al. (1986) also performed a study with some bearing upon retrieval hypotheses for Huntington's disease patients. Their study implied that retrieval deficits may be demonstrated under some conditions but not others. The study has some implications for the conditions under which Huntington's patients may be able to create long-term memories but not use them. The authors tested recognition memory in Huntington's, Alzheimer's, and alcoholic Korsakoff's patients and in normal controls. Memory for position on a board, colors, linear designs, faces, and words were tested. Separate tasks were developed for each type of stimulus. On each trial, a new stimulus was added, and the subject had to point out the new stimulus. Once a stimulus was added to the array, it remained present for the remainder of the task. Alzheimer's and Korsakoff's patients were impaired relative to controls on all five types of stimuli, but Huntington's patients showed impairment relative to controls on four of five stimulus types, with relative preservation of recognition of verbal stimuli.

The authors also asked subjects to recall the words from the words task at 15 seconds and 2 minutes after exposure. All patient groups were impaired relative to normals at 15 seconds; however, only the Alzheimer's patients demonstrated further drop in performance at 2 minutes. Further, Huntington's disease patients remembered more words at the 2-minute recall that they had not remembered at the 15-second recall than did Alzheimer's patients, Korsakoff's patients, or controls. This finding indicates that the Huntington's patients had more information available to them at the 15-second recall than they were able to express. This interpretation is also consistent with the fact that verbal-recognition memory was unimpaired in Huntington's patients relative to controls. The authors suggested that Huntington's patients had difficulty retrieving verbal information from memory stores. However, a retrieval deficit cannot apply to other forms of memory (faces, colors, position, design) because Huntington's disease subjects were equally impaired with the other patient groups on these types of stimuli. Although a primary visuo-spatial impairment could explain deficits on the faces, position, and design stimuli, it cannot explain decreased performance on the color stimuli. One possibility regarding the verbal task which was not mentioned by the authors is that the verbal-memory task relied more on a set of items already represented in semantic memory than did the other tasks. Thus, if an item already exists in semantic memory, then it is more likely to be recognized later than if no preexisting semantic-memory representation is present. Such an explanation is similar to explanations sometimes used in implicit-memory tasks (see below).

Kramer et al. (1988) gave the California Verbal Learning Test (Delis, Kramer, Kaplan, & Ober, 1987) to Huntington's patients, suspected Alzheimer's disease patients, and younger and older controls. The Huntington's patients were divided into mildly demented and moderately-to-severely demented groups. Both Hunting-ton's groups scored worse than normal controls on both recall and recognition measures of verbal memory. However, the moderately-to-severely demented Huntington's patients showed a significant in-crease in false-positive errors on the yes-no recognition trial, whereas the mildly demented Huntington's patients did not demonstrate such errors. This pattern of response on the recognition trial for the moderately-to-severely demented Huntington's patients was similar to that of the Alzheimer's patients. Yet, on delayed-recall trials, the Alzheimer's patients made significantly more intrusion errors than this Huntington's group. The authors attempted to explain this difference between more severely impaired Huntington's and Alzheimer's patients, suggesting that the Huntington's patients search less exten-sively through semantic memory during recall and therefore are less likely to have problems discriminating list from nonlist items. However, when they are presented with options, they have greater difficulty distinguishing list from nonlist items. Such a decreased tendency to search semantic memory could be a cause of retrieval deficits in Huntington's disease. Yet, these results again suggest that more than a retrieval deficit was operative since Huntington's patients performed more poorly than controls on the recognition trial.

Massman, Delis, Butters, Levin, and Salmon (1990) studied memory in Huntington's patients, Parkinson's patients, and controls, again using the California Verbal Learning Test. Although a wide variety of indices were evaluated, the findings have some relevance to retrieval deficit in Huntington's disease. Similarities between Parkin-son's and Huntington's patients included impaired immediate recall, inconsistency of learning across trials, deficient use of semantic clustering, increased intrusions, impaired recognition-memory per-formance, and normal retention of material across a delay. Hunting-ton's patients, however, did demonstrate some unique patterns of performance relative to Parkinson's patients and controls. They demonstrated less learning across trials, greater responding from the more recently presented items during learning trials, and more perseverations during recall. However, it was the Huntington's patients' ability to improve performance on a recognition as opposed to a recall trial that led the authors to conclude that Huntington's patients were showing a greater retrieval deficit than the other groups. They further suggested that the greater responding in the recency range of Huntington's patients reflected a lesser difficulty retrieving items from short-term than long-term memory. Since Huntington's patients have been shown to use cues provided for them (Granholm &

Butters, 1988), the authors surmised that their lack of semantic clustering indicated that the disease interferes with spontaneous utilization of effective encoding strategies. However, this difficulty must be considered unique to Huntington's patients' active application of learning strategies because they also show a normal sensitivity to semantic information in a release-from-proactive-interference paradigm (Beatty & Butters, 1986).

In summary: The best argument supporting the presence of retrieval deficits in Huntington's disease is relative improvement in recognition tasks over recall tasks (Butters et al., 1985; Butters et al., 1986; Kramer et al., 1990). Retrieval demands, of course, are reduced in recognition as opposed to recall tasks. The poor performance of Huntington's patients relative to controls on word-list generation has also been used to support the idea of a retrieval deficit (Butters et al., 1987; Butters et al., 1986). If defective word-list generation (e.g., Butters et al., 1987; Butters et al., 1986) suggests defective retrieval, it also suggests that memory deficits could exist in Huntington's disease without encoding or registration deficits because retrieval deficits exist in word-list generation where subjects are retrieving information from already encoded semantic-memory stores. Indeed, the weight of the evidence suggests that encoding deficits do not occur in Huntington's disease. Nonetheless, a lack of semantic clustering in word-list memory (Massman et al., 1990) means that Huntington's patients fail to use more active encoding strategies. Regarding retrieval, the hypothesis that Huntington's patients use less efficient strategies to search long-term stores (e.g., Butters et al., 1986; Kramer et al., 1988) would be quite consistent with a failure to use active encoding strategies. Since Huntington's patients still performed worse than controls on recognition-memory tasks (Butters et al., 1986; Butters et al., 1985), it must be concluded that other factors in addition to retrieval deficits are active. Some difficulty is preventing the normal amount of material from reaching long-term stores in the first place.

Studies of Procedural Learning

Results of procedural-memory studies with Huntington's disease patients have been somewhat mixed. Whether Huntington's patients show procedural learning may depend upon the nature of the task. Deficient procedural learning appears to be the rule for tasks involving at least some motor component; however, Huntington's patients perform more normally on some more cognitively oriented procedural-learning tasks with minimal motor components. It is unclear if the lack of a motor component or the possibility of declarative-memory mediation allows Huntington's patients to perform at near-normal levels on tasks like the Tower of Hanoi puzzle.

Martone et al. (1984) measured mirror-reading speed of word triads for Huntington's patients, alcoholic Korsakoff's patients, and controls. The idea behind this experiment was that mirror reading was a novel skill at which profiency would have to be acquired. The authors found that Huntington's patients did not improve in mirror-reading speed for novel word triads as much as controls or alcoholic Korsakoff's syndrome patients from the 2nd to the 3rd day of training. However, when word triads were repeated, controls and Huntington's patients seemed to gain a similar advantage, implying that they were able to recognize the repeated triads more easily than the novel ones. In contrast, Korsakoff's patients did not benefit as much from repeated words. Confirming the difference in memory for words, Huntington's patients were superior to Korsakoff's patients in a recognition-memory task for the words used in the mirror-reading task. The authors concluded that procedural learning could be dissociated from explicit memory. Huntington's disease patients had difficulty with procedural learning but not so much difficulty with explicit memory, while Korsakoff's patients had trouble with explicit memory but not procedural learning. The authors noted that the apparent lack of explicit-memory deficit in Huntington's patients was probably due to the use of recognition-memory tasks as opposed to recall tasks where they seem to have greater difficulty.

Butters et al. (1985) used the Tower of Hanoi puzzle to attempt to extend findings regarding procedural learning in patients with Huntington's disease. Because the ability to learn to solve the puzzle had previously been found intact in amnesic subjects, it was thought to be an example of procedural learning. The authors tested patients with early and advanced Huntington's disease, patients with diencephalic amnesia, a patient with amnesia after herpes encephalitis, and controls. Early Huntington's patients improved as much as controls across trials. Further, although advanced Huntington's patients failed to improve to the degree that normals and early Huntington's patients did, amnesic patients also failed to show the expected ability to improve their performance. Since the predicted dissociation in performance between amnesic and Huntington's patients did not materialize, the authors concluded that the Tower of Hanoi puzzle may sometimes be a flawed measure of procedural learning. More specifically, they suggested that impaired problem-solving abilities often associated with frontal lobe dysfunction might also interfere with learning more efficient ways of solving the puzzle. This could explain the failure of the diencephalic amnesics to improve on the task since many show difficulty on problem-solving tasks. However, it does not explain the intact learning of the early Huntington's patients on this task. If caudate degeneration is responsible for impaired procedural learning, then patients with early Huntington's disease should demonstrate some impairment because degeneration begins with the caudate nucleus. Thus, these findings are problematic for the procedural-learning hypothesis of Huntington's disease since this task is more free from motor constraints than the mirror-reading task of Martone et al. (1984).

Heindel, Butters, and Salmon (1988) studied motor learning in Huntington's disease patients, Alzheimer's disease patients, amnesic patients of mixed origin, and controls. The pursuit rotor that they used to perform the experiment requires subjects to keep a stylus on a small target on a rotating turntable. As subjects learn the task, the percent of time the stylus is kept on the target increases. Initial performance between groups was equated by adjusting the speed of the turntable, with the Huntington's patients requiring the slowest rotation. The Alzheimer's, amnesic, and control subjects all demonstrated significant improvement across trials, but the Huntington's patients showed significantly less improvement than the other groups. Since the Huntington's patients showing the least motor impairment and the Huntington's patients showing the most motor impairment demonstrated similar levels of improvement across trials, the authors suggested that motor impairment itself was not responsible for the lack of motor learning in the Huntington's group. Rather, their inability to generate new motor programs may have prevented them from adopting more effective modes of performance.

Heindel, Salmon, Shults, Walicke, and Butters (1989) replicated the findings of Heindel et al. (1988). Huntington's disease patients again showed impaired learning on the pursuit-rotor task, while normal controls and Alzheimer's patients did not show such a defect. There was a significant correlation between the degree of dementia and the lack of learning on the pursuit rotor in Huntington's disease; however, there was no correlation between movement symptoms and pursuit rotor learning in the Huntington's group. According to the authors, this latter finding suggests that difficulties in pursuit rotor learning were not the result of impaired movement per se, but represented a genuine learning difficulty. Demented but not nondemented Parkinson's disease patients also showed difficulty in pursuit-rotor learning.

In summary: The lack of impairment of early Huntington's patients on the Tower of Hanoi puzzle (Butters et al., 1985) suggests that Huntington's patients are not impaired on all procedural learning tasks. It seems safer to say that Huntington's patients have difficulty learning to perform tasks that involve a motor component such as the pursuit rotor (Heindel et al., 1988, 1989). Since the difficulty in motor-skill learning appears to be more closely correlated with severity of dementia as opposed to motor symptoms (Heindel et al., 1989), we must for now conclude that Huntington's patients' difficulty with motor-skill learning is not secondary to motor symptoms. However, even Heindel et al. (1989) could not entirely rule out motor deficits as a causative factor in Huntington's patients' inability to learn the motor skill. Since mirror reading of word triads (Martone et al., 1984) involves eye movements and since eye movements can be impaired in Huntington's disease, mirror reading may be considered to have a motor skill component (Crosson, 1986). This factor may be the common link between mirror reading and the pursuit rotor.

Studies of Implicit Memory

In some places (e.g., Squire, 1987) motor skills, procedural learning, and priming are considered to be variations of the same kind of learning. The fact that acquisition of motor skills and other procedural learning do not necessarily demonstrate similar impairments in Huntington's disease casts some doubt on whether these types of learning all have a similar substrate. Exploration of implicit memory (i.e., priming) for Huntington's disease also will shed some light on the issue of the similarities between these types of learning.

Shimamura, Salmon, Squire, and Butters (1987) studied implicit memory in patients with Alzheimer's disease, Huntington's disease, and alcoholic Korsakoff's syndrome. Each patient group had their own control group. On recall and recognition tests of explicit word-list memory, all patient groups were impaired relative to their respective controls, but the Huntington's patients performed better than the other patient groups on the verbal-recall task. For the stem-completion priming task, on the other hand, only the Alzheimer's group was impaired relative to its respective control group. The Huntington's group demonstrated normal stem-completion priming.

Smith et al. (1988) studied language functions and priming in patients with Huntington's disease. Language tests included word-list generation by letter and category, naming, and vocabulary. On all these tasks, Huntington's patients performed below controls, and in both word-list-generation tasks and the naming task, moderately demented Huntington's patients performed below the level of mildly demented Huntington's patients. The priming task involved judging how closely related word pairs were. Some pairs were related by function, and others were related in that the second was an exemplar of the category represented by the first (e.g., Bird--Robin). For each type of word pair, the words of some pairs were strongly associated, and the words of other pairs were moderately associated. Immediately after rating the word pairs, subjects were required to free-associate to words that included the first word of the word pairs. When findings were collapsed across conditions, all groups primed equally well. However, there was a Group X Strength interaction effect such that the difference in priming effect between strong and moderate associates decreased from controls to mildly demented Huntington's patients and decreased from mildly demented Huntington's patients to moderately demented Huntington's patients. Both groups of Huntington's patients seemed to show increased priming for moderately associated pairs, and the moderately demented Huntington's group showed decreased priming for strongly associated pairs.

The authors (Smith et al., 1988) concluded that their findings could be explained by changes in the Huntington's patients' ability to activate given associations and inhibit competing associations. According to Smith et al. (1988), associations between words that are activated by the priming paradigm also inhibit competing associations. Competing associations also exercise some degree of inhibition over the activated association. If Huntington's patients have a decreased inhibition for other associations, then the strong associations activated by priming will be less able to inhibit competing associations, and a reduction in the priming effects for strong associations would result. For moderate-level associations, some degree of activation from the priming task still leaves these associations in competition with other associations that have a stronger resting level of activation. However, a reduction in the inhibition of the primed association by the other competing associations would increase the net activation for the moderate-level association. Thus, this reduction in inhibition would explain why the gap between the strong and moderate associations decreases in priming for Huntington's disease. It should be noted that this explanation would be consistent with Wallesch and Papagno's (1988) theory of the participation of the striatum in language. The reader will recall that the latter authors hypothesized the role of the striatum in language to be selection of the strongest of parallel, competing associations for final expression (see Chapter 4).

In addition to testing pursuit-rotor performance in several patient groups, Heindel et al. (1989) gave a stem-completion priming task to their subjects. Although patients with Huntington's disease demonstrated impaired explicit memory in both recall and recognition tasks, they demonstrated intact stem-completion priming, replicating the findings of Shimamura et al. (1987). Demented Parkinson's patients did, however, show impaired stem-completion priming, a result I will discuss at greater length in the next section of this chapter.

In summary: Implicit memory in Huntington's disease, as measured by stem-completion priming, remains relatively intact (Heindel et al., 1989; Shimamura et al., 1987). This is true even though Huntington's patients demonstrate impairment in explicit memory. This further suggests that implicit memory may have a different neuroanatomic/neurochemical substrate than motor-skill learning since motor-skill learning is impaired in Huntington's disease but implicit memory is not. However, even though stem-completion priming is intact in Huntington's patients and paired-associates priming is generally at the same level as controls for Huntington's patients, the results of Smith et al. (1988) suggest that priming is not always totally unaffected by Huntington's disease. In paired-associates priming, it may be somewhat more difficult to prime pairs with strong associations but easier to prime pairs with moderate associations relative to normal performance. This finding suggests that for Huntington's disease some forms of priming may be influenced by changes in interactions within semantic networks.

Studies of Remote Memory

Deficits in remote memory have also been explored in Huntington's disease subjects. Although Huntington's patients do show impaired remote memory, they do not demonstrate the temporal gradient for remote memory shown by alcoholic Korsakoff's syndrome. As noted in Chapter 6, Albert et al. (1981) gave three remote-memory tasks to Huntington's patients, alcoholic Korsakoff's patients, and normal controls. The three tests were a task requiring identification of famous faces, a test requiring recall of well-known public events and persons from verbal questions, and a multiple-choice recognition test of famous events and persons. Subjects were tested for decades between the 1930s and the 1970s, inclusive. Korsakoff's patients showed greater impairment in identification of famous faces and in recall of public events for the 1960s and 1970s than for the 1930s and 1940s. This result confirmed a temporal gradient in retrograde amnesia for these patients. More germane to the current discussion, however, is the fact that Huntington's patients were impaired relative to controls, but they did not show a temporal gradient. They were equally impaired across decades for recall of public events and for identification of famous faces. On the latter two tests, when the subject was not able to recall the correct answer, cues were given. The cues alternated between phonemic cues and semantic cues. Both patient groups were helped by the cues less often than controls, but there was no difference between the two patient groups in this respect. All groups were able to use phonemic cues more effectively than semantic cues.

Beatty, Salmon, Butters, Heindel, and Granholm (1988) updated the famous-faces identification test and the public-events recall test of Albert et al. (1981), and they administered the tasks to patients with Huntington's disease, patients with Alzheimer's disease, and normal controls. Findings essentially replicated the findings of Albert et al. Huntington's patients performed significantly below controls, with no difference in impairment between decades. The Alzheimer's patients performed at a level below that of both controls and Huntington's patients. Alzheimer's patients, in contrast to Huntington's patients, did show a temporal gradient with greater difficulty with more recent items. The findings for both groups were similar for both cued and unaided recall, except that a "floor effect" prevented the temporal gradient in unaided recall from being found in Alzheimer's patients without additional analyses to correct for the floor effect. The authors suggested that impaired remote-memory performance for the Huntington's patients may be due to the same retrieval deficits that cause difficulty for new verbal learning and verbal-fluency tests.

Thus, patients with Huntington's disease do show impairment for remote memory; however, there is no temporal gradient in their recall. The importance of these findings is twofold: First, the lack of a temporal gradient distinguishes these patients with degenerative striatal disease from patients with Alzheimer's dementia or alcoholic Korsakoff's syndrome, who do demonstrate temporal gradients in remote memory. Along with data discussed above, this is another finding that suggests that different memory processes may be impaired for Huntington's patients than for Alzheimer's and Korsakoff's patients. Second, the equal impairment across decades has been used to support the hypothesis that Huntington's patients have a retrieval deficit since retrieval problems would be expected to show no difference for time period. However, the fact that Huntington's patients did not receive differential benefits from cueing relative to Korsakoff's patients (Albert et al., 1981) could be seen as problematic for this hypothesis unless Korsakoff's patients also have retrieval deficits. Cueing would provide a strategy with which Huntington's patients could search long-term stores. Since they appear to be deficient at developing their own search strategies (Butters et al., 1986; Kramer et al., 1988), Huntington's patients should have benefited from receiving cues if such a retrieval hypothesis were true.

Conclusions

Based on currently available data, some conclusions regarding the nature of memory deficits in Huntington's disease can be drawn. As noted above, the weight of the evidence does support the existence of a retrieval deficit. On the other hand, the bulk of evidence does not support a blanket encoding deficit; therefore, it is unlikely that retrieval deficits in Huntington's disease result from faulty encoding. Huntington's patients clearly differ from alcoholic Korsakoff's patients and patients with diencephalic infarcts in this respect. An alternative hypothesis is that Huntington's patients either fail to initiate or cannot devise effective strategies for searching long-term memory stores when recall is required, resulting in faulty retrieval. This hypothesis has not been tested sufficiently at this time.

Because Huntington's patients score below controls on recognition-memory tasks where retrieval demands are minimized, it is possible that, in addition to retrieval deficits, they do not store as much information in long-term memory as do neurologically unimpaired persons. The fact that they do not show abnormally rapid forgetting suggests that this is not a consolidation problem, but the fact that they require a greater stimulus exposure to approach normal memory performance on a recognition-memory task implies that initial registration of information into long-term stores is faulty. Whether faulty registration is related to attentional or short-term memory deficits is not clear. Further, inconsistent responding to the same repeated target words in a recognition-memory task may mean that Huntington's patients have trouble accessing information in long-term memory even under recognition conditions. Possible explanations for this phenomenon include weaker strength of long-term traces, attentional deficits, or fluctuating response bias. Further, even though data do not support a blanket encoding deficit, there is some evidence that Huntington's patients may fail to employ more active encoding strategies.

There is some evidence that Huntington's patients show deficient acquisition of motor skills, but this difficulty may be specific to motor skills. This would imply that the basal ganglia may play a role in acquisition of new motor skills. Up to this point in time, priming experiments indicate that the implicit-memory system may be relatively intact for Huntington's patients. Nonetheless, changes in interactions between semantic-memory-system components may have an impact on certain types of priming relying on these interactions, such as paired-associate priming. The fact that priming is disrupted in Alzheimer's patients indicates that this memory system can be impacted by some neurologic processes. Perhaps the relatively widespread involvement of association cortex is the key factor required to disrupt implicit memory.

Finally, it should be reiterated that Huntington's disease cannot be considered an absolute model of basal ganglia dysfunction, especially in the later stages where cortical involvement is clear. Although cortical atrophy does not precede caudate atrophy in Huntington's disease, changes in cortical activity may precede caudate atrophy. This hypothesis is based upon the assumption that caudate neuronal loss may be due to an overabundance of glutamate in the caudate nucleus. Glutamate is known to be the cortico-striatal neurotransmitter. Although cortical oversupply of glutamate to the striatum is just one hypothesis concerning the cause of Huntington's disease, the fact that this hypothesis is active indicates that Huntington's disease cannot be considered a simple model for striatal dysfunction. Even so, data indicate that Huntington's patients do not show memory patterns characteristic of frontal lobe dysfunction; thus, memory problems of Huntington's patients cannot be blamed on frontal deficits.

Memory Deficits in Parkinson's Disease

Although the major neuropathological feature of Parkinson's disease is degeneration of the dopaminergic neurons in pars compacta of the substantia nigra, Parkinson's disease most often has been considered a model for basal ganglia dysfunction. This viewpoint emphasizes the target organ of the nigrostriatal dopaminergic neurons rather than the origin. Since a minimal supply of dopamine is necessary for normal striatal functions, it does not seem unreasonable to focus on the target organ. Further, Parkinson's patients do show increased gliosis relative to controls in the caudate nucleus, putamen, medial and lateral pallidum, and thalamus, while showing a lack of such changes in the cortex (De la Monte, Wells, Hedley-Whyte, and Growdon, 1989).

Nonetheless, the use of Parkinson's disease patients as models of striatal dysfunction still can be questioned. There is some evidence that cognitive decline in Parkinson's disease is related to loss of neurons in the medial substantia nigra pars compacta (Rinne, Rummukainen, Paljarvi, & Rinne, 1989). Subcortically, these neurons project primarily to the caudate nucleus, but they also project to the hippocampus and cerebral cortex. It is unclear if decreased dopamine supply to the cortex could cause cognitive dysfunction without causing gliosis. Another problem relates to separating patients with pure Parkinson's disease from patients with Parkinson's disease plus Alzheimer's disease. Although this feat can be accomplished by doing postmortem examinations of morphological changes (e.g., Chui et al., 1986; De la Monte et al., 1989), such distinctions can be more problematic in the living patient (e.g., Huber et al., 1989). As a result, some patients with Alzheimer's changes in addition to Parkinsonian changes may be included in studies of Parkinson's disease. This unfortunate reality is particularly critical for examining memory problems. Thus, as we examine the literature relating Parkinson's disease and memory function, we must keep in mind these potential flaws in using Parkinson's disease as a model for striatal dysfunction.

In general, Parkinson's patients do show recall deficits relative to normals, but frequently their recognition is equivalent to that of controls. In accordance with the classical interpretations of this pattern, some investigators have taken this pattern as an indication of a retrieval deficit. Parkinson's subjects show differences from alcoholic Korsakoff's patients, including impairment on motor-skill learning and impairment on implicit-memory tasks (i.e., repetition priming). These findings are discussed in greater detail in the following paragraphs.

Flowers, Pearce, and Pearce (1984) tested recognition memory in patients with Parkinson's disease. Two tasks involved recognition memory for objects and histogramlike shapes; these tasks were performed within a multiple-choice recognition format. Two other tasks involved recognition memory for letter combinations, number combinations, and words on one task and recognition memory for abstract pictures on the other task; these latter two tasks were done in a yes-no recognition format. Both immediate and delayed recognition were done on all tasks. The level of performance was virtually identical for controls and Parkinson's patients on all tasks for immediate and delayed recognition. Parkinson's patients were less certain of their correct responses than normal controls. The authors cited a few earlier studies that indicated memory deficits in Parkinson's disease. They believed that the absence of memory deficits on the recognition-memory tasks indicated that Parkinson's patients had a retrieval deficit. They saw recall tasks as involving active manipulation of data and organization of a response, while recognition memory was seen as a more passive endeavor for subjects. Flowers et al. hypothesized these characteristics to be responsible for previous difficulties on some memory tasks for Parkinson's patients but normal recognition memory on their tasks.

One concept with some saliency for Parkinson's disease research is "subcortical dementia." According to Cummings and Benson (1984), subcortical dementia involves memory problems, slowed mentation, decreased problem solving, and an inability to use stored information. Aphasia, apraxia, and agnosia, which are commonly seen in Alzheimer's disease, are not present in subcortical dementia. Huber, Shuttleworth, Paulson, Bellchambers, and Clapp (1986) set out to verify this pattern of subcortical dementia by testing patients with Alzheimer's disease, patients with Parkinson's disease, and controls. Compared to controls, Parkinson's patients did not show impaired language, praxis, and orientation. However, Parkinson's patients did show impairment in memory, visuospatial skills, and depression relative to controls. Alzheimer's patients performed more poorly than Parkinson's patients and controls on all cognitive measures.

Huber, Shuttleworth, and Paulson (1986) made an effort to explore memory patterns in Parkinson's disease. They divided Parkinson's patients into those with impaired cognition, and those without impaired cognition as measured by the Mini Mental State Examination. A control group was also tested. Neither Parkinson's group differed from controls in short-term memory (i.e., digit span). A verbal paired-associate learning task was used to test other memory functions in this study. This test involves presenting words initially in pairs. During the recall phase, the first word of the pair is presented, and subjects are required to recall the second word of the pair. On paired-associate learning, controls performed better than unimpaired Parkinson's disease patients, who performed better than the cognitively impaired Parkinson's group. On remote memory, only the impaired Parkinson's group scored lower than both the unimpaired Parkinson's and control groups. Results imply that memory disorder progresses as Parkinson's disease progresses.

El-Awar, Becker, Hammond, Nebes, and Boller (1987) replicated the findings of Huber, Shuttleworth, and Paulson (1986) for a verbal paired-associates task. Parkinson's patients were impaired relative to normal controls but performed better than patients with Alzheimer's disease. Parkinson's patients also recalled fewer words used in the task after a delay, but they did not lose a greater amount of information across a delay than controls. Parkinson's patients appeared to have a bimodal distribution on the paired-associate task. One group of subjects performed more like the normal control group, and the other performed more like the Alzheimer's patients, though this more severely impaired Parkinson's group still did not lose more information than controls across a delay.

Sahakian et al. (1988) performed several visual-memory tests with Parkinson's patients, Alzheimer's patients, and controls. In general, they confirmed that Parkinson's patients were impaired relative to normals on tests of visual as well as verbal memory. However, it is of interest that Parkinson's patients had trouble matching visual stimuli even when they were presented together, indicating a visual-discrimination deficit. Alzheimer's patients did not show a visual-discrimination deficit. Thus, it was unclear for Parkinson's patients whether difficulty matching visual stimuli after a delay was due to a perceptual deficit or a memory deficit. Parkinson's patients who were later in the course of their illness and medicated also performed below controls on visual-pattern and spatial-recognition-memory tasks, similar to patients with Alzheimer's disease. Parkinson's disease patients who were recently diagnosed and not on medication were unimpaired relative to controls on the pattern and spatial-recognition-memory tasks, indicating that impairment in these tasks most likely progressed as the disease process advanced. Finally, subjects had to remember the position in which an abstract visual figure had been placed. For the most difficult version of this task, late Parkinson's patients showed a learning curve but still performed at below-normal levels. Recently diagnosed Parkinson's patients did not differ from controls on this task. Thus, Parkinson's patients appear to show visual-memory deficits as their disease progresses, but it is uncertain to what extent visual-memory problems might be related to visual-perceptual problems.

Unlike Sahakian et al. (1988), Freedman and Oscar-Berman (1989) found differences in visual and spatial learning between Alzheimer's and demented Parkinson's patients. The latter authors hid monetary rewards in one of two wells covered with lids. In the spatial-learning paradigm, the wells were covered with identical lids, and patients had to learn on which side the reward was placed. Once this learning took place, the side was reversed four times. In the visual-discrimination learning task, the authors hid monetary rewards under one of two lids with different visual patterns. Patients had to learn under which pattern the reward was hidden. After subjects learned this pattern, the pattern signifying reward was reversed four times. In the original spatial learning, there were no significant differences in trials to criterion between groups. However, demented Parkinson's patients and Alzheimer's patients had significantly more trials to criterion on reversal trials than either controls or nondemented Parkinson's patients. On the visual-learning task, Alzheimer's patients were impaired relative to all other groups on both original learning and on reversal trials. But, demented Parkinson's patients did not differ from controls on this task. Thus, demented Parkinson's patients seem to have problems with spatial-reversal learning but not with visual-discrimination learning.

Sagar, Sullivan, Gabrieli, Corkin, and Growdon (1988) showed Parkinson's patients, Alzheimer's patients, and controls 493 nouns. At varying intervals, pairs of words were presented. Sometimes in these pairs, a previously presented word was paired with a new word, and the patient had to recognize which word previously had been presented (content discrimination). Sometimes, two previously presented words were shown, and subjects had to pick the one presented most recently (recency discrimination). These trials were presented with a varying number of stimuli between the previously presented word(s) and the memory trial. Alzheimer's patients were impaired on both content and recency discriminations. In general, Parkinson's patients were impaired on recency but not content discriminations when scores were summed across the intervals between the presentation of a stimulus and its inclusion in a memory trial. However, Parkinson's patients were impaired on content discriminations at the shorter but not the longer intervals. The former deficit, an inability to make temporal-order judgments, was deemed to be due to frontal lobe dysfunction since patients with frontal dysfunction also show this type of deficit. Impaired content discrimination only at shorter intervals was deemed due to bradyphrenia (i.e., slow thinking). According to this hypothesis, registration of material in memory takes a longer time in Parkinson's patients so that content discriminations were normal only after longer intervals when registration increased. The authors suggested that this bradyphrenia was also due to frontal dysfunction.

Levin et al. (1989) gave a number of cognitive measures to Parkinson's patients whose symptom onset was 3 years or less from the testing. These early Parkinson's patients performed worse than normal controls on immedate and delayed recall of paragraphs, cued recall of paragraphs, and visual-recognition memory. Two frontal lobe measures, word-list generation and perseverations on card sorting, were also impaired relative to normal performance. Some measures of visual spatial functioning were also impaired. Measures of verbal and visual memory span and of auditory attention did not differ between Parkinson's patients and controls. Performance of subjects treated with anticholinergics did not differ from those not treated with anticholinergics. These findings were similar to earlier findings of Pillon et al. (1986), who found Parkinson's patients to score lower than controls on immediate paragraph recall, immediate paired-associates recall, and measures of frontal lobe dysfunction. The latter authors suggested that the pattern of performance in Parkinson's disease might be due to loss of striatal functions that in turn had the impact of reducing input to frontal cortex from cortico-striato-pallido-thalamo-cortical loops.

Bradley, Welch, and Dick (1989) found no differences between Parkinson's patients and controls in either verbal- or visual-memory span. However, subjects were also required to make decisions based upon a memorized path between two squares or based upon a memorized phrase. For the path, subjects merely had to indicate right or left turns along the path. For the short phrase, the decision involved the first letters. Both the path and the phrase tasks were thought by the authors to be tapping working memory. Each of these tasks was run under three dual-task-interference conditions: visual interference, auditory interference, and no interference. Parkinson's patients performed significantly below controls on the visual task, but not on the verbal task. The authors interpreted this finding to mean that visual-performance deficits in patients with Parkinson's disease were related to visual-working-memory deficits. Contrary to expectations, interference type had no effect on performance of the two groups.

As noted above, Kramer et al. (1989) studied memory in Huntington's, Parkinson's, and Alzheimer's patients using the California Verbal Learning Test. Parkinson's patients had a more rapid rate of forgetting than Huntington's subjects, but Huntington's patients had more repeated items (perseverations). Alzheimer's disease patients made more intrusions than either Huntington's or Parkinson's patients, had a more rapid rate of forgetting than Huntington's patients, and made more perseverations than the Parkinson's group. The authors concluded that Parkinson's and Huntington's patients demonstrated different patterns of verbal-memory deficit, suggesting that the underlying differences in neuropathology may be important for this aspect of cognition.

Studies of memory processes have not been as prevalent with Parkinson's disease as they have been with alcoholic Korsakoff's syndrome and Huntington's disease. Nonetheless, a few studies of Parkinson's patients have explored retrieval, motor and procedural learning, implicit memory, and temporal gradient in the retrograde memory compartment.

For example, as noted above, Massman et al. (1990) studied memory in Huntington's patients, Parkinson's patients, and controls using the California Verbal Learning Test. Similarities between Parkinson's and Huntington's patients included impaired immediate recall, inconsistency of learning across trials, deficient use of semantic clustering, increased intrusions, impaired recognition-memory performance, and normal retention of material across a delay. Huntington's patients, however, did demonstrate some impairments in performance relative to Parkinson's patients and controls. They demonstrated less learning across trials, greater responding from the more recently presented items during learning trials, and more perseverations during recall. Huntington's patients also demonstrated greater improvement in performance on the recognition trial as opposed to the recall trial. The authors surmised, however, that the differences between Parkinson's and Huntington's patients were differences of magnitude, not of kind. Thus, they assumed that Parkinson's patients had a less severe retrieval deficit than Huntington's patients.

Heindel et al. (1989) did incidental recall and recognition for separate lists on which subjects had rated their liking of items. These tasks were performed as a part of a larger experiment on stem-completion priming. Patients with Huntington's and Alzheimer's diseases were impaired relative to controls on both tasks. Nondemented Parkinson's patients equalled controls on both; however, demented Parkinson's patients were worse on recall but not recognition. This latter pattern of performance is further evidence of a retrieval deficit in Parkinson's disease. It is also evidence that the demented Parkinson's patients in this study were not merely cases of Alzheimer's plus Parkinson's disease.

Studies in procedural and motor learning and implicit memory have also been applied to patients with Parkinson's disease. For example, Heindel et al. (1989) studied stem-completion priming and pursuit-rotor performance for Huntington's, Parkinson's, and Alzheimer's patients. As noted above, Huntington's patients were impaired on pursuit-rotor learning but not on stem-completion priming. Alzheimer's patients showed the opposite pattern: impairment on stem-completion priming and intact pursuit-rotor performance relative to controls. Demented Parkinson's patients, on the other hand, demonstrated impaired performance for both the motor-learning and priming tasks. Nondemented Parkinson's patients did not differ from controls on either task. Pursuit-rotor performance was correlated with level of dementia, not with motor symptoms. The initial speed of the turntable, which was individually determined for each subject, was not a factor in motor learning. Because Alzheimer's patients had difficulty with stem-completion priming, this task was considered cortically mediated, and since Huntington's patients had difficulty with motor learning on the pursuit rotor, this task was considered to be mediated by the basal ganglia. Since demented Parkinson's patients differed from Alzheimer's patients on other dimensions, the most logical explanation for these findings is that both cortical and basal ganglia systems were affected by loss of dopaminergic input.

Crawford, Henderson, and Kennard (1989) investigated saccadic (rapid) eye movements from a central fixation point to a peripheral target. Targets and fixation points consisted of light-emitting diodes. Offset of the fixation diode was the signal for subjects to move their eyes. In one condition, the target was illuminated at the offset of the fixation diode. In another condition, there was some temporal overlap between the onset of the target and the offset of the fixation point. In the final condition, the target diode flashed briefly while the fixation diode remained illuminated, and subjects had to saccade to the location where they remembered the target to have been. Eye movements elicited by the peripheral targets did not differ between Parkinson's patients and controls. However, saccades to the to-be-remembered target were dysmetric in Parkinson's patients relative to controls, that is, the initial (primary) saccade tended to "undershoot" the target location, and a greater number of subsequent saccades was necessary to reach the proper location. Since Parkinson's subjects did reach the remembered position as accurately as normals after the larger number of saccades, the dysmetria was not due to a loss of information about target location. One hypothesis offered by the authors was that Parkinson's patients have greater difficulty when saccades have to be internally generated (to a remembered position) than when they are elicited by an external stimulus. This hypothesis is consistent with recent hypotheses about the role of the supplementary motor area, anterior cingulate, and basal ganglia in movement and cognition (Brown & Marsden, 1988a, 1988b; Early et al., 1989b; Goldberg, 1985). Although one should be careful about extending this paradigm to standard memory studies, it could be conjectured that recall paradigms are more difficult in basal ganglia dysfunction because they require generation of a response from an internal data base, whereas recognition memory simply requires response to an external stimulus. (This hypothesis will be explored further in the next chapter.)

Finally, remote-memory functions have been investigated in Parkinson's disease. Freedman, Rivoira, Butters, Sax, and Feldman (1984) gave the famous-faces task to demented and nondemented Parkinson's patients as well as to controls. Demented Parkinson's patients were impaired relative to controls, but there was no evidence of a temporal gradient across decades. On the other hand, Sagar, Cohen, Sullivan, Corkin, and Growdon (1988) performed a rather complex study of remote memory with different findings. Subjects were shown pictures of well-known public events in the five decades from the 1940s through the 1980s. In a "yes-no" recognition task, they simply had to distinguish the well-known events from nonfamous events. In the recall task, subjects had to identify the event, its general content, its specific scenario, and its date. In the multiple-choice recognition format, subjects merely had to distinguish the event from two other possibilities. There was also a multiple-choice verbal questionnaire about public events during these decades. Further, personal remote memory was tested by having subjects give and date a memory that they associated with each of ten common nouns. For the yes-no recognition of pictures, Parkinson's patients were impaired relative to controls only for the

1980s events, but Alzheimer's subjects were impaired on other decades as well. For recall of event-related information, Parkinson's patients were impaired for only the 1970s and the 1980s, while Alzheimer's subjects showed impairment for all five decades. However, for dating the events, both patient groups showed impairment across all decades. For the multiple-choice format, Parkinson's patients were unimpaired in recognizing the content of events, but they were impaired in recognizing the dates. No temporal gradient existed for the date recognition. Both Parkinson's and Alzheimer's patients demonstrated at least some deficit in generating personal memories, and more memories came from earlier decades for both patient groups. Both groups also showed inconsistency in dating personal memories when retested. The severity of remote-memory deficit was correlated with the severity of dementia. Thus, in this latter study, Parkinson's patients did show a temporal gradient in recall for well-known events and in recall of personal events. Since the deficits did not exist for recognition of content of events, the authors surmised that there was a retrieval deficit that selectively affected the most recent memories. The authors also concluded that the consistent difficulty of Parkinson's subjects to date memories was related to temporal judgments and sequencing of information, which are impaired with frontal lobe dysfunction.

Conclusions

Parkinson's patients generally demonstrate intact memory span, but other verbal- and visual-memory tasks yield deficits. To some degree, visual-memory deficits may be related to deficits in visual perception. Memory deficits are more severe when cognition is impaired enough to warrant a diagnosis of dementia. Some have interpreted this latter finding as indicating progression of memory deficit during the course of the disease; however, this interpretation does not take into account the possibility that demented and nondemented Parkinson's patients may be separate groups, and that the nondemented patients may never develop dementia. The fact that Parkinson's patients demonstrate a normal degree of information loss over delays indicates that their memory problems are not due to a consolidation deficit. Evidence for a retrieval deficit has been found. One hypothesis states that this retrieval deficit is due to parkinsonian patients' inability to generate responses based upon an internal data base.

Like Huntington's patients, demented Parkinson's patients demonstrate difficulty in motor learning. This motor-learning deficit is more closely related to ratings of dementia than to ratings of motor dysfunction. Unlike Huntington's patients, on the other hand, Parkinson's patients are also impaired on stem-completion priming. This fact may mean that both cortical and subcortical dysfunction are present in Parkinson's disease with dementia. Finally, results considering a temporal gradient in remote memory for Parkinson's subjects were equivocal.

Memory Deficits in Other Basal Ganglia Disorders

Memory functions have been examined in other disorders involving the basal ganglia. Progressive supranuclear palsy was prominent in early conceptualizations of subcortical dementias, where forgetfulness was listed as one symptom (Albert, Feldman, & Willis, 1974). Occasional studies have investigated memory deficits in Wilson's disease and after subcortical stroke.

Progressive supranuclear palsy is a degenerative disease involving the basal ganglia, the cerebellum, and brain-stem nuclei. Deficits include defects of ocular gaze, axial dystonia and rigidity, spasticity of the face, bradykinesia and rigidity, frontal lobe signs, and postural instability with a tendency to fall backward (Lees, 1990). Although Albert et al. (1974) noted forgetfulness to be a part of the cognitive syndrome, Litvan, Grafman, Gomez, and Chase (1989) noted there has been some controversy regarding the impairment of memory in this disorder. For example, Maher, Smith, and Lees (1985) found memory deficits in only 37% of their population, but they did not test age- and education-matched controls. Two other recent studies have shown clear evidence of memory impairment in this disorder.

Pillon, Dubois, Lhermitte, and Agid (1986) studied memory and other deficits in patients with progressive supranuclear palsy, Parkinson's disease patients, Alzheimer's disease patients, and controls. Progressive supranuclear palsy patients were impaired in paragraph memory and paired-associate learning. They were the only patient group to show a lower digit-span test than normals; however, it was the impairment on frontal lobe tasks that was the most significant nonmemory change. This is consistent with a finding by Maher et al. (1985) that approximately 70% of their patients demonstrated impairment on frontal tasks.

Litvan et al. (1989) compared the performance of progressive supranuclear palsy patients to that of controls on memory tasks. The patients demonstrated deficits relative to controls in memory for both paragraphs and lists. The progressive supranuclear palsy patients were worse than controls in recalling word triads after distraction-filled intervals of up to 36 seconds, and their recognition memory for these words was also worse than controls. The authors interpreted these findings to represent defective consolidation of information. However, their use of the term *consolidation* is different than the usage in this volume. A failure of memory in such a short period of time more likely represents defective registration of information in long-term memory. This issue will be discussed further in the next chapter. Although recognition memory for a 15-word list was also worse than controls, Litvan et al. found the patients' performance to be better on recognition memory than recall (p. 676). Further, patients had impaired word-list generation. The authors took the latter two facts to mean progressive supranuclear palsy patients have impaired retrieval of information from long-term memory. While this conclusion seems reasonable, the fact that recognition was still significantly impaired means that initial registration was probably impaired as well. Of further interest is that scanning of information held in short-term memory appeared intact. Subjects saw sets of 1 to 6 digits shown for 200 msec per digit. Then they were presented a single probe digit and were required to respond as to whether it had been a member of the previously displayed set. Although patients were slower in reacting, mean reaction times did not increase significantly more for patients compared to controls when the number of digits in the set increased. This means that the increased reaction times were more a function in differences in output than in processing speed. Thus, the data of Litvan and colleagues indicate that progressive supranuclear palsy patients have deficits in initial registration of material in long-term memory and in subsequent retrieval of information from long-term stores. The fact that retrieval from semantic-memory stores was also impaired indicates that the retrieval deficit was not merely a function of deficient encoding since this type of retrieval does not depend upon recent encoding operations.

Wilson's disease is another entity affecting basal ganglia functions. It is an autosomal recessive hereditary disorder. Because symptoms result from a genetic abnormality in the liver's excretion of copper in the diet, Wilson's disease is also known as hepatolenticular degeneration. Copper diffuses from the blood to many organs, including the brain, where it affects the basal ganglia. Most frequently, the disease can be controlled pharmacologically (Medalia, Isaacs-Glaberman, & Scheinberg, 1988).

Medalia et al. (1988) compared cognitive functioning in symptomatic Wilson's disease patients, Wilson's disease patients whose symptoms were controlled by medication, and neurologically normal controls. Standard clinical neuropsychological measures were used. Symptomatic Wilson's disease patients had lower Wechsler Memory Quotients than both asymptomatic patients and controls; however, there were no group differences in the paired-associates, paragraph-memory, and geometric-designs subtests. It should be noted that delayed recall was not tested; therefore, the authors did not have a sensitive measure of long-term memory. The symptomatic group was also lower than controls on nonverbal intelligence, visuo-motor speed, and a dementia scale. No group differences existed on verbal intelligence, naming, word-list generation by category, or a conceptual task thought to reflect frontal lobe functioning. The authors suggested that motor functions and memory deficits accounted for the group differences, but differences on the Wechsler Memory Scale could have come from attentional or short-term memory deficits.

Unfortunately, studies of memory functions after vascular lesion of the basal ganglia have been far less prolific than studies of language function or even neglect after these lesions. A recent study by Weiller, Ringlestein, Reiche, Thron, and Buell (1989) focusing on cerebral blood flow and cognitive deficits after striato-capsular infarcts is an example of a study that focused on language deficits and neglect, but not on memory. Of course, the existence of aphasia and neglect after basal ganglia lesions would complicate memory testing. For verbal memory, the ability to recall material would be confounded with language expression, and the ability to encode and register verbal material would be confounded with the ability to linguistically decode the material in the first place. Likewise, neglect could interfere with the ability to accurately perceive visual patterns, resulting in distorted visual-memory encoding. Neglect could further prevent accurate production of designs from memory. As noted in Chapter 2, a further complication in interpreting data from vascular lesions of the basal ganglia is that they typically damage surrounding white matter pathways that could be involved in transmitting information or regulatory functions between different centers.

Nonetheless, a few studies of basal ganglia vascular lesions have provided information relevant to memory functions. For example, Risse, Rubens, and Jordan (1984) studied verbal-memory span and list learning in 20 patients with aphasia. Ten patients had either basal ganglia or frontal lobe lesions, and ten had posterior lesions involving at least portions of the posterior language cortex. Although many of the former had a nonfluent aphasia acutely, all but one patient in both groups were fluent at the time of testing. Testing was done in the chronic phase. List learning was tested using a nine-item version of the selective reminding task, and memory span was tested using multiple versions of digit-span tests. On list learning, patients with posterior lesions showed adequate learning though their performance was below that of controls. Patients with frontal and/or basal ganglia lesions showed virtually no learning curve, starting with an average of approximately three items and ending learning trials with an average of approximately four items. They tended to rely upon memory for items that had just been given to them, as opposed to long-term storage. They performed below the posterior aphasic patients and controls after a 60-minute delay, but did not differ from either group when a recognition memory procedure was used. On the memory-span tests, results were reversed, with posterior aphasic patients demonstrating a deficit and the frontal and/or basal ganglia patients showing no difference from controls. The importance of these results are twofold. The authors hypothesized that the frontal/basal ganglia lesions disconnected the frontal lobes from the hippocampal-diencephalic memory complex. Given evidence discussed above, a more adequate hypothesis might be that the frontal cortex and basal ganglia are together involved in circuitry having a bearing upon retrieval functions. The second conclusion from these results is that earlier suggestions that short-term and long-term memory systems could be anatomically and functionally dissociated (e.g., Warrington & Shallice, 1969) were confirmed.

Pozzilli, Passafiume, Bastianello, D'Antona, and Lenzi (1987) studied two cases of caudate lesion. The first case had bilateral hemorrhages of the head of the caudate nucleus extending into the anterior limb of the internal capsule, and, on the left side, laterally into the putamen and medially into the lateral ventricle. At discharge 4 weeks after stroke, he evidenced abulic behavior (i.e., emotional flatness, decreased spontaneity, and decreased motivation and initiation). Sixteen months later, his scores on verbal and nonverbal memory span, verbal memory, and visual memory were all within normal limits. His SPECT scan demonstrated decreased blood flow in the frontal cortex, particularly marked in the left hemisphere. The second case had a unilateral hemorrhage of the left head of the caudate nucleus with medial extension into the lateral ventricle. Although his verbal and nonverbal memory span and his visual memory were roughly equal to that of controls, his story memory, paired-associates memory, and his verbal-list generation were below that of controls. Language was relatively preserved; therefore, his memory deficits appeared to be in the realm of long-term memory, perhaps with a retrieval deficit. His decreased blood flow was present in the frontal lobe like the first case who had no memory deficit, but the second case also had decreased blood flow in the left temporal and parietal lobes. Perhaps these latter changes were a prerequisite for the existence of chronic long-term memory deficits. Both vascular lesion studies cited herein point to at least a retrieval component to memory dysfunction after vascular lesion of the basal ganglia.

Conclusions

Thus, results of studies of progressive supranuclear palsy, Wilson's disease, and vascular lesions of the basal ganglia add some support to the notion that the basal ganglia are involved in memory. This evidence is important since it comes from divergent pathological entities. Because none of the entities affecting the human basal ganglia are limited to these structures, evidence of memory disturbance from one source alone can be questioned because of the involvement of other structures. However, when considering structures other than the basal ganglia, each of these disease entities (Huntington's disease, Parkinson's disease, progressive supranuclear palsy, Wilson's disease, vascular lesion) involves different cortical or subcortical structures in different ways, leaving the disturbance of basal ganglia functions the most salient common factor between them. In this sense, the weight of the evidence does suggest basal ganglia involvement in memory.

More importantly, there is a common thread running throughout studies of the basal ganglia. This thread points to deficits in the retrieval of information from long-term memory stores. Retrieval deficits were suggested in progressive supranuclear palsy (Litvan et al., 1989) and in vascular lesion (Pozzilli et al., 1987; Risse et al., 1984), adding to similar evidence in Huntington's and Parkinson's diseases, as discussed above. Another common thread in progressive supranuclear palsy (Maher et al., 1985; Pillon et al., 1986) and vascular lesion (Pozzilli et al., 1987) was the presence of deficits on frontal lobe tasks, similar to those found in Huntington's and Parkinson's diseases. However, the existence of such frontal lobe deficits in Wilson's disease has been questioned (Medalia et al., 1988). Risse and colleagues' (1984) data suggests that retrieval functions might be linked to the cortico-striato-pallido-thalamo-cortical loops, which are partially closed by thalamic projections back to the frontal cortex. However, the data of Pozzilli et al. (1987) suggests that input of posterior cortical areas into these loops may be involved in memory as well.

Findings on short-term memory are not so clear. Pillon et al. (1986) found decreased verbal memory span for progressive supranuclear palsy patients. Yet, Litvan and colleagues (1989) found normal scanning of short-term memory in the same population of patients. Vascular lesion studies (Pozzilli et al., 1987; Risse et al., 1984) also suggest that memory span may be relatively intact in cases of basal ganglia lesion. Studies using brief distraction-filled intervals may be more an indication of long-term memory registration, as discussed in the next chapter; therefore, these later studies cannot be used to assess short-term memory. Future studies should investigate both short-term memory functioning and long-term memory processes more.

8

Subcortical Functions and Memory Theories

It is interesting to compare the role of theory in the study of subcortical language functions versus its role in the study of subcortical memory functions. Much of the literature on subcortical language functions has amounted primarily to clinical descriptions of language after subcortical lesions; studies from this literature that have been theoretically driven are the exception. Nonetheless, the concept of thalamic participation in semantic processing has arisen from these clinical observations. Conversely, the literature on subcortical memory functions frequently has been derived from theoretical concepts. Most often these concepts have been borrowed from the cognitive literature, with the implicit memory literature being a possible exception.

The existence of adequate numbers of patients with subcortical involvement and memory deficits, such as patients with alcoholic Korsakoff's syndrome, Huntington's disease, or Parkinson's disease, is one factor making a more theoretically driven approach to memory possible. Extensive theoretically oriented studies have been accomplished, especially on the former two populations. The recent subcortical language literature, in contrast, consists primarily of patients with subcortical cerebral vascular accidents. Because of the unpredictability of the latter events, it is difficult to organize an extended line of research around such patients.

It is curious, then, that unified theories of subcortical participation in language have been developed (e.g., Crosson, 1985; Crosson & Early, 1990; Wallesch & Papagno, 1988), while no comprehensive theories of subcortical participation in memory have been developed. In other words, we lack a theory regarding the problem of how temporal lobe structures, diencephalic structures, basal ganglia structures, and basal forebrain structures function together to create permanent memories and later retrieve them. At least two reasons account for this lack of a unified theory of subcortical memory processes. First, there is no widely accepted theory of cortical involvement in memory upon which to build. It is obvious that subcortical structures do not perform memory or language functions in isolation from cortical activity. Indeed, in many respects, subcortical functions may subserve cortical functions, at least according to some theoretical accounts (e.g., Crosson, 1985). The fact that cortical theories of language functions have been developed and debated back to the time of Broca and Wernicke has provided a context in which to consider subcortical functions in language. No such context has existed in memory. Second, theorists concerned with memory face a daunting complexity of issues concerning memory. Issues regarding multiple versus single stores, the nature of short-term memory, and the structure and operation of long-term memory are still hotly debated, and the underlying concepts are still in the process of formulation. Thus, it is difficult to apply the knowledge generated by the subcortical-memory literature to a set of concepts that are currently not entirely adequate and still in flux.

Whereas in Chapter 4 on language theory I spent most of the space discussing subcortical language theories, such a discussion obviously will not be possible in the current chapter. An attempt to develop a unified theory of subcortical memory functions would be premature. Rather, it seems appropriate here to ask the question: What do subcortical studies tell us about memory theory? In order to answer this question, in the first portion of this chapter I will cover two theories of memory function. One "multiple-stores" approach to memory (Atkinson & Shiffrin, 1968) has had substantial influence on studies of subcortical memory functions; the other (Cowan, 1988) is a more recent attempt to bring memory theory into agreement with the cognitive literature on memory. One focus of this discussion will be the relationship of short-term and long-term memory processes. After I review these theories, I will discuss them in light of the subcortical-memory literature. Subsequently, I will discuss long-term memory processes. In particular, I shall explore levels of processing (Craik & Lockhart, 1972) and how the concepts of attention and intention (e.g., Heilman, Bowers, Valenstein, & Watson, 1987; Heilman & Watson, 1989; Watson et al., 1981) may be applied to memory. After summarizing the theoretical import of the subcortical literature for memory theory, I will make a few closing remarks, and draw some parallels between memory and language.

Two Cognitive Models of Memory

Many of the concepts and models used to study memory disturbance were originally developed in cognitive psychology. One early influential model was that of Broadbent (1958). He distinguished different types of memory stores that operated sequentially to eventually produce a more lasting record of incoming information. This information was first held in a brief store of very limited duration. From there it was passed through a limited-capacity filter, and from this filter, selected information was passed into long-term storage. Atkinson and Shriffrin (1968) presented a similar but more elaborate model, as I shall discuss momentarily. The Atkinson and Shiffrin model involved multiple stores: a brief sensory register, a short-term store, and a long-term store, with only the latter providing a lasting record of the input. Since 1968 much of the cognitive literature has focused on questions related to this model, such as: Is there one memory store or multiple stores? Does information have to be sequentially processed through different stores? What other processes might be necessary to explain memory phenomena? One recent alternative model by Cowan (1988) proposes that short-term memory is the subset of long-term memory which contains currently activated features. Both the Atkinson and Shriffrin (1968) and Cowan (1988) models are discussed below.

The Atkinson and Shriffrin (1968) Model

Atkinson and Shiffrin's model can be seen as an elaboration of Broadbent's (1958) model. The essentials have been represented in Figure 8-1. Atkinson and Shiffrin postulate three types of stores: a sensory register, a short-term store, and a long-term store. Within each store reside certain control processes that determine how memory is processed within that particular store and how it is passed on to the next level of storage. Incoming information is first processed in single modality (i.e., auditory, visual, tactile) sensory stores. These sensory stores can hold large quantity of information for a very brief period of time. Control processes for the sensory register include selection of which sensory-input channel(s) to attend to, selection of parts of the information array for transfer to the short-term store, and transfer of information to the short-term store.

Information from these sensory buffers next feeds into a short-term store that probably has a limited capacity. A number of control processes reside within short-term memory; these processes affect the probability that information will be stored and the way in which it is stored in long-term memory. For example, rehearsal is a means by

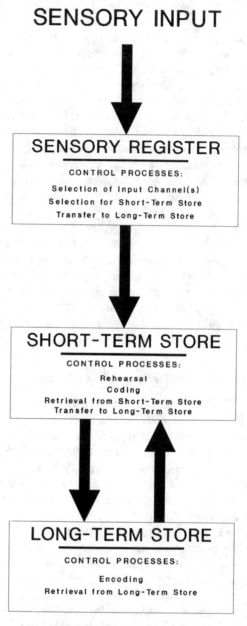

Figure 8-1. Diagram of Atkinson and Shiffrin's memory model. Note that the only access to long-term memory is through short-term memory. Note also that various processes by which information in short-term memory is manipulated are assumed to reside within short-term memory.

which information can be held in short-term memory for a longer period of time, preventing decay. According to the model, the probability of long-term storage is increased if items can be held in short-term storage longer. Another control process involves coding, that is, the alteration of information in the short-term store in accordance with other information retrieved from the long-term store. Two other control processes involve search and retrieval of information from short-term storage, and transfer of information to long-term storage.

Atkinson and Shiffrin only elaborated on one route for accessing long-term stores through short-term memory. Information must first be processed by short-term memory before it can be placed into long-term (permanent) storage. If impairment of short-term memory limits or prevents information from being held in short-term storage, then that information will be blocked for the most part from reaching long-term memory. Since items also are retrieved from long-term stores into short-term memory, short-term memory is the first place where incoming information can interact with information from long-term memory. Such material from long-term stores is often important for interpreting incoming information and for encoding the new information for long-term memory. Control processes in the long-term store determine how the information is stored (i.e., encoding) and guide searches of long-term memory during retrieval.

Baddeley (1990) has discussed some of the difficulties with the Atkinson and Shriffrin model of memory: (1) For example, he cited evidence that the amount of time information is held in short-term memory does not always increase the probability that it will be transferred to long-term storage. (2) Baddeley and Hitch (1977) had subjects who were being tested on free recall for a list of unrelated words recite sets of digits. The recitation of digits interfered with primacy but not recency effects. Recency effects refer to the greater probability for items at the end of a list to be recalled than items in the middle of the list, and this effect is assumed to be due to the fact that words at the end of the list can be held in short-term as well as long-term memory. According to the Atkinson and Shiffrin model, the digits should have competed with recent list items for short-term memory capacity. Thus, their model would have predicted a reduction or abolition of the recency effect. Instead, recitation of digits interfered with recall of the items at the beginning of the list, which should have been kept in long-term storage. (3) Finally, the fact that patients with reduced memory spans can show normal long-term retention (Risse et al., 1984; Shallice & Warrington, 1970) calls into question the proposition that short-term memory processing is the only road to long-term storage.

Baddeley (1990) noted that when problems with the Atkinson and Shiffrin model became apparent, the field of memory research became fragmented, and multiple models of short-term memory were developed. Occasionally, a paradigm such as Craik and Lockhart's (1972) levels of processing would draw significant interest, but general agreement on the nature and relationship of memory processes is still lacking. Most models of memory that have arisen since Atkinson and Shiffrin's influential theory still have some flaws.

The Cowan Model

One attempt to integrate cognitive literature into a more current memory model was produced by Cowan (1988). This schema of memory maintains the same basic concepts as the Atkinson and Shiffrin paradigm, but suggests considerably different relationships between components. Cowan's ideas have some distinct advantages over those of Atkinson and Shiffrin, but I can only discuss them briefly. Readers wishing to peruse the evidence behind Cowan's model are referred to the original article.

Cowan's model is represented in Figure 8-2. According to Cowan, short-term memory is the subset of long-term memory, consisting of the items within long-term memory that are in a heightened state of activation. Short-term memory has the same limited capacity that is frequently assumed in works written over the last few decades. However, unlike the creators of many other conceptualizations during this time, Cowan did not equate the contents of awareness with short-term memory. Instead, Cowan postulated that the focus of awareness at any one point in time is a subset of short-term memory (i.e., a subset of those items in a heightened state of activation). The contents of the focus of awareness may be limited to two or three items, whereas the contents of short-term memory may be limited to approximately seven items.

The first brief stage of sensory memory is considered to be separate from short-term and long-term memory. Previous models such as Atkinson and Shiffrin's (1968) suggested that specific bits of information were selected from sensory memory for further processing. In Cowen's model, instead of active selection of information from sensory memory for further processing, unwanted channels of information are assumed to be habituated, and therefore unattended. How, then, can information enter the focus of awareness? This can happen in several ways: In one way, a change in a habituated channel will call attention temporarily to that channel. Habituation is assumed to occur because the system builds a model of the unattended channel.

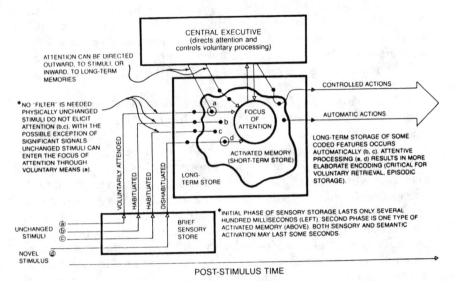

Figure 8-2. Schematic representation of Cowan's (1988) model. Short-term memory is assumed to be a subset of items within long-term memory, and the focus of attention is assumed to be a subset of items within short-term memory. Brief sensory memory processes and the central executive are assumed to be distinct from long-term memory. From "Evolving Conceptions of Memory Storage, Selective Attention, and Their Mutual Constraints within the Human Information-Processing System," by N. Cowan, 1988, *Psychological Bulletin, 104*: 180. Copyright by the American Psychological Association. Reprinted by permission.

As long as information on a channel is consistent with the internal model, habituation continues. However, a mismatch between information in a channel and the internal model causes orientation to the channel. This is how novel information will demand attention. In a second way, a stimulus of predetermined importance to the organism (e.g., one's own name) enters a channel, and then demands active attention. In a third way, attention can be voluntarily directed to a channel of information.

This voluntary direction of attention is accomplished by a central executive, conceptualized by Cowan as a conglomeration of related processes that not only direct attention, but also control voluntary processing of information. According to this model, attentive processing (i.e., processing within the focus of attention) results in more elaborate encoding of information which is critical for what Cowan calls voluntary retrieval (i.e., explicit recall). Attention can be directed to external or internal stimuli. The central executive can scan short-term memory to select items to which attention may be directed. In addition to voluntarily directing attention, the central executive performs at least the following functions: maintenance of information in short-term memory through rehearsal, search of long-term memory to accomplish more elaborate storage of items in short-term memory, and problem-solving activities.

The relationships between long-term memory, short-term memory, and the focus of attention in this model are critical. First, it should be noted that information occurring in habituated (i.e., nonattended) channels does enter short-term memory even though it does not become the focus of attention. Information entering short-term memory without being the deliberate focus of attention might provide the basis for what this volume calls implicit memory. As just noted, information that does enter the focus of attention (i.e., becomes the subject of effortful processing) can become available to explicit (as well as implicit) recall at a later point in time. Thus, amnesias such as those created in diencephalic lesion are seen as defects in an effortful processing system that admits information into the focus of attention. In Cowan's model, implicit memory can be maintained because it does not require this effortful processing.

It should also be noted that information directed toward the focus of attention either from external sources or from the central executive will activate related information already in long-term storage, thereby bringing the relevant information from long-term storage into short-term memory, and potentially into the focus of attention. Thus, in contrast to the Atkinson and Shiffrin (1968) model, relevant information in long-term stores is activated prior to the beginning of effortful processing.

Two kinds of actions can be generated from short-term (i.e., activated) memory. In general, actions result from the "activation of premotor and motor pathways in short-term storage." In the case of voluntary actions, the necessary information has been activated through the central executive. In the case of automatic (i.e., involuntary) actions, the impetus is spontaneous activation in long-term storage. Sometimes, both involuntary and voluntary actions can occur simultaneously, in some instances causing errors in output.

Comparison of the Atkinson and Shiffrin and Cowan Models

Both models of memory discussed above focused on the relationship between short-term and long-term memory. Indeed, a major distinction between the two models is that the Atkinson and Shiffrin model considered short-term memory as a separate entity controlling access to long-term memory. Cowan, in contrast, considered short-term memory to be the subset of items in long-term memory that are in a heightened state of activation. A further distinction can be made on the basis of processing functions. Atkinson and Shiffrin assumed many of these functions to reside within the short-term and long-term stores, whereas Cowan placed many of the same functions in the central executive, which lies outside the realm of both short-term and long-term memory. A third distinction between the two models is that incoming information in the Cowan model activates related items in long-term memory, which by virtue of the increased activation become a part of short-term memory. In the Atkinson and Shiffrin model, incoming information must first be registered in the short-term store before short-term memory retrieves related information from long-term memory. Finally, Cowan indicated that some information in a heightened state of activation (i.e., in short-term storage) becomes the focus of effortful processing (i.e., within the focus of attention) while other information does not. As I shall discuss further below, this distinction is important for procedural and implicit memory. Atkinson and Shiffrin made no such distinction within short-term memory.

What the Subcortical Literature Indicates about Models of Memory

Prior to exploring the implications of the subcortical literature for these theories of memory, I need to make a few preliminary remarks. Although not necessarily intended by the authors of either theory, when these models are proliferated, there is some tendency to reify processes into entities. For the purposes of translating these cognitive theories into neuropsychological constructs, the distinction between process and entity should be made clear. The brain structures involved in memory (diencephalic and basal forebrain structures, basal ganglia, hippocampus, amygdala, cortical structures), of course, fall into the category of entity. Upon autopsy, these structures can be found, examined microscopically, etc. In the sense that memories stored for brief or longer periods can be accessed by the person storing them, such memories might also be considered a kind of cognitive entity. However, when we talk about sensory, short-term, or long-term memory, these are best conceptualized as processes that produce specific memories rather than entities.

If we avoid the reification of these processes into entities, then we can focus on how different components of a system work together during the process of short-term or long-term memory. This may seem like a trivial distinction, but consider the following. If one conceptualizes short-term and long-term memory as entities, then one begins to look for the neuroanatomic correlates of these entities. If the entities are distinct, logic dictates a corresponding neuroanatomic distinction. However, if one considers short-term and long-term memory as processes, one begins to examine how various neuroanatomic systems perform these processes. It is no longer necessary to look for anatomic separation. Short-term and long-term memories could be stored within the same anatomic unit, but might be the result of different neurochemical, electrophysiologic, and/or structural change processes. This distinction between cognitive processes and cognitive entities should be kept in mind while perusing the remainder of this chapter.

Since both theories (Atkinson & Shiffrin, 1968; Cowan, 1988) deal with the concept of short-term memory, one issue that can be explored is what the subcortical data say about short-term memory. Actually, the literature on alcoholic Korsakoff's syndrome is marked by a contradiction regarding short-term memory. The fact that these patients usually demonstrate a tested memory span within normal limits (e.g., Talland, 1965) had been taken by some as an indication that short-term memory was intact for this population. But, impairment at the longer intervals in the Peterson and Peterson (1959) paradigm (Butters et al., 1973; Cermak et al., 1971; Samuels et al., 1971) had been interpreted by some as demonstrating impaired short-term memory for this population. The latter interpretation seems to fit the Atkinson and Shiffrin model which would assume that the distraction-filled delay would prevent information from entering long-term memory by minimizing any operations performed on such information by short-term memory. Thus, according to the Atkinson and Shiffrin model, the Peterson and Peterson paradigm would measure primarily short-term memory. Why, then, would patients with alcoholic Korsakoff's syndrome show intact memory span but impaired short-term memory under other circumstances? One possibility is that span of apprehension and sustaining items in short-term stores represent related but dissociable processes. However, the Atkinson and Shiffrin model gives no theoretical reason to presume such a dissociation.

Another possibility (as mentioned in Chapter 6) is that recall at the longer intervals in the Peterson and Peterson paradigm allows the use of long-term as well as short-term memories. Actually, based upon an analysis of proactive interference effects, Cowan (1988) had suggested that long-term as well as short-term memory processes were active during Peterson and Peterson–type experiments. Thus, the impairment of alcoholic Korsakoff's patients at the longer intervals would be caused by their inability to establish long-term memories and make use of them at the longer intervals as short-term memory begins to decay. We might conclude, accordingly, that since Cowan's model is more compatible with the simultaneous activity of short-term and long-term processes when rehearsal is prevented, it is more adequate than the Atkinson and Shiffrin model to account for the impairment of alcoholic Korsakoff's subjects on Peterson and Peterson tasks. One piece of data that does not fit this explanation is the fact that Baddeley and Warrington (1970) found a group of amnesic patients whose performance on a Peterson and Peterson–type task was not impaired. (The latter work was not reviewed in this volume because it was not possible to separate the results of the subcortical patients from the results of other patients in their study.)

The dissociation of short-term memory performance (i.e., memory span) from long-term memory performance presents problems for the Atkinson and Shiffrin model (see Baddeley, 1990). Such a dissociation was seen in the study of Risse et al. (1984), where aphasics with frontal and basal ganglia lesions showed impairment of long-term recall but not of memory span, and aphasics with posterior cortical lesions showed impairment of memory span but not of long-term memory. The Atkinson and Shiffrin model might predict impairment of long-term memory without impairment of memory span, but under the assumptions of their model, impairment of memory span (i.e., short-term memory) without impairment of long-term performance would be impossible. Thus, their model cannot account for the Risse et al. data. Cowan (1988), on the other hand, suggests that impaired memory span may be indicative of dysfunction in one of the control processes (i.e., in the central executive) as opposed to impairment of actual short-term memory processes per se.

One other advantage of Cowan's model over the Atkinson and Shiffrin model is that the former can account for implicit memory. According to Cowan (1988), those items that have been the subject of short-term memory processing without being effortfully processed (i.e., as the focus of attention) enter procedural memory, but only effortfully processed information becomes available for explicit memory. In a sense, then, becoming available to procedural memory (by being the subject of short-term memory processing) is a prerequisite for explicit (i.e., effortful) memory processing. The Atkinson and Shiffrin model cannot account for implicit memory. Although Cowan's model can account for implicit memory, his attempt at an explanation falls short. The fact that motor-skill learning is impaired in Huntington's disease (Heindel et al., 1988, 1989) but stem-completion priming is not (Heindel et al., 1987, 1989) indicates that motor-skill learning, procedural memory, and implicit memory (indicated by performance on priming tasks) cannot be explained by a single unitary phenomenon. Thus, Cowan's model needs to be extended to differentiate between types of memory at this level, though such a differentiation does not seem to be too much of a reach for the model.

The fact that Cowan's model could allow for the interaction of implicit and explicit memory is a strength. A reevaluation of the evidence on proactive interference suggests that such an interaction actually does occur in patients with alcoholic Korsakoff's syndrome (Cermak & Butters, 1972; Cermak et al., 1974; Squire, 1982) and in some patients with diencephalic amnesia (Graff-Radford et al., 1990). The buildup of proactive interference occurs across trials in experiments that exceed the time frame and the span for short-term memories. Yet, proactive interference continues to build. Patients with alcoholic Korsakoff's syndrome or diencephalic amnesia are just as sensitive to proactive interference and probably more so than are neurologically intact subjects. As noted above, this effect cannot be due to short-term memory, and for the amnesic patients, the effect cannot be due to explicit long-term memory, because the devastation of their explicit long-term memory would be expected to considerably weaken effects with which it is associated. The buildup of proactive interference, then, is most likely due to the implicit memory of prior items interfering with explicit recall. In Cowan's model, incoming items would activate prior items from long-term procedural (implicit) memory, thereby causing interference, but in the case of amnesics, the items activated from implicit memory are somehow prevented from becoming the focus of effortful attention during recall in explicit-memory tasks.

The more troubling aspect of Cowan's model is its inability to account for amnesic syndromes, such as alcoholic Korsakoff's syndrome or diencephalic amnesia, in the first place. If short-term memory is a subset of long-term memory, then registration of information in short-term memory means that it has de facto been entered into long-term memory. Since amnesics can access information in their short-term memory, one would have to assume under Cowan's model that the information has been entered into long-term memory. Further, the fact that they can access the information indicates that it can be effortfully processed within short-term memory. But, if the information is entered into long-term memory under conditions of effortful processing, then, according to Cowan's model, it *should* be available to explicit long-term recall. If that latter assumption were correct, then where is the defect in amnesics' memory? Actually, the fact that amnesics with alcoholic Korsakoff's syndrome can demonstrate normal long-term recognition memory under some recognition conditions if given adequate exposure time (Huppert & Piercy, 1978; Martone et al., 1986; Squire, 1981) suggests that Cowan's model may be too simple. Since amnesics do not require the extra time to demonstrate adequate short-term memory (i.e., memory span) performance, then registration of a long-term memory cannot be equated to registration of a short-term memory. Cowan might suggest that the difference lies in the way in which the central executive facilitates long-term storage, but, as we shall shortly see, this explanation is not entirely convincing. It should be noted that it was not Cowan's purpose to provide extensive explanations of long-term memory functioning. Nonetheless, such issues are critical to our consideration of subcortical memory functions, and I will now turn to a consideration of long-term memory.

Subcortical Data and Long-Term Memory Processes

Long-term memory issues are critical to our discussion of subcortical memory dysfunctions because the major deficit in diencephalic amnesias appears to be in the registration of long-term memories. The following discussion will focus on four issues regarding long-term memory and subcortical functions in memory. The first issue deals with Craik and Lockhart's (1972) assumption that the "more deeply" items are processed, the more likely they are to be stored as long-term memories. This concept had a major influence on some studies of memory functions in alcoholic Korsakoff's syndrome. The second issue addresses the differences and similarities between diencephalic, bitemporal, and basal forebrain amnesias. The third issue deals with a person's ability to respond to external stimuli versus their ability to generate responses based upon an internal frame of reference. During this latter discussion, data from movement in Parkinson's disease and from akinetic mutism will be applied to memory processes. Finally, the anatomical confluence of systems involved in long-term memory processes will be considered.

Levels of Processing

Craik and Lockhart (1972) suggested that the probability of information being stored in long-term memory depended upon how deeply it was processed. The deeper the level of processing, the more likely an item was to be stored. For verbal information, semantic analysis was felt to be the deepest level of processing. Processing of words by their sound (i.e., phonemic processing) was less deep than semantic processing. Processing written words by their visual characteristics was an even more superficial means. Thus, words processed semantically were more likely to reach long-term storage than words processed by the more superficial means.

This levels-of-processing paradigm influenced neuropsychological research. As the discussion in Chapter 6 revealed, for example, patients with alcoholic Korsakoff's syndrome were more likely to make false-positive recognitions for items that were homonyms and associates of target items than they were for items that were synonyms of target items (Cermak et al., 1973). As another example, alcoholic Korsakoff's patients failed to show improved recognition under semantic-processing conditions versus visual- or phonemic-processing conditions, whereas controls did show such improvement (Wetzel & Squire, 1980). These findings indicated that patients with alcoholic Korsakoff's syndrome either failed to attend to semantic characteristics or were unable to use them for encoding long-term memories. Further, alcoholic Korsakoff's patients' failure to release from proactive interference with shifts in semantic categories (Cermak et al., 1974; Squire, 1982) also was taken to indicate that these subjects were not processing the semantic features of the words they were presented. According to the levels-of-processing paradigm, this inability to attend to the semantic aspects of stimuli was responsible for their deficits in long-term memory storage. If applied to Cowan's (1988) model, this finding might be taken as a sign of a defect in the central executive and its resultant influence on the processing of short-term memories.

This explanation has a problem: the coexistence of semantic-processing deficits and severe memory problems does not necessarily mean that the semantic-processing deficits caused the memory deficits. It is possible that both semantic-processing and memory deficits were caused by some third factor. Or, alternatively, each disturbance might be caused by separate factors that frequently coexist in certain types of amnesic patients. A third explanation is that memory deficits might somehow reduce the efficiency of semantic processing.

The study by Squire (1982) gave some insight into these issues. He demonstrated that at least one subject with diencephalic lesions and memory disturbance, patient N.A., had no failure to release from proactive interference. This finding was taken as a dissociation of a memory deficit from semantic-processing difficulties. In other words, a deficit in semantic processing does not seem to be a necessary condition for the long-term memory disturbance that accompanies some diencephalic lesions. Rather, Squire found such problems to be correlated with deficits in tests normally indicating frontal lobe dysfunction.

On the other hand, Graff-Radford et al. (1990) and Winocur et al. (1984) did find a failure to release from proactive interference with semantic-category shifts collectively in three patients with diencephalic amnesia and no indication of structural changes in the frontal lobes. This leaves us with a question: Are semantic-processing deficits dissociable from severe memory deficits in at least some cases of diencephalic amnesias as indicated by Squire's case? A review of the anatomy of the dorsal medial nucleus (Carpenter & Sutin, 1983; Jones, 1985) suggests this is at least a possibility. The magnocellular (medial) division is the portion of the nucleus that receives fibers from the amygdala and possibly the nucleus basalis. By virtue of these connections, the magnocellular division would be expected to be the portion involved in memory. However, it is the parvicellular (lateral) division that makes connections with the dorsolateral frontal cortex and could be expected to be associated with cognitive functions normally related to frontal lobe functioning.

Thus, while this possibility of dissociation between memory and semantic-processing deficits after medial thalamic lesions exists, it would be comforting if a case other than that of Squire (1982) could be found. Because medial thalamic lesions must involve both the dorsal medial nucleus and/or its input from the amygdala, and some portion of Papez' circuit (i.e., the mammillothalamic tract) (Cramon et al., 1985; Graff-Radford et al., 1990) to create an amnesic syndrome, it is unlikely that vascular lesions will produce such dissociations. The reader will recall that medial thalamic lesions causing diencephalic amnesia typically involve both the mammillothalamic tract and the thalamic continuation of the ventral amygdalofugal pathway which terminates in the dorsal medial nucleus. Since these lesions typically also involve the lateral portion of the dorsal medial nucleus, it is impossible to separate the effects of interrupting the mammillothalamic tract and the ventral amygdalofugal pathway from the effects of damaging the part of the dorsal medial nucleus projecting to the dorsolateral frontal lobe. Since Squire's (1982) case sustained a penetrating wound, the topography is different than that created by the typical infarct. (The reader will recall, however, that the lesion did involve both the dorsal medial nucleus and the mammillary bodies, that is, a portion of Papez' circuit in addition to the dorsal medial nucleus [Squire et al., 1989].) To reiterate, lesions that allow for the possible separation of diencephalic pathways related to memory from diencephalic areas related to the frontal lobes will be rare and not vascular in origin.

Diencephalic versus Basal Forebrain versus Bitemporal Amnesia

At this point, it is worth reviewing the similarities and differences between memory deficits associated with diencephalic, basal forebrain, and bitemporal lesions. Such a review could render some idea as to the role of these different structures in long-term memory processes.

At one point (Squire, 1981), it was thought that diencephalic and bitemporal amnesics differed on at least one dimension. The work of Huppert and Piercy (1979) had suggested that no matter how it was presented, the long-term memory of the bitemporal patient H. M. would decay abnormally rapidly over a period of a few days. On the other hand, alcoholic Korsakoff's patients will demonstrate a normal rate of forgetting in certain recognition-memory paradigms when given extra time to process stimuli (e.g., Huppert & Piercy, 1978). These findings suggested that the hippocampus and amygdala versus diencephalic structures were involved in different memory processes. The temporal lobe structures were thought to be involved in consolidation of materials into long-term memories while diencephalic structures might be involved in encoding processes. However, the data on H. M. of Huppert and Piercy (1979) have recently been called into question; it appears that H. M. may simply require an even greater length of exposure than that of diencephalic amnesics in order to demonstrate a normal rate of forgetting on recognition memory (Freed et al., 1987). This leaves us with a question: Are diencephalic and bitemporal amnesias simply variations of the same syndrome? In other words, are the structures involved in the same basic long-term memory process, or are they involved in distinct processes? The fact that H. M. can show normal decay of recognition memory with even longer exposure intervals than alcoholic Korsakoff's patients suggests that H. M. has a similar but more severe deficit to that of the alcoholic Korsakoff's patients.

Graff-Radford and colleagues (1990) also noted a similarity between diencephalic and basal forebrain amnesias. Both types of amnesia produced difficulty in temporal orientation and temporal sequencing of events in memory. Further, both types of patients can improve recollection during interview if given cues to assist recall. If DeLuca and Cicerone (1989) were correct, confabulation in both types of amnesia may be related to direct damage to frontal cortex (accompanying basal forebrain lesion) or damage to structures related to frontal cortex (within the diencephalon). More process-oriented testing of memory functions in patients with basal forebrain amnesias would be useful in making distinctions and drawing similarities between this group and patients with diencephalic amnesias.

Thus, the question just asked concerning patients with diencephalic and bitemporal amnesias also can be applied to the basal forebrain: Do these forms of amnesia represent impairment of distinct memory functions, or do these forms of amnesia represent impairment of the same, unitary memory function? In other words, are the differences in these forms of amnesia a matter of *type* of dysfunction or *degree* of dysfunction? Since the mesial temporal, diencephalic, and basal forebrain structures are all interconnected, there is some possibility that they all may play some role in the same basic process. Since many long-term memories remain after damage to these structures, it is clear that they are not the site of permanent storage. Yet, it is equally obvious that they do play a role in the establishment of long-term memories.

Squire (1987) reviewed the evidence for the neocortex as the site of long-term storage and found it convincing for at least some types of information. Indeed, information may be stored in those neocortical areas responsible for analyzing or integrating the information. For example, there is evidence that some inferior temporal areas responsible for processing visual information may also be the site where that information is stored (e.g., Mishkin, 1966). Squire (1987) also seemed to lean toward an explanation of morphological synaptic changes as the neuronal mechanism of storage. Perhaps the temporo-diencephalic-basal forebrain system provides some prerequisite for such morphological changes. It is tempting to speculate that acetylcholine might play such a role, though there are certainly other processes at work as well.

Intentional and Attentional Systems in Memory

With the exception of research on implicit memory, most neuropsychological memory research has borrowed heavily from the cognitive literature on memory. It has been rare that conceptual paradigms for explicit memory have been neuropsychologically driven. The importance of neuropsychological literature for ultimate understanding of memory should be obvious: since the brain as the organ of memory provides processing systems for and constraints upon cognitive operations, we will have to understand more about the organ before we can hope to understand memory processes. Since there have been few neuropsychologically driven models for memory processes, we must look to other areas of neuropsychology to ascertain if we can find any concepts that will help us understand the role of subcortical structures in memory. The concepts of sensory processing versus activation and preparation to respond as discussed by Watson et al. (1981) may have some utility in this respect. In particular, the idea of endo-evoked versus exo-evoked intentional operations (Heilman & Watson, 1989) may be applicable to retrieval problems and basal ganglia dysfunction.

First, it should be noted that what the literature has called explicit memory in experimental paradigms is the long-term storage of information gathered through some sensory modality or modalities. As just noted, there is evidence that long-term memories may actually be stored in sensory cortex or cortex very closely associated with sensory processes (see Squire, 1987, for discussion). Also just noted, the role of the septal-diencephalic-hippocampal system may be to provide some prerequisite for this type of storage. Watson et al. (1981) have distinguished between the sensory-processing system and an intentional system involved in motor activation and preparation to respond. According to their model, the intentional system involves the basal ganglia, the prefrontal cortex, and—for the most part—a different set of structures than the sensory-processing system. It would seem to be a logical extension of Watson and colleagues' model that the intentional system or closely related structures are involved in motor-skill learning. Thus, the association of the intentional system, including the basal ganglia, with motor-skill learning would explain impaired motor learning in patient's with Huntington's and Parkinson's diseases (Heindel et al., 1988, 1989).

An extension of the concept of intentional system into cognitive operations has the potential to explain other memory phenomena. Such a cognitive-intentional system could be involved in the conscious organization of sensory information for the purpose of remembering, for example. In other words, the cognitive-intentional and sensory-processing systems might interact for the purposes of explicit memory. While sensory-processing systems are involved in long-term storage, intentional systems might assist in invoking useful associations which would aid in categorizing the information for long-term storage (i.e., encoding). This could be the reason Huntington's patients fail to use active encoding strategies (e.g., Massman et al., 1990).

Further, Squire (1982) suggested that sensitivity to semantic categories may be a function of frontal lobe processing, implying that the frontal lobes may be involved in encoding. If this interpretation of the data is correct, this type of encoding may facilitate long-term retrieval by establishing associations but may not be absolutely necessary for long-term storage because it does not interrupt storage in sensory cortex. The facts that Huntington's patients do not show a failure to release from proactive interference with semantic-category shifts (Beatty & Butters, 1986), and do not preferentially use more superficial forms of encoding (Butters et al., 1976), indicates that the basal ganglia are not involved in this type of encoding, even though the frontal lobes may be involved.

However, one potentially even more useful extension of intention into the cognitive realm involves the concepts of endo-evoked and exo-evoked activation. According to Heilman and Watson (1989), exo-evoked movements are actions evoked by stimuli external to an organism. In contrast, endo-evoked movements are actions evoked by stimuli internal to the organism, such as primary drives, emotions, or internally set goals. Akinesias are failures to move under some circumstances that are not caused by weakness or paralysis. Although endo-evoked and exo-evoked akinesias often coexist, it is sometimes possible to see an akinesia that is primarily endo- or exo-evoked. For example, a patient might not spontaneously move a limb but might do so when properly stimulated.

In his discussion of the structure and function of the supplementary motor area (i.e., medial premotor cortex), Goldberg (1985) noted similar distinctions. He discussed two motor-programming systems. In the "projectional" system, action is derived from an internal model that permits prediction of a future state of affairs. This action is similar to Heilman and Watson's (1989) endo-evoked behavior driven by internally set goals. According to Goldberg, the supplementary motor area, the basal ganglia, and the portion of the ventral lateral nucleus receiving pallidal input are involved in this projectional system. In the "responsive" system, action is based upon an explicit external input. This system correlates motivational significance with external objects. It bears some similarity to Heilman and Watson's (1989) exo-evoked behavior. The responsive system is associated with the lateral premotor cortex, the cerebellum, and the portion of the ventral lateral nucleus receiving cerebellar input.

Heilman and Watson's (1989) analysis of two forms of akinesia is of interest here. Akinetic mutism involves a lack of spontaneous movement and speech. Those actions or that speech that can be seen in akinetic mutism are evoked by external stimuli. Thus, Heilman and Watson classify akinetic mutism as primarily an endo-evoked akinesia. The fact that akinetic mutism is usually associated with lesions of the anterior cingulate cortex and/or the supplementary motor area is consistent with Goldberg's analysis of the involvement of the supplementary motor area in the projectional system. Further, Heilman and Watson (1989) suggested that the akinesia associated with Parkinson's disease is also endo-evoked because these patients can at times respond much more quickly to external stimuli than their spontaneous movement would suggest to be possible. This analysis of Parkinson's disease is consistent with Goldberg's analysis that the basal ganglia participate in the projectional system.

In their model of schizophrenia, Early et al. (1989b) made an attempt to apply the concepts from Goldberg (1985) to cognition. Instead of focusing upon the supplementary motor area for movement, they focused on the anterior cingulate for "intentional cognitive activity." Indeed, Early and colleagues emphasized the loop from limbic areas through the ventral striatum, the globus pallidus, the dorsal medial thalamus, and back to the anterior cingulate in cognition. According to their theory, the role of the anterior cingulate loop in cognition is driven by "an internally selected, internally represented goal." Thus, there is precedent for applying the division between internally and externally evoked actions to cognition.

For the purposes of this work, the terms *endo-evoked* and *exo-evoked* will be applied to cognition. To the extent that cognition involves self-initiated access to, generation of, or motivation by an internal data base, model, or goal, it can be considered endo-evoked. To the extent that cognition is driven by external stimuli, it can be considered exo-evoked. For example, in Chapter 3, I briefly considered the possibility of applying these concepts to language. Repetition of oral language was considered to be exo-evoked because it primarily involves responding to (i.e., reproducing) external stimuli. Semantic operations were considered to be endo-evoked because they involve access to internally stored representations.

While explicit-memory storage can be conceptualized as involving information derived from sensory systems, accessing stored information can be considered to involve intention in the cognitive realm. Further, because it involves self-initiated processes to access long-term memories, retrieval is more endo-evoked than exo-evoked. On the other hand, because recognition memory involves responding to an external stimulus, it is more of an exo-evoked than an endo-evoked process. According to Cowan's (1988) model, an incoming stimulus in a recognition-memory paradigm would activate related episodic information in long-term memory, and subjects would simply have to use such activated episodic information to make the response called for by the recognition paradigm. By comparison, recall paradigms require the subject to initiate retrieval processes.

The understanding that retrieval of long-term memories is an endo-evoked cognitive process would explain why patients with basal ganglia dysfunction have retrieval deficits. In other words, because the basal ganglia are involved in endo-evoked cognition, such patients will have problems with retrieval as one type of endo-evoked cognition.

This explanation would take cognitive dysfunction as parallel to some types of motor dysfunction in basal ganglia disorders. For example, Parkinson's patients often show little spontaneous behavior even though they can be incited to action by external stimulation. Retrieval deficits in Parkinson's disease patients (Flowers et al., 1984; Massman et al., 1990; Sugar, Sullivan, Gabrieli, Corkin, & Growdon, 1989) would be seen as a cognitive equivalent to endo-evoked akinesia.

This analysis bears some similarity to Flowers and colleagues' (1984) conclusion that Parkinson's patients could perform well on recognition-memory tasks that primarily involved "passive" reception of information, but they would perform poorly on tasks requiring more active organization and retrieval of information. However, the present interpretation involves parallels between movement and cognition. Saint-Cyr, Taylor, Lang, and Trepanier (1989) also have emphasized that the striatum participates in various memory processes carried out implicitly using internal rather than external cues. The reliance upon internal versus external cues is similar to the endo- versus exo-evoked cognition distinction. However, the current application suggests that explicit retrieval is also affected because of its greater demands on accessing an internal data base.

Since the current analysis proposes that Parkinson's patients demonstrate an endo-evoked deficit in the cognitive as well as the movement realm, it would be more convincing if differences in responding to external stimuli versus internal models could be shown in other cognitive processes independent of memory. Actually, Cools, Van den Bercken, Horstink, van Spaedonck, & Berger (1984) had concluded that Parkinson's patients demonstrated deficits on tasks not directed by external sensory information. Taylor, Saint-Cyr, Lang, and Kenny (1986) have examined tasks upon which Parkinson's patients are impaired or not impaired and came to the conclusion that they are unable to generate planning specific to tasks. Brown and Marsden (1988b) also suggested that Parkinson's patients were impaired on tasks in which there were no external cues to direct attention, but unimpaired on tasks in which such external cues were available. These same authors actually manipulated the availability of external cues within a single task and confirmed relative impairment for Parkinson's patients but not controls on the task without external cues (Brown & Marsden, 1988a).

Brown (Brown, 1989; Brown & Marsden, 1988a) has suggested that the difference between tasks with and without external cues is that tasks with external cues require less processing resources than tasks without external cues. He suggested that Parkinson's patients simply have fewer processing resources within their supervisory attentional systems (similar to Cowan's [1988] central executive) than do normal controls. Brown links this deficit to decreased frontal functioning created by dysfunction in cortico-striato-pallido-thalamo-cortical loops. For reasons too detailed to explore in this volume, Brown's data with respect to limited processing resources in Parkinson's disease are not entirely convincing. I suggested above that it is the nature of the endo-evoked versus the exo-evoked processes that determines impaired retrieval in patients with Parkinson's disease. In other words, the basal ganglia may participate in endo-evoked but not exo-evoked processes, as demonstrated by the nature of their akinesia. To compare concepts, Brown sees decreased performance as a matter of distribution of processing resources, but the present extension of Heilman and Watson's (1989) model suggests differences in types of processing and underlying systems. A further distinction is the emphasis on attention in the former model, but an emphasis on the interaction of intentional and attentional systems in the latter. Nonetheless, there is a precedent that endo-evoked cognitive processes other than memory may be impaired in Parkinson's disease while exo-evoked cognitive processes tend not to be as impaired. The existence of these findings supports the idea of retrieval deficits as endo-evoked.

The Anatomical Confluence of Basal Ganglia and Temporal Lobe Systems

Thus, the basal ganglia and related structures may perform different processes in memory than the mesial temporal lobes and related subcortical structures. It is important to look at the anatomical confluence of these systems for two reasons. First, overlap in the systems at some point could indicate possible interaction of the two systems at that point. Second, in places where the two systems are anatomically proximate to one another, though not necessarily overlapping, there may be implications for lesion studies. Since vascular lesions respect vascular territories but not neural system boundaries, infarcts may affect two systems at once when the two systems are located in close proximity.

One major point of confluence is within the dorsal medial thalamus. The magnocellular (medial) division receives input from the amygdala via the ventral amygdalofugal pathway (Carpenter & Sutin, 1983; Jones, 1985). According to the analysis of Alexander et al. (1986), the magnocellular division also receives input from the portion of the globus pallidus associated with an orbitofrontal cortico-striato-pallido-thalamo-cortical loop. The implication for orbitofrontal cortex in direct memory processes is uncertain, though DeLuca and Cicerone (1989) have suggested that the frontal cortex may have to be involved before confabulation is seen in basal forebrain lesions.

However, if my analysis and the analysis of Early et al. (1989b) is correct, the anterior cingulate loop may be the basal ganglia loop involved in memory. This is not only consistent with the retrieval deficits in basal ganglia disorders (Butters et al., 1985, 1986; Flowers et al., 1984; Massman et al., 1990; Risse et al., 1984) and the idea of basal ganglia involvement in endo-evoked cognition, it is consistent with the case study of Lhermitte and Signoret (1976) showing retrieval deficit in anterior cingulate lesion. According to Alexander et al. (1986), the portion of the globus pallidus that is a part of the anterior cingulate cortico-striato-pallido-thalamo-cortical loop projects into the posterior medial portion of the dorsal medial nucleus. This latter location would appear to be a posterior portion of the magnocellular division. Thus, this anatomical confluence may provide a means for the interaction of basal ganglia and temporal lobe systems. If not, the anatomical proximity suggests that both systems may be involved in some lesions.

Thus, lesions in the posterior magnocellular area may be implicated in retrieval processes in addition to processes related to the amygdala. This could explain some evidence for retrieval deficits in patients with alcoholic Korsakoff's syndrome since the portion of the dorsal medial nucleus involved in the anterior cingulate loop could be damaged. It also indicates the importance of testing patients with more posterior lesions in the dorsal medial nucleus for retrieval deficits, even if they do not exhibit profound amnesias (e.g., see Cramon et al., 1985; Graff-Radford et al., 1990).

Summary

A brief summary will help to crystallize applications of subcortical research to memory theory. This volume has discussed two theories. The multiple-stores model of Atkinson and Shiffrin (1968) was unable to explain many phenomena in the literature. The model of Cowan (1988) was found to have some advantages. Cowan proposed that short-term memory was a subset of long-term memory consisting of those items from long-term memory in a heightened state of activation. Items in short-term memory that were the subject of effortful processing are a separate subset of short-term memory, referred to as the focus of attention. All items entering short-term memory were later available to "procedural" memory, but only those that are effortfully processed were available to explicit memory. Brief sensory memory, which has a less limited capacity than short-term memory, is distinct from short-term memory but feeds information into short-term memory. The central executive, a conglomerate of processes, is also distinct from long-term memory but controls effortful processing.

An examination of Cowan's model in light of the subcortical literature revealed some advantages. First, it allowed for the simultaneous activation of short-term and long-term memory processes in spite of distraction. Second, its constructs allow for a type of memory other than explicit, though Cowan's use of the term *procedural* to cover all nondeclarative (i.e., nonexplicit) memory is not adequate. Further articulation of such memory functions is necessary. Third, the model allows for some interaction between explicit and implicit memory, which research on buildup of proactive interference in amnesic patients indicates is desirable. One disadvantage must also be noted: Cowan's model does not account well for the type of amnesia seen in diencephalic or bitemporal amnesia. The ability of amnesic patients to effortfully process short-term memories in the face of an inability to form long-term memories indicates that registration of an explicit short-term memory does not necessarily imply registration of the same item as a long-term memory. Thus, some distinction between short-term and long-term registration processes is necessary for a viable theory.

A levels-of-processing model does not seem adequate to account for the lack of long-term memories in diencephalic amnesias. In at least one instance of diencephalic lesion (Squire, 1982), severe memory problems existed without difficulty in processing semantic features of words. The core difficulty in diencephalic amnesia appears to be a difficulty in registration of material as a long-term memory (see Chapter 6). At least for recognition memory, the deficit in registration for diencephalic amnesia can be overcome by additional exposure time (e.g., Huppert & Piercy, 1978; Squire, 1981).

The current question regarding diencephalic and basal forebrain amnesias is: Do they represent types of memory problems separate from bitemporal amnesias, or are they similar dysfunctions? The interconnection of the amygdala, the dorsal medial thalamus, and the septal region and of the hippocampal formation, the mammillary bodies, and the nucleus of the diagonal band suggests that temporal lobe structures, diencephalic structures, and basal forebrain structures may collaborate in creating the necessary conditions for long-term storage. However, further research would be quite useful in making any distinctions possible between amnesias precipated by lesions in these two sets of divergent but interconnected areas. There is a particular paucity of information on disrupted processes in basal forebrain amnesias.

A consideration of literature on attention and intention suggests that some concepts developed in these areas might be useful for understanding memory. To the degree explicit memory involves recollection of sensory information, it seems logical that long-term storage processes may ultimately involve sensory cortices. Morphological changes at the level of the synapse may be a part of the substrate for long-term memories. The temporo-diencephalic-basal forebrain system may somehow be involved in creating the necessary conditions for such storage. Given that increased exposure time can lead to normal forgetting curves, initial registration of a long-term memory is a critical process in which diencephalic centers are involved.

Intentional systems, on the other hand, involve the basal ganglia (Early et al., 1989b; Goldberg, 1985; Heilman & Watson, 1989; Watson et al., 1981). Conceptually at least, it seems likely that intentional systems are involved in encoding processes and in providing some associations for incoming information; however, it seems likely that this process generally involves the frontal cortex but not the basal ganglia. The involvement of the basal ganglia may be more specific to active application of encoding strategies. Further, with respect to the basal ganglia, the most useful application of intentional concepts to memory may be the concepts of endo-evoked and exo-evoked cognition. Because retrieval of long-term memories involves deliberately accessing internal stores of information, it can be considered an endo-evoked process. If cognition and movement are parallel functions, it would make sense that patients having trouble with endo-evoked movements also would have trouble with endo-evoked cognition. Thus, Parkinson's patients who have an endo-evoked akinesia may have trouble with retrieval because it is an endo-evoked process. Recognition-memory paradigms may involve more exo-evoked cognition. If Cowan (1988) was right that incoming information items activate related long-term memories, then recognition-memory procedures may simply involve explicitly using the activated information to make the necessary discrimination. The concept of recognition memory as exo-evoked would explain why Parkinson's patients have less trouble with recognition tasks.

Conclusions

Finally, a few concluding remarks are in order. First, I will address the status of memory theory. I will ask the reader to consider the proposition that memory theory should be driven to some degree by the desire for a greater understanding of how brain systems produce memory. Second, discussion will turn to a few parallels between language and memory theory. Third, I will consider future directions.

Memory Theory and the Subcortical Literature

As already noted, subcortical research has most frequently borrowed models and paradigms from cognitive research. The most notable exception to this trend has been in the area of implicit memory, where the demonstration of intact implicit learning in patients with profound explicit-memory deficit has driven interest in implicit-memory studies. In general, the cognitive literature has provided a great service by loaning its concepts and paradigms to subcortical studies. The Peterson and Peterson (1959) paradigm, Craik and Lockhart's levels-of-processing paradigm (1972), Broadbent's (1958) model, and Atkinson and Shiffrin's (1968) later extension of this model are examples. Indeed, the influence of the Atkinson and Shiffrin model, as well as these other concepts, is still a major impetus in the subcortical-memory literature. This volume also has attempted to show the applicability of Cowan's (1988) model to issues raised in the subcortical-memory literature.

In spite of the tremendous advantages of borrowing concepts and paradigms from the cognitive literature, there is at least one major disadvantage in doing so. For the most part, these models and concepts have been developed outside the realm of neurobehavioral research, in the absence of neurobehavioral concepts. Frequently, they do not directly take into account the constraints that brain systems would imply for cognitive processing. Further, they do not have as a goal the ultimate explanation of how the brain produces behavior. The danger with borrowing heavily from the purely cognitive literature and with more modest information flow moving in the opposite direction is that our understanding of brain systems will not develop adequately.

What is needed is a more even information flow in both directions. Indeed, purely cognitive studies are actually studying the brain to the extent cognitive tasks are the end result of complex brain functions and limited by the types and capacities of brain processing. At the very least, cognitive models should be modified on the basis of what neuropsychological studies say about the processes, capacities, and limitations of brain systems. For example, Cowan's (1988) model has some promising characteristics from a neuropsychological standpoint. But it needs to be modified to account for different types of nondeclarative memory and to account for long-term-memory deficits in the face of focused processing in short-term memory, as suggested by the neuropsychological literature. Whether Cowan's model could endure with such changes is a matter for future conceptualization and research. On the other hand, it is possible that memory models may need to be developed out of a neurobehavioral research base. Such models would have to account for phenomena detailed in the subcortical literature.

This analysis implies that we must carefully reconsider time-honored concepts from the memory literature. Some concepts may need to be modified or replaced. For example, I have suggested in this volume that registration of material as a long-term memory and encoding of material for long-term memory may be at least partially separable processes. In the past, many have considered these processes to be the same. The concepts of consolidation and retrieval should be similarly examined. The controversy over H. M.'s rate of forgetting suggests that consolidation may be dependent upon the strength of original registration. Is a separate concept of consolidation justified?

These issues are not merely semantic games. Our ability to understand the neural substrates of memory depends upon our ability to adequately conceptualize the processes of memory. If we have inadequately conceptualized the processes, our concepts will act as a hindrance in attempting to ascertain the neural substrates of memory. We will be looking for evidence of neural processes to explain memory phenomena that may not actually happen. This would be a bit like the man who loses a $100 bill in a dark area, but looks for it down the street under a street lamp because that is where the light is.

Examples of blending cognitive and neurobehavioral literature exist. Brown's (1989) examination of the reasons why Parkinson's patients respond better with external cues is one good example. Heilman and colleagues' (Heilman et al., 1987; Heilman & Watson, 1989; Watson et al., 1981) analysis of the subtypes of attention and intention is another good example of conceptualization that is driven by neurobehavioral phenomena. It looks as though memory research also can become more driven by neurobehavioral evidence, such as that from the subcortical literature.

Parallels between Memory and Language

In this volume, I have treated the issues of subcortical participation in language and memory functions as separate issues. One might ask whether there are any common characteristics between subcortical functions in language and subcortical functions in memory.

One set of concepts briefly mentioned in both Chapter 3 on the thalamus in language and the current chapter is endo- versus exo-evoked cognition. The reader will recall that for language repetition was conceptualized as exo-evoked cognition since it involves response to an external stimulus. In other words, the model for language production was externally derived. Semantic processes were seen as endo-evoked because they involved internal symbolic representation. In other words, semantic processes involve accessing the internal data base for symbolic representation. I suggested that the thalamus was involved in endo-evoked language because semantic processes seemed impaired after thalamic lesion while repetition is relatively intact. For memory, on the other hand, I suggested that retrieval involves accessing internal data bases, that is, endo-evoked cognition, while recognition-memory paradigms represent more response to external stimulation.

The problem with application of the concepts of endo-evoked versus exo-evoked cognition to both memory and language is that the implicated structures for language versus memory are not the same. For language, I suggested that the thalamic nuclei might be involved in endo-evoked cognition, but for memory, I suggested that the basal ganglia was involved since retrieval deficits were commonly found in patients with basal ganglia disorders. One might use the idea of cortico-striato-pallido-thalamo-cortical loops to explain why the thalamus seems to be involved for language but the basal ganglia seem to be involved for memory. Perhaps the basal ganglia are also involved for language and the thalamus is also involved for memory.

However, this explanation has problems. First, repetition is not always unimpaired for dominant basal ganglia lesions the way it is for dominant thalamic lesions, suggesting that the thalamus and the basal ganglia cannot be considered functionally unified in language. Further, patients with pulvinar lesions (e.g., Crosson et al., 1986) show the pattern of impaired semantic processes with intact repetition. The pulvinar does not receive input from the basal ganglia. Finally, the parallel between endo-evoked versus exo-evoked akinesia and cognition suggests that the basal ganglia might fit a model of endo-evoked cognition better since Parkinson's patients show endo-evoked akinesia. In other words, the idea of endo-evoked cognition seems to fit retrieval deficits in basal ganglia disorders better than it fits thalamic involvement in language.

Actually, a different parallel between thalamic aphasias and diencephalic amnesias lies in the disruption of semantic processing for language and memory, respectively. It will be recalled that patients with diencephalic amnesias, including alcoholic Korsakoff's syndrome, exhibit failure to release from proactive interference and failure to process semantic attributes (Cermak et al., 1973, 1974; Cermak & Reale,

1978; Graff-Radford et al., 1990). It could be that the thalamus is generally involved in semantic processing across both cognitive processes, but different nuclei are involved for memory versus language.

There are also problems with this suggestion, however. First, Squire (1982) indicated that not all patients with diencephalic memory problems demonstrate failure to release from proactive interference, and Wetzel and Squire (1980) demonstrated that not all diencephalic patients fail to increase performance when using semantic processing. These findings suggest that inattentiveness to semantic characteristics may not be a necessary condition for diencephalic amnesia. Second, the prevailing thought regarding amnesias created by medial thalamic infarcts is that they must interrupt systems related to both the hippocampal formation and the amygdala to create severe memory problems. There is no evidence that difficulties in semantic processing arise when these temporal lobe structures are lesioned. Squire (1982) suggested that memory and frontal processing systems may be dissociated in at least some cases.

One final possible parallel between subcortical functions in language and memory should be mentioned. Regarding language, Crosson's (1985) model suggested that the basal ganglia were involved in regulating the release of sequential language segments but not in decision-making processes regarding semantic content. Crosson (1989) and Crosson and Early (1990) have since suggested that basal ganglia functions in language are based upon quantitative, not patterned, neuronal activity. Processing semantic information could only take place on the basis of patterned activity. Wallesch and Papagno (1988), on the other hand, have suggested that the basal ganglia do perform information-processing functions, choosing the best of multiple lexical alternatives. This latter suggested role would involve patterned neuronal activity. Thus, Crosson's model suggests that the basal ganglia are involved in regulating output based on cortical activity, while Wallesch and Papagno's model suggests that processing of semantic information can take place at the level of the basal ganglia as well as at the level of the cortex.

The question of whether the basal ganglia are involved in information-processing versus neuroregulatory functions in language is a question for future research. However, one also wonders to what extent this question could also be asked in memory. Does the evidence regarding retrieval deficits in basal ganglia disorders suggest that the basal ganglia interpret informational patterns or regulate cortical functions somehow? Application of the endo-evoked-cognition concept to retrieval suggests that the basal ganglia may regulate access to internal data bases as opposed to actually processing complex informational patterns.

To summarize: Our discussion of parallels for subcortical functions in language and memory has raised more questions than it has answered. Can the concepts of endo-evoked and exo-evoked cognition be applied to the subcortical literature? If so, is the concept more appropriate as it applies to the participation of the basal ganglia in memory or to the participation of the thalamus in language? Are there parallels in semantic processing at the thalamic level for language and memory? Are various subcortical structures involved in regulatory functions or in the generation, modification, and transfer of informational content within the nervous system? These questions could be important for future research, which leads to discussion of the final topic: future directions in research.

Future Research

The above discussion suggests a number of future directions for research. The issues can be divided into three areas: model-building issues, more specific theoretical concerns, and research methodology. The following paragraphs will discuss these three areas.

With respect to broad theoretical issues, development of a model of memory consistent with data from the subcortical literature and other neuropsychological data should be given some priority as a long-term goal. Such a model should provide an integrated idea of how different brain structures function together to produce a permanent record of events as well as how different areas work together to access the permanent record at a later time. Such a model should not be constrained by current concepts. For example, modification of current concepts of registration, encoding, consolidation, and retrieval, or even the introduction of new concepts, may be one step to developing a comprehensive model. Further, inclusion of information about morphological changes and neurochemical processes at the cellular and systems level will be important. Continued development in some areas of basic research may be critical for the eventual development of a comprehensive model, and certainly a high level of integration between basic neuroscience and neuropsychological research will be necessary.

What would an adequate neuropsychological model of memory look like? There are several essential characteristics: (1) Such a model would break memory down into an orderly series of processes necessary for establishing and accessing permanent records of events, knowledge, or procedures. In this volume, I have already questioned whether current concepts of memory are adequate for a comprehensive neuropsychological model. At the very least, such concepts must undergo rigorous reconsideration. (2) An adequate model must carefully specify which memory processes it is attempting to explain and to what memory processes it does not apply. For example, differences between declarative memory, motor skills, and other forms of procedural learning will be areas in which distinctions are made. (3) An acceptable model must specify which brain structures are involved in creating and accessing permanent records. At the present time, it appears that temporal lobe, diencephalic, and basal forebrain structures will all be involved in establishing declarative memories. (4) An adequate model must specify how the different structures involved in some type of memory participate in the various steps of the process. For example, exactly what are the contributions of temporal lobe, diencephalic, and basal forebrain structures to memory? (5) Finally, an adequate model must emphasize how various structures are anatomically connected and how they interact to create some kind of permanent record. Understanding of neurotransmitter systems and their impact on target structures will be necessary to understand memory processes completely.

Thus, the development of a reasonable neural systems model may be possible only in the more distant future. However, this does not mean that attempts at modeling should be put off until we are absolutely certain about *every* detail at *all* levels of information processing. Indeed, one heuristic purpose of theory is to develop research hypotheses. Confirmation or rejection of such hypotheses then leads to further refinement of a model or development of alternative models. Whatever direction future theoretical research takes, it is obvious that focusing upon memory processes and avoiding reification of processes into entities will be necessary.

At a somewhat less global level, there are more specific theoretical issues suggested by the above discussion. For example, what is the relationship between short-term and long-term memory processes? To what degree can Cowan's (1988) conceptualizations be useful, or to what extent is an alternative model with greater distinction between short-term and long-term processes necessary? Also, the relationship between implicit and explicit memory will need to be mapped more completely. Cowan's (1988) model suggests that implicit memory may be a prerequisite for explicit memory, but others would suggest that implicit and explicit systems are more separate. Evidence on proactive interference (e.g., Cermak & Butters, 1972; Cermak et al., 1974; Graff-Radford et al., 1990), as mentioned above, indicates that these two types of memory at least interact even if the neural substrates are more separate. (The reader will recall it was hypothesized that proactive interference across trials must be based on implicit recollection of previous trials in amnesics since explicit recollections are absent.)

The questions of what types of memory processes exist and what systems are responsible for these processes lead to some more specific questions. Can involvement of the basal ganglia in retrieval be confirmed? If so, what are the neurochemical and neurophysiologic correlates of this process? Are temporal lobe structures, diencephalic structures, and basal forebrain structures involved in a single memory process or multiple memory processes? One step to answering this question will be more complete description of memory disturbance in a number of basal forebrain lesions cases. It will be particularly important to more completely assess the similarities and differences between basal forebrain memory disturbances, on the one hand, and mesial temporal and diencephalic disturbances, on the other hand.

Definition of the role of the basal ganglia in memory also leads to some specific questions. Can the concepts of endo-evoked and exo-evoked cognition be useful in explaining retrieval deficits in basal ganglia disturbance? To what extent are cortico-striato-pallido-thalamo-cortical loops involved in memory? And, if they are involved in memory, what are the implications of dysfunction at different levels of the loops? Is disruption of the loop at the level of the basal ganglia the same as disruption of the loop at the level of the thalamus? What are the neural substrates of such similarities or differences? Other than retrieval, can a role for the basal ganglia in long-term registration or active application of encoding strategies be confirmed? Finally, regarding the basal ganglia, is the neurophysiological substrate of basal ganglia participation in memory related to quantitative (i.e., neuroregulatory) processes or patterned activity (i.e., processing of specific informational content)?

The subcortical literature clearly indicates the necessity for distinguishing between declarative (explicit) memory and other forms of memory. What are the different distinguishable types of nondeclarative memory and what are the relationships between these forms of memory? For example, the Huntington's literature (e.g., Heindel et al., 1988, 1989; Shimamura et al., 1987; Smith et al., 1988) indicates that motor skill-learning and implicit memory can be dissociated in this population. But it is not clear to what extent nonmotoric-procedural memory correlates with either of these two processes.

The context in which these questions must be answered presents a major obstacle to future research. The major source of data for Chapters

6 and 7 has been alcoholic Korsakoff's syndrome and degenerative disorders of the basal ganglia, respectively. The problem with alcoholic Korsakoff's syndrome is that involved structures outside the diencephalon (e.g., Arendt et al., 1983; Roche et al., 1988; Shimamura et al., 1988; Victor et al., 1971) may have effects on memory directly or on the paradigms used to study memory. For example, patients with frontal lobe lesions demonstrate a failure to release from proactive interference (Squire, 1982) and alcoholic Korsakoff's patients demonstrate frontal lobe changes. Degenerative diseases of the basal ganglia like Huntington's and Parkinson's diseases also affect other areas of the brain, including the frontal lobes. It is particularly obvious in Parkinson's disease that degeneration of dopaminergic neurons projectioning from the substantia nigra and ventral tegmental area affect systems other than the striatum. Thus, confirmation of diencephalic memory dysfunction in populations other than alcoholic Korsakoff's syndrome and confirmation of basal ganglia memory dysfunction in populations other than Parkinson's and Huntington's diseases patients is necessary.

One major candidate for such an alternative population is cases of subcortical infarct. Complications with such a population have been mentioned in previous chapters. Not the least of these complications with basal ganglia cases is that they typically involve surrounding white matter, making the assumption of exclusive damage impossible in all but a very small number of cases. When taking this limitation into account, the number of basal ganglia and thalamic infarct cases appropriate for study is quite small. The lack of general availability of such cases in a single center presents a major logistical barrier for research. It is quite difficult to accumulate enough cases to conclude that one's results apply across the majority of patients in a population. Further, it would seem a waste of time to construct an extensive memory battery to administer to a series of subcortical patients when only a few such patients will probably be seen within a center even over a period of years. Nonetheless, the construction of such batteries should be accomplished; it simply will take time to accumulate enough data to ascertain which results can be applied across the majority of groups with specific types of lesions. In the meantime, other approaches to the study of subcortical structures in memory must be attempted.

While the simple study of cognitive processes in normals by itself cannot provide the type of data necessary to develop neural systems models, the development of cerebral blood flow– and metabolism-imaging techniques provides an opportunity to study normal subjects. In the area of language, advances in using these techniques in activation studies with neurologically normal subjects have been made (e.g., Petersen et al., 1988; Wallesch et al., 1985). Activation studies during different memory processes are also possible and would provide valuable data. However, such studies necessitate some understanding of memory processes in order to be successful. Thus, it will be necessary to integrate research regarding memory processes in cases of subcortical lesion with PET and SPECT activation studies. If this can be done, our understanding of memory processes as they relate to brain systems will be greatly enhanced.

The challenges in understanding the way subcortical structures participate in neural memory systems are considerable. These challenges exist on a conceptual as well as a practical, logistical level. The magnitude of effort required to answer the important questions will deter many researchers. However, those who decide to make a commitment in the area will be rewarded by creating a critical link in our ultimate understanding of brain functions. We cannot hope to truly understand the way the brain controls cognition without understanding the systems to which subcortical structures contribute.

EPILOGUE

The Link between Language and Memory: Subcortical Implications

It is appropriate at this point to add a few final thoughts regarding the relationship between language and memory as applied to subcortical functions. As I mentioned in Chapter 8, there are many parallels between subcortical language and subcortical memory functions. Further exploration and delineation of these parallels would advance our knowledge in both areas. In addition, there are compelling reasons to consider relationships between these functions. Notably, language and verbal memory are interdependent in several ways.

Most obviously, verbal memory is dependent upon language functions to at least some degree. Before an item can be stored in long-term verbal memory, it must be decoded and recognized as a linguistic item with phonological and/or semantic characteristics. The ability to retrieve an item from verbal memory depends upon access to the verbal representation(s) of the item. Thus, language is the medium through which these lasting impressions are conveyed at a later time.

One obvious way in which language is dependent on verbal memory is that vocabulary is learned via verbal-memory functions. The acquisition of a new word and its meaning requires the use of verbal memory to enter the item into more permanent semantic storage. However, in a much more fundamental way, the language system is a form of remote memory. Our vocabulary is a form of remote, verbal-semantic memory. When we recall a word, we are retrieving it from a remote lexical storage in which the contextual aspects of the original learning have been lost or are irrelevant. Thus, our vocabulary is a type of long-term memory, and therefore inseparable from memory processes.

This thinking can also be extended to grammar. Morphology is the set of rules that governs the structure and interrelationships of words; syntax is the set of rules that governs the combination and ordering of words to convey a meaningful idea. Further, for most speakers who have not studied grammar extensively, morphological and syntactic rules are implicit: these rules are routinely applied without explicit conscious awareness of them. In this sense, grammar can be conceived of as a form of remote procedural memory for how to combine linguistic symbols into meaningful units (Hirst, Phelps, Johnson, & Volpe, 1988).

If cases of subcortical language or memory deficit are considered separately, it seems as though there is no relationship between language and memory at the subcortical level. For example, cases of alcoholic Korsakoff's syndrome or other cases of diencephalic amnesia are characterized by severe problems entering new information into long-term memory and relatively intact language. As long as memory and language are seen as separate cognitive compartments, cases of diencephalic amnesia suggest that language and memory can be separated. From the standpoint of remote memory, one might say that persons with diencephalic lesions that cause amnesia may demonstrate a temporal gradient in episodic remote memories (though, as noted in Chapter 6, this is not a necessary condition for diencephalic amnesia) and that semantic memory is unaffected by diencephalic lesion.

On the other hand, as just noted, language and memory processes can be seen as different facets of the same function. Sometimes these facets converge and sometimes one is a necessary component of the other. For example, word finding is the retrieval of information from long-term semantic storage; in this case, memory and language converge. As another example, one must understand the language of another before it can be remembered. In this case, language comprehension subserves verbal memory. Yet language input can only be decoded by reference to the set of symbols held in semantic memory and by the set of rules governing the various aspects of grammar. Thus, language comprehension involves both remote semantic stores and remote procedural (grammatical) memory.

Taking this perspective, verbal-memory deficit after diencephalic lesion impairs not only a patient's ability to use language for the purpose of storing new information, but also may have a bearing on a patient's ability to acquire new linguistic symbols. Yet it is clear that the relationship between amnesic syndromes and the ability to acquire new vocabulary has not been satisfactorily worked out. On the one hand, Squire (1987) suggested that amnesic patients show impairment of semantic memory knowledge when that knowledge is dependent upon events that have happened during patients' period of retrograde amnesia or in the time since the onset of the amnesia. On the other hand, Warrington and McCarthy (1988) found a patient who maintained vocabulary obtained during this period of retrograde amnesia for personal events. Furthermore, Hirst et al. (1988) discussed an amnesic patient who could acquire the vocabulary of a foreign language in addition to its grammatical rules. The ability to acquire vocabulary items in diencephalic and basal forebrain amnesias might be a fruitful area for future research. Similarly, semantic deficits in thalamic aphasia are not merely word-finding problems: They are the loss of or loss of access to remote semantic information. Thus, diencephalic lesion can cause disruption of one form of long-term semantic memory.

Viewing language and verbal memory from this standpoint raises several interesting questions. For example, Chapter 7 discusses the probable difficulty patients with basal ganglia dysfunction (i.e., Huntington's disease or Parkinson's disease) have acquiring new procedural skills. But what is the impact of basal ganglia dysfunction on remote procedural skills? If grammar is considered to be a form of remote procedural memory, it is possible that grammatical rules or access to them might be lost in addition to difficulty acquiring new procedural skills. In fact, the most consistent evidence regarding language and Huntington's and Parkinson's diseases points to some difficulty with complex syntax (see Chapter 2).

Does this phenomenon represent a loss of procedural memory or a loss of access to procedural memories? One way to test this hypothesis would be to find other remote procedural memory systems and test them in patients with Huntington's and Parkinson's diseases. For example, would loss of procedural memory in some common skill, such as driving, correlate with the subtle syntactic deficits in patients with basal ganglia disorders?

Theoretically, at least, a similar question could be asked with respect to semantic deficits during thalamic aphasia. Would thalamic lesions cause loss of or loss of access to remote semantic memory systems other than language? Functionally, this is a more difficult question to answer. Other than language symbols, it is difficult to imagine what remote semantic memory system a dominant thalamic lesion might affect. Perhaps one way to address this question is to ask if a nondominant thalamic lesion might affect a spatial "semantic" memory system.

A third type of function overlapping with both language and memory is attention. Rafal and Posner (1987) have shown that lesions of the pulvinar can affect attention. Ojemann (e.g., 1977) has invoked attentional mechanisms to account for why subjects remember the name for stimuli better if they are presented during dominant ventral lateral thalamic stimulation but have greater difficulty remembering if asked to recall the name of stimuli during dominant ventral lateral stimulation. The fact that responses were different during dominant pulvinar as opposes to dominant ventral lateral stimulation suggests that ventral lateral and pulvinar attentional mechanisms may differ.

The relationship between language and verbal memory, on the one hand, and attention, on the other, may be conceptualized in at least two different ways. First, attentional processes may be seen as a necessary prerequisite for language and especially memory. If one does not attend to an item, chances are that it will not be remembered explicitly (e.g., see Cowan, 1988). As with language and memory, however, we cannot assume at this time that attention is that separable from other cognitive functions. For example, if Ojemann is correct that there is a specific dominant thalamic mechanism causing us to pay attention to linguistic information in our environment, then this attentional mechanism is a part of the language/verbal memory system. Thus, the second way of conceptualizing attentional mechanisms is to see them as a part of various cognitive systems as opposed to a separate cognitive compartment supporting other functions.

Thus, scientific investigation could turn some consideration to the question of how separable attentional mechanisms are from other cognitive functions. In other words, are there attentional mechanisms specific to language and memory, or are attentional mechanisms generally separate and distinct from language and memory? This question may be the most extraordinarily challenging question to ask from a neuropsychological standpoint. The latter proposition would imply that attentional mechanisms could remain intact if the language or memory systems were dysfunctional. But, if attention is not entirely separable from language, for example, then how does one separate language processing from attentional mechanisms specific to language? If reaction times to language symbols increase, how does one know whether it is due to attentional difficulties or to language-processing difficulties?

This question focuses attention on another issue. Over the last few decades, there has been a trend toward greater compartmentalization of cognitive functions in research and in our conceptualizations.

Memory is considered as one system, language as a different system, and attention as still a third system. This compartmentalization tends to deemphasize the points of convergence of the language, memory, and attentional systems. I do not mean to suggest that attention, verbal memory, and language are totally inseparable. However, I do suggest that compartmentalization has been assumed but infrequently subjected to empirical investigation. This state of affairs is in part due to our attempts to break down cognition into component parts using laboratory paradigms with finer and finer distinctions. While such experiments serve a valuable purpose, what has been lost is the integration of divergent lines of inquiry into meaningful functional neurobiological systems. Yet just such integration is needed to tell us how humans function on a day-to-day basis, not just in the experimental laboratory.

The future role of research into subcortical functions could be crucial in providing a vehicle for integrating different lines of research. First, investigating the role of subcortical structures in cognition forces us to think in terms of neuroanatomic systems. Since it is obvious that much of the cognitive processing takes place at the cortical level, subcortical structures must be working in concert with cortical structures in cognition. Second, critical work in the morphology and neurochemistry of subcortical systems is taking place. The increasing sophistication provided by this work can act as a catalyst and a database for improving models of subcortical functions. Third, subcortical structures may act as points of anatomic convergence for cognitive systems such as language, memory, and attention (e.g., see Graff-Radford et al., 1985, regarding polar artery lesions), forcing us to look at the relationships between them. Thus, progress in understanding the role of subcortical structures in cognition will not only inform us about functional brain systems, it also is likely to yield information regarding the relationship between language, verbal memory, and attention.

In closing, I hope that this volume has made some contribution to the consideration of neurobiological systems in language and memory. Future empirical studies and theoretical contributions in the area should help us to discover how complex brain systems work. In many respects, an understanding of subcortical functions in cognition is one critical link to developing further knowledge about these systems.

References

Aggleton, J. P. (1986). Memory impairments caused by experimental thalamic lesions in monkeys. *Revue Neurologique, 142,* 418–424.

Albert, M. L., Bachman, D. L., Morgan, A., & Helm-Estabrooks, N. (1988). Pharmacotherapy for aphasia. *Neurology, 38,* 877–879.

Albert, M. L., Feldman, R. G., & Willis, A. L. (1974). The "subcortical dementia" of progressive supranuclear palsy. *Journal of Neurology, Neurosurgery, and Psychiatry, 37,* 121–130.

Albert, M. S., Butters, N., & Brandt, J. (1981). Patterns of remote memory in amnesic and demented patients. *Archives of Neurology, 38,* 495–500.

Albert, M. S., Butters, N., & Levin, J. (1979). Temporal gradients in retrograde amnesia of patients with alcoholic Korsakoff's disease. *Archives of Neurology, 36,* 211–216.

Alexander, G. E., DeLong, M. R., & Strick, P. L. (1986). Parallel organization of functionally segregated circuits linking basal ganglia cortex. *Annual Review of Neuroscience, 9,* 357–381.

Alexander, M. P. (1989, September). *Nonthalamic subcortical lesions and aphasia: CT and PET studies.* Paper presented at the Meeting on Neuropsychological Disorders Associated with Subcortical Lesions, Como, Italy.

Alexander, M. P., & Freedman, M. (1983). Amnesia after anterior communicating artery aneurysm rupture. *Neurology, 34*(Supp. 2), 104.

Alexander, M. P., & LoVerme, S. R. (1980). Aphasia after left hemispheric hemorrhage. *Neurology, 30,* 1193–1202.

Alexander, M. P., Naeser, M. A., & Palumbo, C. L. (1987). Correlations of subcortical CT lesion sites and aphasia profiles. *Brain, 110,* 961–991.

Allen, C. M., Turner, J. W., & Gadea-Ciria, M. (1966). Investigations into speech disturbances following stereotaxic surgery for parkinsonism. *British Journal of Communication Disorders, 1,* 55–59.

Aram, D. M., Rose, D. F., Rekate, H. L., & Whitaker, H. A. (1983). Acquired capsular/striatal aphasia in childhood. *Archives of Neurology, 40,* 614–617.

Archer, C. R., Ilinsky, I. A., Goldfader, P. R., & Smith, K. R. (1981). Aphasia in thalamic stroke: CT stereotactic localization. *Journal of Computer-Assisted Tomography, 5,* 427–432.

Ardila, A., & Lopez, M. V. (1984). Transcortical motor aphasia: One or two aphasias? *Brain and Language, 22,* 350–353.

Arendt, T., Bigl, V., Arendt, A., & Tennstedt, A. (1983). Loss of neurons in the nucleus basalis of Meynert in Alzheimer's disease, paralysis agitans, and Korsakoff's disease. *Acta Neuropathologica, 61,* 101–108.

Asanuma, C., Andersen, R. A., & Cowan, W. M. (1985). The thalamic relations of the caudal inferior parietal lobule and the lateral prefrontal cortex in monkeys: Divergent cortical projections from cell clusters in the medial pulvinar nucleus. *Journal of Comparative Neurology, 241,* 357–381.

Asanuma, C., Thach, W. T., & Jones, E. G. (1983a). Anatomical evidence for segregated focal groupings of efferent cells and their terminal ramifications in the cerebellothalamic pathway of the monkey. *Brain Research Review, 5,* 267–297.

Asanuma, C., Thach, W. T., & Jones, E. G. (1983b). Cytoarchitectonic delineation of the ventral lateral thalamic region in monkeys. *Brain Research Review, 5,* 219–235.

Asanuma, C., Thach, W. T., & Jones, E. G. (1983c). Distribution of cerebellar terminations and their relation to other afferent terminations in the thalamic ventral lateral region of the monkey. *Brain Research Review, 5,* 237–265.

Asso, D., Crown, S., Russell, J. A., & Logue, V. (1969). Psychological aspects of the stereotactic treatment of parkinsonism. *British Journal of Psychiatry, 115,* 541–553.

Atkinson, R. C., & Shiffrin, R. M. (1968). Human memory: A proposed system and its control process. In K. W. Spence & J. T. Spence (Eds.), *Advances in the psychology of learning and motivation research and theory* (Vol. 2, pp. 89–195). New York: Academic Press.

Bachevalier, J., Parkinson, J. K., & Mishkin, M. (1985). Visual recognition in monkeys: Effects of separate vs. combined transection of fornix and amygdalofugal pathways. *Experimental Brain Research, 57,* 554–561.

Baddeley, A. D. (1990). *Human memory: Theory and practice.* Needham Heights, MA: Allyn and Bacon.

Baddeley, A. D., & Hitch, G. (1977). Recency re-examined. In S. Dornic (Ed.), *Attention and performance* (Vol. 6, pp. 647–667). Hillsdale, NJ: Lawrence Erlbaum.

Baddeley, A. D., & Warrington, E. K. (1970). Amnesia and the distinction between long- and short-term memory. *Journal of Verbal Learning and Verbal Behavior, 9,* 176–189.

Baddeley, A. D., & Warrington, E. K. (1973). Memory coding and amnesia. *Neuropsychologia, 11,* 159–165.

Bannister, R. (1985). *Brain's clinical neurology* (6th ed.). New York: Oxford University Press.

Baron, J. C., D'Antona, R., Pantano, P., Serdaru, M., Samson, Y., & Bousser, M. G. (1986). Effects of thalamic stroke on energy metabolism of the cerebral cortex: A positron tomography study in man. *Brain, 109,* 1243–1259.

Bartus, R. T., Flicker, C., Dean, R. L., Pontecorvo, M., Figueiredo, J. C., & Fisher,

S. K. (1985). Selective memory loss following nucleus basalis lesions: Long-term behavioral recovery despite persistent cholinergic deficiencies. *Pharmacology, Biochemistry, and Behavior, 23,* 125–135.

Basso, A., Sala, S. D., & Farabola, M. (1987). Aphasia arising from purely deep lesions. *Cortex, 23,* 29–44.

Bayles, K. A., & Tomoeda, C. K. (1983). Confrontation naming impairment in dementia. *Brain and Language, 19,* 98–114.

Beatty, W. W., & Butters, N. (1986). Further analysis of encoding in patients with Huntington's disease. *Brain and Cognition, 5,* 387–398.

Beatty, W. W., Salmon, D. P., Butters, N., Heindel, W. C., & Granholm, E. L. (1988). Retrograde amnesia in patients with Alzheimer's disease or Huntington's disease. *Neurobiology of Aging, 9,* 181–186.

Bell, D. S. (1968). Speech functions of the thalamus inferred from the effects of thalamotomy. *Brain, 91,* 619–636.

Beninger, R. J., Jhamandas, K., Boegman, R. J., & El-Defrawy, S. R. (1986a). Effects of scopolamine and unilateral lesions of the basal forebrain on T-maze spatial discrimination and alternation in rats. *Pharmacology, Biochemistry, and Behavior, 24,* 1353–1360.

Beninger, R. J., Jhamandas, K., Boegman, R. J., & El-Defrawy, S. R. (1986b). Kynurenic acid-induced protection of neurochemical and behavioral deficits produced by quinolinic acid injections into the nucleus basalis of rats. *Neuroscience Letters, 68,* 317–321.

Benson, D. F. (1979). *Aphasia, alexia, and agraphia.* New York: Churchill-Livingstone.

Benson, D. F. (1985). Aphasia. In K. M. Heilman & E. Valenstein (Eds.), *Clinical neuropsychology* (pp. 17–47). New York: Oxford University Press.

Bhatnager, S. C., Andy, O. J., Korabic, E. W., Tikofsky, R. S., Saxena, V. K., Hellman, R. S., Collier, B. D., & Krohn, L. D. (1989). The effect of thalamic stimulation in processing of verbal stimuli in dichotic listening tasks: A case study. *Brain and Language, 36,* 236–251.

Bird, T. D., Stranahan, S., Sumi, S. M., & Raskind, M. (1983). Alzheimer's disease: Choline acetyltransferase activity in brain tissue from clinical and pathological subgroups. *Annals of Neurology, 14,* 284–293.

Bladin, P. F., & Berkovic, S. F. (1984). Striatocapsular infarction: Large infarcts in the lenticulostriate arterial territory. *Neurology, 34,* 1423–1430.

Blumstein, S. E. (1981). Neurolinguistic disorders: Language-brain relationships. In S. B. Filskov & T. J. Boll (Eds.), *Handbook of clinical neuropsychology* (pp. 227–256). New York: Wiley.

Blumstein, S. E., Goodglass, H., Statlender. S., & Biber, C. (1983). Comprehension strategies determining reference in aphasia: A study of reflexivization. *Brain and Language, 18,* 115–127.

Bogousslavsky, J., Miklossy, J., Deruaz, J. P., & Regli, F. (1988). Thalamic aphasia. *Neurology, 38,* 1662.

Bogousslavsky, J., Regli, F., & Assal, G. (1986). The syndrome of unilateral tuberothalamic artery territory infarction. *Stroke, 17,* 434–441.

Bogousslavsky, J., Regli, F., & Uske, A. (1988). Thalamic infarcts: Clinical syndromes, etiology, and prognosis. *Neurology, 38,* 837–848.

Bos, J., & Benevento, L. A. (1975). Projections of the medial pulvinar to orbital cortex and frontal eye fields in the rhesus monkey. *Experimental Neurology,* *49,* 487–496.

Botez, M. I., & Barbeau, A. (1971). Role of subcortical structures, and particularly the thalamus, in mechanisms of speech and language. *International Journal of Neurology, 8,* 300–320.

Bowers, D., Verfaellie, M., Valenstein, E., & Heilman, K. M. (1988). Impaired acquisition of temporal information in retrosplenial amnesia. *Brain and Cognition, 8,* 47–66.

Bradley, V. A., Welch, J. L., & Dick, D. J. (1989). Visuospatial working memory in Parkinson's disease. *Journal of Neurology, Neurosurgery, and Psychiatry, 52,* 1228–1235.

Brandt, J., & Butters, N. (1986). The neuropsychology of Huntington's disease. *Trends in Neurosciences, 9,* 118–120.

Brandt, J., Folstein, S. E., & Folstein, M. F. (1988). Differential cognitive impairment in Alzheimer's disease and Huntington's disease. *Annals of Neurology, 23,* 555–561.

Broadbent, D. E. (1958). *Perception and communication.* London: Pergamon Press.

Broadbent, G. (1872). *On the cerebral mechanisms of speech and thought.* London. (Cited by Wallesch & Papagno, 1988.)

Brooks, D. N., & Baddeley, A. D. (1976). What can amnesic patients learn? *Neuropsychologia, 14,* 111–122.

Brown, G. G., Kieran, S., & Patel, S. (1989). Memory functioning following a left medial thalamic hematoma. *Journal of Clinical and Experimental Neuropsychology, 11,* 206–218.

Brown, J. W. (1975). On the neural organization of language: Thalamic and cortical relationships. *Brain and Language, 2,* 18–30.

Brown, J. W. (1977). Thalamic mechanisms in language. In M. J. Gazzaniga (Ed.), *Handbook of behavioral neurobiology: Vol. 2. Neuropsychology* (pp. 215–237). New York: Plenum Press.

Brown, J. W., Riklan, M., Waltz, J. M., Jackson, S., & Cooper, I. S. (1971). Preliminary studies of language and cognition following surgical lesions of the pulvinar in man. *International Journal of Neurology, 8,* 276–299.

Brown, R. G. (1989, September). *Processing resources and dual task performance in patients with Parkinson's disease.* Paper presented at the Meeting on Neuropsychological Disorders Associated with Subcortical Lesions, Como, Italy.

Brown, R. G., & Marsden, C. D. (1988a). Internal versus external cues and the control of attention in Parkinson's disease. *Brain, 111,* 323–345.

Brown, R. G., & Marsden, C. D. (1988b). An investigation into the phenomenon of "set" in Parkinson's disease. *Movement Disorders, 3,* 152–161.

Brunner, R. J., Kornhuber, H. H., Seemuller, E., Suger, G., & Wallesch, C. W. (1982). Basal ganglia participation in language pathology. *Brain and Language, 16,* 281–299.

Bruyn, R. P. M. (1989). Thalamic aphasia: A conceptual critique. *Journal of Neurology, 230,* 21–25.

Buckingham, H. W., Jr., & Hollien, H. (1978). A neural model for language and speech. *Journal of Phonetics, 6,* 283–297.

Bucy, P. C. (1942). The neural mechanisms of athetosis and tremor. *Journal of Neuropathology and Experimental Neurology, 1,* 224–231.

Bugiani, O., Coforto, C., & Sacco, G. (1969). Aphasia in thalamic hemorrhage. *Lancet, 1,* 1052.

Buschke, H. (1973). Selective reminding for analysis of memory and learning. *Journal of Verbal Learning and Verbal Behavior, 12*(12), 543–550.

Butters, N. (1985). Alcoholic Korsakoff's syndrome: Some unresolved issues concerning etiology, neuropathology, and cognitive deficits. *Journal of Clinical and Experimental Neuropsychology, 7,* 181–210.

Butters, N., & Cermak, L. S. (1980). *Alcoholic Korsakoff's syndrome: An information-processing approach to amnesia.* New York: Academic Press.

Butters, N., Granholm, E., Salmon, D. P., Grant, I., & Wolfe, J. (1987). Episodic and semantic memory: A comparison of amnesic and demented patients. *Journal of Clinical and Experimental Neuropsychology, 9,* 479–497.

Butters, N., Lewis, R., Cermak, L. S., & Goodglass, H. (1973). Material-specific memory deficits in alcoholic Korsakoff patients. *Neuropsychologia, 11,* 291–299.

Butters, N., Miliotis, P., Albert, M. S., & Sax, D. S. (1984). Memory assessment: Evidence of the heterogeneity of amnesic symptoms. In G. Goldstein (Ed.), *Advances in clinical neuropsychology* (Vol. 1, pp. 127–159). New York: Plenum Press.

Butters, N., Sax, D., Montgomery, K., & Tarlow, S. (1978). Comparison of the neuropsychological deficits associated with early and advanced Huntington's disease. *Archives of Neurology, 35,* 585–589.

Butters, N., & Stuss, D. T. (1989). Diencephalic amnesia. In F. Boller & J. Grafman (Eds.), *Handbook of neuropsychology* (Vol. 3, pp. 107–148). Amsterdam: Elsevier.

Butters, N., Tarlow, S., Cermak, L. S., & Sax, D. (1976). A comparison of the information processing deficits of patients with Huntington's chorea and Korsakoff's syndrome. *Cortex, 12,* 134–144.

Butters, N., Wolfe, J., Granholm, E., & Martone, M. (1986). An assessment of verbal recall, recognition, and fluency abilities in patients with Huntington's disease. *Cortex, 22,* 11–32.

Butters, N., Wolfe, J., Martone, M., Granholm, E., & Cermak, L. S. (1985). Memory disorders associated with Huntington's disease: Verbal recall, verbal recognition, and procedural memory. *Neuropsychologia, 23,* 729–743.

Caine, E. D., Ebert, M. H., & Weingartner, H. (1977). An outline for the analysis of dementia: The memory disorder of Huntington's disease. *Neurology, 27,* 1087–1093.

Cairns, H., & Mosberg, W. H. (1951). Colloid cyst of the third ventricle. *Surgery, Gynecology, and Obstetrics, 92,* 545–570.

Cambier, H., Elghozi, D., & Graveleau, P. (1982). *Neuropsychologie des lesions du thalamus.* Rapport de Neurologie. Congres de Psychiatrie et de Neurologie de langue francaise. (Cited by Demonet, 1987)

Caplan, L. R., Schmahmann, J. D., Kase, C. S., Feldmann, E., Baquis, G., Greenberg, J. P., Gorelick, P. B., Helgason, C., Hier, D. B. (1990). Caudate infarcts. *Archives of Neurology, 47,* 133–143.

Cappa, S. F., Cavallotti, G., Guidotti, M., Papagno, C., & Vignolo, L. A. (1983). Subcortical aphasia: Two clinical-CT scan correlation studies. *Cortex, 19,* 227–241.

Cappa, S. F., Papagno, C., Vallar, G., & Vignolo, L. A. (1986). Aphasia does not always follow left thalamic hemorrhage: A study of five negative cases. *Cortex, 22,* 639–647.

Cappa, S. F., & Vallar, G. (1989, September). *Neuropsychological disorders after subcortical lesions and neural models of language and spatial attention.* Paper presented at the Meeting on Neuropsychological Disorders Associated with Subcortical Lesions, Como, Italy.

Cappa, S. F., & Vignolo, L. A. (1979). "Transcortical" features of aphasia following left thalamic hemorrhage. *Cortex, 15,* 121–130.

Carpenter, M. B., & Sutin, J. (1983). *Human neuroanatomy* (8th ed.). Baltimore: Williams and Wilkins.

Casamenti, F., Bracco, L., Bartolini, L., & Pepeu, G. (1985). Effects of ganglioside treatment in rats with a lesion of the cholinergic forebrain nuclei. *Brain Research, 338,* 45–52.

Castaigne, P., Lhermitte, F., Buge, A., Escourolle, R., Hauw, J. H., & Lyon-Caen, O. (1981). Paramedian thalamic and midbrain infarcts: Clinical and neuropathological study. *Annals of Neurology, 10,* 127–148.

Cermak, L. S. (1984). The episodic-semantic distinction in amnesia. In L. R. Squire & N. Butters (Eds.), *Neuropsychology of memory* (pp. 55–62). New York: Guilford Press.

Cermak, L. S., & Butters, N. (1972). The role of interference and encoding in the short-term memory deficits of Korsakoff patients. *Neuropsychologia, 10,* 89–95.

Cermak, L. S., Butters, N., & Gerrein, J. (1973). The extent of the verbal encoding ability of Korsakoff patients. *Neuropsychologia, 11,* 85–94.

Cermak, L. S., Butters, N., & Goodglass, H. (1971). The extent of memory loss in Korsakoff patients. *Neuropsychologia, 9,* 307–315.

Cermak, L. S., Butters, N., & Moreines, J. (1974). Some analyses of the verbal encoding deficit of alcoholic Korsakoff patients. *Brain and Language, 1,* 141–150.

Cermak, L. S., Lewis, R., Butters, N., & Goodglass, H. (1973). Role of verbal mediation in performance of motor tasks by Korsakoff patients. *Perceptual and Motor Skills, 37,* 259–262.

Cermak, L. S., & Reale, L. (1978). Depth of processing and retention of words by alcoholic Korsakoff patients. *Journal of Experimental Psychology: Human Learning and Memory, 4,* 165–174.

Cermak, L. S., Talbot, N., Chandler, K., & Wolbarst, L. R. (1985). The perceptual priming phenomenon in amnesia. *Neuropsychologia, 23,* 615–622.

Chesson, A. L. (1983). Aphasia following a right thalamic hemorrhage. *Brain and Language, 19,* 306–316.

Choi, D., Sudarsky, L., Schachter, S., Biber, M., & Burke, P. (1983). Medial thalamic hemorrhage with amnesia. *Archives of Neurology, 40,* 611–613.

Chui, H. C., Mortimer, J. A., Slager, U., Zarow, C., Bondareff, W., & Webster, D. D. (1986). Pathologic correlates of dementia in Parkinson's disease. *Archives of Neurology, 43,* 991–995.

Chusid, J. G. (1985). *Correlative neuroanatomy and functional neurology* (19th ed.). Los Altos, CA: Lange Medical Publications.

Ciemans, V. A. (1970). Localized thalamic hemorrhage: A cause of aphasia. *Neurology, 20,* 776–782.

Cofer, C. N. (1976). An historical perspective. In C. N. Cofer (Ed.), *The structure of human memory* (pp. 1–14). San Francisco: W. H. Freeman.

Cohen, J. A., Gelfer, C. E., & Sweet, R. D. (1980). Thalamic infarction producing aphasia. *Mount Sinai Journal of Medicine, 47,* 398–404.

Cohen, N. J., & Squire, L. R. (1980). Preserved learning and retention of pattern-analyzing skill in amnesia: Dissociation of knowing how and knowing that. *Science, 210,* 207–210.

Cools, A. R., van den Bercken, J. H. L., Horstink, M. W. I., van Spaedonck, K. P. M., & Berger, H. J. C. (1984). Cognitive and motor shifting aptitude disorder in Parkinson's disease. *Journal of Neurology, Neurosurgery, and Psychiatry, 47,* 443–453.

Cooper, I. S. (1958). Chemopallidectomy and chemothalamectomy for parkinsonism and dystonia. *Proceedings of the Royal Society of Medicine, 52,* 47–60.

Cooper, I. S., Riklan, M., Stellar, S., Waltz, J. M., Levita, E., Ribera, V. A., & Zimmerman, J. (1968). A multidisciplinary investigation of neurosurgical rehabilitation in bilateral parkinsonism. *Journal of the American Geriatrics Society, 16,* 1177–1306.

Corkin, S. (1968). Acquisition of motor skill after bilateral medial temporal lobe excision. *Neuropsychologia, 6,* 255–265.

Cote, L., & Crutcher, M. D. (1985). Motor functions of the basal ganglia and diseases of transmitter metabolism. In E. R. Kandel & J. H. Schwartz (Eds.), *Principles of neural science* (2nd ed., pp. 523–536). New York: Elsevier.

Cowan, N. (1988). Evolving conceptions of memory storage, selective attention, and their mutual constraints within the human information-processing system. *Psychological Bulletin, 104,* 163–191.

Coyle, J. T., Price, D. L., & DeLong, M. R. (1983). Alzheimer's disease: A disorder of cortical cholinergic innervation. *Science, 219,* 1184–1190.

Craik, F. I. M., & Lockhart, R. S. (1972). Levels of processing: A framework for memory research. *Journal of Verbal Learning and Verbal Behavior, 11,* 671–684.

Cramon, D. Y. von. (1989, September). *Focal cerebral lesions damaging (subcortical) fiber projections related to memory and learning functions in man.* Paper presented at the Meeting on Neuropsychological Disorders Associated with Subcortical Lesions, Como, Italy.

Cramon, D. Y. von, Hebel, N., & Schuri, U. (1985). A contribution to the anatomical basis of thalamic amnesia. *Brain, 108,* 993–1008.

Cramon, D. Y. von, Hebel, N., & Schuri, U. (1986). Is vascular thalamic amnesia a disconnection syndrome? In K. Poeck, H. J. Freund, & H. Ganshirt (Eds.), *Neurology* (pp. 195–203). Berlin: Springer-Verlag.

Cramon, D. Y. von, Hebel, N., & Schuri, U. (1988). Verbal memory and learning in unilateral posterior cerebral infarction: A report on 30 cases. *Brain, 111,* 1061–1077.

Crawford, T. J., Henderson, L., & Kennard, C. (1989). Abnormalities of nonvisually guided eye movements in Parkinson's disease. *Brain, 112,* 1573–1586.

Crosson, B. (1981, August). *The thalamic feedback loop in aphasia: A tentative model.* Paper presented at the annual meeting of the American Psychological Association, Los Angeles.

Crosson, B. (1984). Role of the dominant thalamus in language: A review. *Psychological Bulletin, 96,* 491–517.

Crosson, B. (1985). Subcortical functions in language: A working model. *Brain and Language, 25,* 257–292.

Crosson, B. (1986). On localization versus systemic effects in alcoholic Korsakoff's syndrome: A comment on Butters (1985). *Journal of Clinical and Experimental Neuropsychology, 8,* 744–748.

Crosson, B. (1989, September). *Is the striatum involved in language?* Paper presented at the Meeting on Neuropsychological Disorders Associated with Subcortical Lesions, Como, Italy.

Crosson, B., & Early, T. S. (1990). *A theory of subcortical functions in language: Current status.* Unpublished manuscript.

Crosson, B., & Hughes, C. W. (1987). Role of the thalamus in language: Is it related to schizophrenic thought disorder: *Schizophrenia Bulletin, 13,* 605–621.

Crosson, B., Novack, T. A., & Trenerry, M. R. (1988). Subcortical language mechanisms: Window on a new frontier. In H. A. Whitaker (Ed.), *Phonological processes and brain mechanisms* (pp. 24–58). New York: Springer-Verlag.

Crosson, B., Parker, J. C., Warren, R. L., Kepes, J. J., Kim, A. K., & Tulley, R. C. (1986). A case of thalamic aphasia with post mortem verification. *Brain and Language, 29,* 301–314.

Crosson, B., Parker, J. C., Warren, R. L., LaBreche, T., & Tully, R. (1983, August). *Dominant thalamic lesion with and without aphasia.* Paper presented at the meeting of the American Psychological Association, Anaheim, CA.

Cudeiro, J., Gonzalez, F., Perez, R., Alonso, J. M., & Acuña, C. (1989). Does the pulvinar-LP complex contribute to motor programming? *Brain Research, 484,* 367–370.

Cummings, J. L. & Benson, D. F. (1984). Subcortical dementia: Review of an emerging concept. *Archives of Neurology, 41,* 874–879.

Cummings, J. L., Benson, D. F., Hill, M. A., & Read, S. (1985). Aphasia in dementia of the Alzheimer type. *Neurology, 35,* 394–397.

Cummings, J. L., Darkins, A., Mendez, M., Hill, M. A., & Benson, D. F. (1988). Alzheimer's disease and Parkinson's disease: Comparison of speech and language alterations. *Neurology, 38,* 680–684.

Damasio, A. R., Damasio, H., Rizzo, M., Varney, N., & Gersh, F. (1982). Aphasia with nonhemorrhagic lesions in the basal ganglia and internal capsule. *Archives of Neurology, 39,* 15–20.

Damasio, A. R., Eslinger, P. J., Damasio, H., Van Hoesen, G. W., & Cornell, S. (1985a). Multimodal amnesic syndrome following bilateral temporal and basal forebrain damage. *Archives of Neurology, 42,* 252–259.

Damasio, A. R., Graff-Radford, N. R., Eslinger, P. J., Damasio, H., & Kassell, N. (1985b). Amnesia following basal forebrain lesions. *Archives of Neurology, 42,* 263–271.

Darley, F. L., Brown, J. R., & Swenson, W. M. (1975). Language changes after neurosurgery for parkinsonism. *Brain and Language, 2,* 65–69.

Davidoff, D., Butters, N., Gerstman, L., Zurif, E., Paul, I., & Mattis, S. (1984). Affective-motivational factors in the recall of prose passages by alcoholic Korsakoff patients. *Alcohol, 1,* 63–69.

Davis, K. L., & Yamamura, H. I. (1978). Cholinergic underactivity in human memory disorders. *Life Sciences, 23,* 1729–1734.

DeCroix, J. P., Graveleau, P., Masson, M., & Cambier, J. (1986). Infarction in the territory of the anterior choroidal artery: A clinical and computed tomographic study of 16 cases. *Brain, 109,* 1071–1085.

De la Monte, S. M., Wells, S. E., Hedley-Whyte, E. T., & Growdon, J. H. (1989). Neuropathological distinction between Parkinson's dementia and Parkinson's plus Alzheimer's disease. *Annals of Neurology, 26,* 309–320.

Delis, D. C., Kramer, J. H., Kaplan, E., & Ober, B. A. (1987). *California Verbal Learning Test.* San Antonio, TX: Psychological Corporation.

Deloche, G., Andreewsky, E., & Desi, M. (1982). Surface dyslexia: A case report and some theoretical implications to reading models. *Brain and Language, 15,* 12–31.

DeLuca, J. (1990). Predicting behavioral patterns following anterior communicating artery aneurysm. *Archives of Physical Medicine and Rehabilitation, 71,* 828.

DeLuca, J., & Cicerone, K. (1989). Cognitive impairments following anterior communicating artery aneurysm. *Journal of Clinical and Experimental Neuropsychology, 11,* 47.

DeLuca, J., & Cicerone, K. D. (in press). Confabulation following aneurysm of the anterior communicating artery. *Cortex.*

Demeurisse, G., Derouck, M., Coekaerts, M. J., Deltenre, P., Van Nechel, C., Demol, O., & Capon, A. (1979). Study of two cases of aphasia by infarction of the left thalamus without cortical lesion. *Acta Neurologica Belgica, 79,* 450–459.

Demonet, J.-F. (1987). *Les Aphasies sous-corticales: Etude linguistique, radiologique et hemodynamique de 31 observations.* These Pour le Doctorat D'Etat en Medicine, Universite Paul Sabatier-Toulouse III, Facultes de Medecine.

Demonet, J.-F., Celsis, P., Puel, M., Cardebat, D., Marc-Vergnes, J. P., & Rascol, A. (1989, September). *A SPECT approach of subcortical thalamic and nonthalamic aphasia.* Paper presented at the Meeting on Neuropsychological Disorders Associated with Subcortical Lesions, Como, Italy.

Direnfeld, L. K., Albert, M. L., Volicer, L., Langlais, P. J., Marquis, J., & Kaplan, E. (1984). Parkinson's disease: The possible relationship of laterality to dementia and neurochemical findings. *Archives of Neurology, 41,* 935–941.

Divak, I. (1984). The neostriatum viewed orthogonally. In D. Evered & M. O'Connor (Eds.), *Functions of the basal ganglia. Proceedings of Ciba Foundation Symposium 107* (pp. 201–215). Summit, NJ: Ciba.

Divac, I., Oberg, G. E., & Rosenkilde, C. E. (1987). Patterned neural activity: Implications for neurology and neuropharmacology. In J. S. Schneider & T. I. Lidsky (Eds.), *Basal ganglia and behavior: Sensory aspects of motor functioning* (pp. 61–67). Lewiston, NY: Hans Huber.

Drachman, D. A. (1977). Memory and cognitive function in man: Does the cholinergic system have a specific role? *Neurology, 27,* 783–790.

Du Cros, J. T., & Lhermitte, F. (1984). Neuropsychological analysis of ruptured saccular aneurysms of the anterior communicating artery after radical therapy (32 cases). *Surgical Neurology, 22,* 353–359.

Dunnett, S. B. (1985). Comparative effects of cholinergic drugs and lesions of nucleus basalis or fimbria-fornix on delayed matching in rats. *Psychopharmacology, 87,* 357–363.

Early, T. S., Posner, M. I., Reiman, E. M., & Raichle, M. E. (1989a). Hyperactivity of the left striato-pallidal projection: 1. Lower level theory. *Psychiatric Developments, 2,* 85–108.

Early, T. S., Posner, M. I., Reiman, E. M., & Raichle, M. E. (1989b). Left striato-pallidal hyperactivity in schizophrenia: 2. Phenomenology and thought disorder. *Psychiatric Developments, 2,* 109–121.

Early, T. S., Reiman, E. M., Raichle, M. E., & Spitznagel, E. L. (1987). Left globus pallidus abnormality in never-medicated patients with schizophrenia. *Proceedings of the National Academy of Sciences* (USA), *84,* 561–563.

Eccles, J. C. (1977). Part II: Chapters E1–E8. In K. R. Popper & J. C. Eccles (Eds.), *The self and its brain* (225–421). New York: Springer.

El-Awar, M., Becker, J. T., Hammond, K. M., Nebes, R. D., & Boller, F. (1987). Learning deficit in Parkinson's disease: Comparison with Alzheimer's disease and normal aging. *Archives of Neurology, 44,* 180–184.

Faber-Langendoen, K., Morris, J. C., Knesevich, J. W., LaBarge, E., Miller, J. P., & Berg, L. (1988). Aphasia in senile dementia of the Alzheimer type. *Annals of Neurology, 23,* 365–370.

Fasanaro, A. M., Spitaleri, D. L. A., Valiani, R., Postiglione, A., Soricelli, A., Mansi, L., & Grossi, D. (1987). Cerebral blood flow in thalamic aphasia. *Journal of Neurology, 234,* 421–423.

Fazio, C., Sacco, G., & Bugiani, O. (1973). The thalamic hemorrhage. An anatomo-clinical study. *European Neurology, 9,* 30–43.

Fensore, C., Lazzarino, L. G., Nappo, A., & Nicolai, A. (1988). Language and memory disturbances from mesencephalothalamic infarcts: A clinical and computed tomography study. *European Neurology, 28,* 51–56.

Ferro, J. M., Martins, I. P., Pinto, F., & Castro-Caldas, A. (1982). Aphasia following right striato-insular infarction in a left-handed child: A clinico-radiological study. *Developmental Medicine and Child Neurology, 24,* 173–178.

Fisher, C. M. (1979). Capsular infarcts: The underlying vascular lesions. *Archives of Neurology, 36,* 65–73.

Fisher, J. M., Kennedy, J. L., Caine, E. D., & Shoulson, I. (1983). Dementia in Huntington disease: A cross-sectional analysis of intellectual decline. In R. Mayeux & W. G. Rosen (Eds.), *The dementias* (pp. 229–238). New York: Raven Press.

Fisher, W., Kerbeshian, J., & Burd, L. (1986). A treatable language disorder: Pharmacological treatment of pervasive developmental disorder. *Developmental and Behavioral Pediatrics, 7(2),* 73–76.

Flicker, C., Dean, R. L., Watkins, D. L., Fisher, S. K., & Bartus, R. T. (1983). Behavioral and neurochemical effects following neurotoxic lesions of major cholinergic input to the cerebral cortex in the rat. *Pharmacology, Biochemistry, and Behavior, 18,* 973–981.

Flowers, K. A., Pearce, I., & Pearce, J. M. S. (1984). Recognition memory in Parkinson's disease. *Journal of Neurology, Neurosurgery, and Psychiatry, 47,* 1174–1181.

Freed, D. M., Corkin, S., & Cohen, N. J. (1987). Forgetting in H. M.: A second look. *Neuropsychologia, 25,* 461–471.

Freedman, M., & Oscar-Berman, M. (1989). Spatial and visual learning deficits in Alzheimer's and Parkinson's disease. *Brain and Cognition, 11,* 114–126.

Freedman, M., Rivoira, P., Butters, N., Sax, D. S., & Feldman, R. G. (1984). Retrograde amnesia in Parkinson's disease. *Canadian Journal of Neurological Sciences, 11,* 297–301.

Fried, I., Ojemann, G. A., & Fetz, E. B. (1981). Language-related potentials specific to human language cortex. *Science, 212,* 353–355.

Fromm, D., Holland, A. L., Swindell, C. S., & Reinmuth, O. M. (1985). Various consequences of subcortical stroke: Prospective study of 16 consecutive cases. *Archives of Neurology, 42,* 943–950.

Fuster, J. M. (1980). *The prefrontal cortex.* New York: Raven Press.

Gade, A. (1982). Amnesia after operations on aneurysms of the anterior communicating artery. *Surgical Neurology, 18,* 46–49.

Gamper, E. (1928). Zur frage der polioencephalitis haemorrhagic der chronischen alcoholiker. Anatomische befunde beim alkoholischen Korsakov undihre Beziehungen zum klinischen bild. *Deutsche Zeitschrift fur Nervenheilkunde, 102,* 122–129. (Cited by Wallesch & Papagno, 1988)

Garcia Bengochea, F., de la Torre, O., Esquivel, O., Vieta, R., & Fernandez, C. (1954). The section of the fornix in the surgical treatment of certain epilepsies: A preliminary report. *Transactions of the American Neurological Association, 79,* 176–178.

Gardner, H., Boller, F., Moreines, J., & Butters, N. (1973). Retrieving information from Korsakoff patients: Effects of categorical cues and reference to task. *Cortex, 9,* 165–175.

Gentilini, M., De Renzi, E., & Crisi, G. (1987). Bilateral paramedian thalamic artery infarcts: Report of eight cases. *Journal of Neurology, Neurosurgery, and Psychiatry, 50,* 900–909.

Gerfen, C. R. (1985). The neostriatal mosaic. 1. Compartmental organization of projections from the striatum to the substantia nigra in the rat. *Journal of Comparative Neurology, 236,* 454–476.

Geschwind, N. (1972). Language and the brain. *Scientific American, 226(4),* 78–83.

Gillingham, F. J., Watson, W. S., Donaldson, A. A., & Naughton, J. A. L. (1960). The surgical treatment of parkinsonism. *British Medical Journal, 2,* 1395–1402.

Glass, A. L., & Butters, N. (1985). The effect of associations and expectations on lexical decision making in normals, alcoholics, and alcoholic Korsakoff patients. *Brain and Cognition, 4,* 465–476.

Globus, M., Mildworf, B., & Melamed, E. (1985). Cerebral blood flow and cognitive impairment in Parkinson's disease. *Neurology, 35,* 1135–1139.

Glosser, G., Kaplan, E., & LoVerme, S. (1982). Longitudinal neuropsychological report of aphasia following left-subcortical hemorrhage. *Brain and Language, 15,* 95–116.

Goldberg, G. (1985). Supplementary motor area structure and function: Review and hypotheses. *Behavioral and Brain Sciences, 8,* 567–615.

Goldenberg, G., Wimmer, A., & Maly, J. (1983). Amnesic syndrome with a unilateral thalamic lesion: A case report. *Journal of Neurology, 229,* 79–86.

Goldman-Rakic, P. S. (1984). Modular organization of the prefrontal cortex. *Transactions in the Neuroscieces, 7,* 419–424.

Goldman-Rakic, P. S., & Selemon, L. D. (1986). Topography of corticostriatal projections in nonhuman primates and implications for functional parcellation of the neostriatum. In E. G. Jones & A. Peters (Eds.), *Cerebral cortex: Vol. 5. Sensory-motor areas and aspects of cortical connectivity* (pp. 447–466). New York: Plenum Press.

Goodglass, H., & Kaplan, E. (1972). *The assessment of aphasia and related disorders.* Philadelphia: Lea and Febiger.

Goodglass, H., & Kaplan, E. (1983). *The assessment of aphasia and related disorders* (2nd ed.). Philadelphia: Lea and Febiger.

Gordon, W. P., & Illes, J. (1987). Neurolinguistic characteristics of language production in Huntington's disease: A preliminary report. *Brain and Language, 31,* 1–10.

Gorelick, P. B., Hier, D. B., Benevento, L., Levitt, S., & Tan, W. (1984). Aphasia after left thalamic infarction. *Archives of Neurology, 41,* 1296–1298.

Graf, P., & Schacter, D. L. (1985). Implicit and explicit memory for new associations in normal and amnesic subjects. *Journal of Experimental Psychology: Learning, Memory, and Cognition, 11,* 501–518.

Graf, P., Squire, L. R., & Mandler, G. (1984). The information that amnesic patients do not forget. *Journal of Experimental Psychology: Learning, Memory, and Cognition, 10,* 164–178.

Graff-Radford, N. R., Damasio, H., Yamada, T., Eslinger, P. J., & Damasio, A. R. (1985). Nonhaemorrhagic thalamic infarction: Clinical, neuropsychological, and electrophysiological findings in four anatomical groups defined by computerized tomography. *Brain, 108,* 485–516.

Graff-Radford, N. R., Eslinger, P. J., Damasio, A. R., & Yamada, T. (1984). Nonhemorrhagic infarction of the thalamus: Behavioral, anatomic, and physiologic correlates. *Neurology, 34,* 14–23.

Graff-Radford, N. R., Tranel, D., Van Hoesen, G. W., & Brandt, J. P. (1990). Diencephalic amnesia. *Brain, 113,* 1–25.

Grafman, J., Salazar, A. M., Weingartner, H., Vance, S. C., & Ludlow, C. (1985). Isolated impairment of memory following a penetrating lesion of the fornix cerebri. *Archives of Neurology, 42,* 1162–1168.

Granholm, E., & Butters, N. (1988). Associative encoding and retrieval in Alzheimer's and Huntington's disease. *Brain and Cognition, 7,* 335–347.

Granholm, E., Wolfe, J., & Butters, N. (1985). Affective-arousal factors in the recall of thematic stories by amnesic and demented patients. *Developmental Neuropsychology, 1,* 317–333.

Grant, D. A., & Berg, E. A. (1948). A behavioral analysis of degree of reinforcement and ease of shifting to new responses in a Weigl-type card-sorting problem. *Journal of Experimental Psychology, 38,* 404–411.

Graybiel, A. M. (1984). Neurochemically specified subsystems in the basal ganglia. In D. Evered & M. O'Connor (Eds.), *Functions of the Basal Ganglia. Proceedings of Ciba Foundation Symposium, 107* (pp. 114–149). Summit, NJ: Ciba.

Graybiel, A. M., Baughman, R. W., & Eckenstein, F. (1986). Cholinergic neuropil of the striatum observes striosomal boundaries. *Nature, 323,* 625–627.

Groves, P. M. (1983). A theory of the functional organization of the neostriatum and the neostriatal control of voluntary movement. *Brain Research Reviews, 5,* 109–132.

Haines, D. E. (1987). *Neuroanatomy: An atlas of structures, sections, and systems.* Baltimore: Urban and Schwarzenberg.

Haroutunian, V., Mantin, R., & Kanof, P. D. (1990). Frontal cortex as the site of action of physostigmine in nbM-lesioned rats. *Physiology and Behavior, 47,* 203–206.

Hayashi, M. M., Ulatowska, H. K., & Sasanuma, S. (1985). Subcortical aphasia with deep dyslexia: A case study of a Japanese patient. *Brain and Language, 25,* 293–313.

Heilman, K. M., Bowers, D., Valenstein, E., & Watson, R. T. (1987). Hemispace and hemispatial neglect. In M. Jeannerod (Ed.), *Neurophysiological and neuropsychological aspects of spatial neglect* (pp. 115–150). Amsterdam: Elsevier.

Heilman, K. M., & Sypert, G. W. (1977). Korsakoff's syndrome resulting from bilateral fornix lesions. *Neurology, 27,* 490–493.

Heilman, K. M., & Watson, R. T. (1989, November). *Intentional-Activation disorders.* Paper presented at the 15th Annual Course in Behavioral Neurology and Neuropsychology of the Florida Society of Neurology and the Center for Neuropsychological Studies, Tampa, FL.

Heindel, W. C., Butters, N., & Salmon, D. P. (1988). Impaired learning of a motor skill in patients with Huntington's disease. *Behavioral Neuroscience, 102,* 141–147.

Heindel, W. C., Salmon, D. P., Shults, C. W., Walicke, P. A., & Butters, N. (1989). Neuropsychological evidence for multiple implicit memory systems: A comparison of Alzheimer's, Huntington's, and Parkinson's disease patients. *Journal of Neuroscience, 9,* 582–587.

Helper, D. J., Olton, D. S., Wenk, G. L., & Coyle, J. T. (1985). Lesions in nucleus basalis magnocellularis and medial septal area of rats produce qualitatively similar memory impairments. *Journal of Neuroscience, 5,* 866–873.

Hermann, K., Turner, J. W., Gillingham, F. J., & Gaze, R. M. (1966). The effects of destructive lesions and stimulation of the basal ganglia on speech mechanisms. *Confinia Neurologica, 27,* 197–207.

Hier, D. B., Davis, K. R., Richardson, E. P., & Mohr, J. P. (1977). Hypertensive putaminal hemorrhage. *Annals of Neurology, 1,* 152–159.

Hirose, G., Kosoegawa, H., Saeki, M., Kitagawa, Y., Oda, R., Kanda, S., & Matsuhira, T. (1985). The syndrome of posterior thalamic hemorrhage. *Neurology, 35,* 998–1002.

Hirst, W., Phelps, E. A., Johnson, M. K., & Volpe, B. T. (1988). Amnesia and second language learning. *Brain and Cognition, 8,* 105–116.

Horenstein, S., Chung, G., & Brenner, S. (1978). Aphasia in two verified cases of left thalamic hemorrhage. *Annals of Neurology, 4,* 177.

Hori, S., & Suzuki, J. (1979). Early and late results of intracranial direct surgery of anterior communicating artery aneurysms. *Journal of Neurosurgery, 50,* 433–440.

Huber, S. J., Shuttleworth, E. C., Christy, J. A., Chakeres, D. W., Curtin, A., & Paulson, G. W. (1989). Magnetic resonance imaging in dementia of Parkinson's disease. *Journal of Neurology, Neurosurgery, and Psychiatry, 52,* 1221–1227.

Huber, S. J., Shuttleworth, E. C., & Paulson, G. W. (1986). Dementia in Parkinson's disease. *Archives of Neurology, 43,* 987–990.

Huber, S. J., Shuttleworth, E. C., Paulson, G. W., Bellchambers, M. J. G., & Clapp, L. E. (1986). Cortical vs. subcortical dementia: Neuropsychological differences. *Archives of Neurology, 43,* 392–394.

Huppert, F. A., & Piercy, M. (1976). Recognition memory in amnesic patients: Effect of temporal context and familiarity of material. *Cortex, 12,* 3–20.

Huppert, F. A., & Piercy, M. (1977). Recognition memory in amnesic patients: A defect in acquisition? *Neuropsychologia, 15,* 643–652.

Huppert, F. A., & Piercy, M. (1978). Dissociation between learning and remembering in organic amnesia. *Nature, 275,* 317–318.

Huppert, F. A., & Piercy, M. (1979). Normal and abnormal forgetting in organic amnesia: Effect of locus of lesion. *Cortex, 15,* 385–390.

Illes, J. (1989). Neurolinguistic features of spontaneous language production dissociate three forms of neurodegenerative disease: Alzheimer's, Huntington's, and Parkinson's. *Brain and Language, 37,* 628–642.

Irle, E., & Markowitsch, H. J. (1987). Basal forebrain-lesioned monkeys are severely impaired in tasks of association and recognition memory. *Annals of Neurology, 22,* 735–743.

Iversen, S. D. (1984). Behavioral effects of manipulation of basal ganglia neurotransmitters. In D. Evered & M. O'Connor (Eds.), *Functions of the Basal Ganglia. Proceedings of Ciba Foundation Symposium, 107* (pp. 183–200). Summit, NJ: Ciba.

Jaffe, P. G., & Katz, A. N. (1975). Attenuating anterograde amnesia in Korsakoff's psychosis. *Journal of Abnormal Psychology, 84,* 559–562.

Jason, G. W., Pajurkova, E. M., Suchowersky, O., Hewitt, J., Hilbert, C., Reed, J., & Hayden, M. R. (1988). Presymptomatic neuropsychological impairment in Huntington's disease. *Archives of Neurology, 45,* 769–773.

Jenkyn, L. R., Alberti, A. R., & Peters, J. D. (1981). Language dysfunction, somasthetic inattention, and thalamic hemorrhage in the dominant hemisphere. *Neurology, 31,* 1202–1203.

Jones, E. G. (1985). *The thalamus.* New York: Plenum Press.

Josiassen, R. C., Curry, L. M., & Mancall, E. L. (1983). Development of neuropsychological deficits in Huntington's disease. *Archives of Neurology, 40,* 791–796.

Jurko, M. F., & Andy, O. J. (1973). Psychological changes correlated with thalamotomy site. *Journal of Neurology, Neurosurgery, and Psychiatry, 36,* 846–852.

Jurko, M. F., & Andy, O. J. (1977). Verbal learning dysfunction with combined centre median and amygdala lesions. *Journal of Neurology, Neurosurgery, and Psychiatry, 40,* 695–698.

Kahn, E. A., & Crosby, E. C. (1972). Korsakoff's syndrome associated with surgical lesions involving the mammillary bodies. *Neurology, 22,* 117–125.

Kameyama, M. (1976/1977). Vascular lesions of the thalamus on the dominant and nondominant side. *Applied Neurophysiology, 39,* 171–177.

Karabelas, G., Kalfakis, N., Kasvikis, I., & Vassilopoulos, D. (1985). Unusual features in a case of bilateral paramedian thalamic infarction. *Journal of Neurology, Neurosurgery, and Psychiatry, 48,* 186.

Kawahara, N., Sato, K., Muraki, M., Tanaka, K., Kaneko, M., & Uemura, K. (1986). CT classification of small thalamic hemorrhages and their clinical implications. *Neurology, 36,* 165–172.

Kemp, J. M., & Powell, T. P. S. (1970). The cortico-striate projection in the monkey. *Brain, 93,* 525–546.

Kennedy, J., Fisher, J., Shoulson, I., & Caine, E. (1981). Language impairment in Huntington disease. *Neurology, 31,* 81–82.

Kertesz, A. (1989, September). *Agraphia in subcortical lesions.* Paper presented at the Meeting on Neuropsychological Disorders Associated with Subcortical Lesions, Como, Italy.

Kessler, J., Markowitsch, H. J., & Sigg, G. (1986). Memory related role of the posterior cholinergic system. *International Journal of Neuroscience, 30,* 101–119.

Kirshner, H. S., & Kistler, K. H. (1982). Aphasia after right thalamic hemorrhage. *Archives of Neurology, 39,* 667–669.

Knopman, D. S., Selnes, O. A., Niccum, N., & Rubens, A. B. (1984). Recovery of naming in aphasia: Relationship to fluency, comprehension, and CT findings. *Neurology, 34,* 1461–1470.

Knowlton, B. J., Wenk, G. L., Olton, D. S., & Coyle, J. T. (1985). Basal forebrain lesions produce a dissociation of trial-dependent and trial-independent memory performance. *Brain Research, 345,* 315–321.

Kocsis, J. D., Sugimori, M., & Kitai, S. T. (1977). Convergence of excitatory synaptic inputs to caudate spiny neurons. *Brain Research, 124,* 403–413.

Kopelman, M. D. (1985). Rates of forgetting in Alzheimer-type dementia and Korsakoff's syndrome. *Neuropsychologia, 23,* 623–638.

Kramer, J. H., Delis, D. C., Blusewicz, M. J., Brandt, J., Ober, B. A., & Strauss, M. (1988). Verbal memory errors in Alzheimer's and Huntington's dementias. *Developmental Neuropsychology, 4,* 1–15.

Kramer, J. H., Levin, B. E., Brandt, J., & Delis, D. C. (1989). Differentiation of Alzheimer's, Huntington's, and Parkinson's disease patients on the basis of verbal learning characteristics. *Neuropsychology, 3,* 111–120.

Kritchevsky, M., Graff-Radford, N. R., Damasio, A. R. (1987). Normal memory after damage to medial thalamus. *Archives of Neurology, 44,* 959–962.

Kussmaul, A. (1877). *Die Storungen der Sprache.* Leipzig: Vogel. [Cited in Wallesch & Papagno, 1988].

Kwo-On-Yuen, P. F., Mandel, R., Chen, A. D., & Thal, L. J. (1990). Tetrahydroaminoacridine improves the spatial acquisition deficit produced by nucleus basalis lesions in rats. *Experimental Neurology, 108,* 221–228.

Laplane, D., Baulac, M., Widlocher, D., & Dubois, B. (1984). Pure psychic akinesia with bilateral lesions of basal ganglia. *Journal of Neurology, Neurosurgery, and Psychiatry, 47,* 377–385.

Larsell, O. (1951). *Anatomy of the nervous system.* New York: Appleton-Century-Crofts.

Lees, A. J. (1990). Progressive supranuclear palsy (Steele-Richardson-Olszewski syndrome). In J. L. Cummings (Ed.), *Subcortical dementia* (pp. 123–131). New York: Oxford University Press.

Lees, A. J., & Smith, E. (1983). Cognitive deficits in the early stages of Parkinson's disease. *Brain, 106,* 257–270.

Leonard, C. M. (1969). The prefrontal cortex of the rat: 1. Cortical projection of the mediodorsal nucleus. 2. Efferent connections. *Brain Research, 12,* 321–343.

Levin, B. E., Llabre, M. M., & Weiner, W. J. (1989). Cognitive impairments associated with early Parkinson's disease. *Neurology, 39,* 557–561.

Lezak, M. D. (1983). *Neuropsychological assessment* (2nd ed.). New York: Oxford University Press.

Lhermitte, F., & Signoret, J.-L. (1976). The amnesia syndromes and the hippocampal-mammillary system. In M. R. Rosenzweig & E. L. Bennett (Eds.), *Neural mechanisms of learning and memory* (pp. 49–56). Cambridge, MA: MIT Press.

Lichtheim., L. (1885). On aphasia. *Brain, 7,* 433–484.

Lieberman, R. R., Ellenberg, M., & Restum, W. H. (1986). Aphasia associated with verified subcortical lesions: Three case reports. *Archives of Physical Medicine and Rehabilitation, 67,* 410–414.

Lindqvist, G., & Norlen, G. (1966). Korsakoff's syndrome after operation on ruptured aneurysm of the anterior communicating artery. *Acta Psychiatrica Scandinavica, 42,* 24–34.

Litvan, I., Grafman, J., Gomez, C., & Chase, T. N. (1989). Memory impairment in patients with progressive supranuclear palsy. *Archives of Neurology, 46,* 765–767.

Logue, V., Durward, M., Pratt, R. T. C., Piercy, M., & Nixon, W. L. B. (1968). The quality of survival after rupture of an anterior cerebral aneurysm. *British Journal of Psychiatry, 114,* 137–160.

Ludlow, C. L., Rosenberg, J., Fair, C., Buck, D., Schesselman, S., & Salazar, A. (1986). Brain lesions associated with nonfluent aphasia fifteen years following penetrating head injury. *Brain, 109,* 55–80.

Luria, A. R. (1973). *The working brain.* (Translated by B. Haigh). New York: Basic Books.

Luria, A. R. (1977). On quasi-aphasic speech disturbances in lesions of the deep structures of the brain. *Brain and Language, 4,* 432–459.

Luria, A. R. (1980). *Higher cortical functions in man.* (Translated by B. Haigh). New York: Basic Books.

Magariños-Ascone, C., Buño, W., & Garcia-Austt, E. (1988). Monkey pulvinar units related to motor activity and sensory response. *Brain Research, 445,* 30–38.

Maher, E. R., Smith, E. M., & Lees, A. J. (1985). Cognitive deficits in the Steele-Richardson-Olszewski syndrome (progressive supranuclear palsy). *Journal of Neurology, Neurosurgery, and Psychiatry, 48,* 1234–1239.

Mair, W. G. P., Warrington, E. K., & Weiskrantz, L. (1979). Memory disorder in Korsakoff's psychosis: A neuropathological and neuropsychological investigation of two cases. *Brain, 102,* 749–783.

Maiuri, F., Signorelli, C., Colella, G., & Gangemi, M. (1983). Aphasia and left thalamic hemorrhage. *Acta Neurologica, 5,* 20–24.

Marie, P. (1906). Revision de la question de l'aphasie: Que faut-il penser des aphasies sous-corticales (aphasies pures)? *La Semaine Medicale,* no. 42, 17 October, 1906. [Cited in Demonet, 1987].

Markowitsch, H. J. (1982). Thalamic mediodorsal nucleus and memory: A critical evaluation of studies in animals and man. *Neuroscience and Biobehavioral Reviews, 6,* 351–380.

Marsden, C. D. (1984). Function of the basal ganglia as revealed by cognitive and motor disorders in Parkinson's disease. *Canadian Journal of the Neurological Sciences, 11,* 129–135.

Martone, M., Butters, N., Payne, M., Becker, J. T., & Sax, D. S. (1984). Dissociations between skill learning and verbal recognition in amnesia and dementia. *Archives of Neurology, 41,* 965–970.

Martone, M., Butters, N., & Trauner, D. (1986). Some analyses of forgetting pictorial material in amnesic and demented patients. *Journal of Clinical and Experimental Neuropsychology, 8,* 161–178.

Massman, P. J., Delis, D. C., Butters, N., Levin, B. E., & Salmon, D. P. (1990). Are all subcortical dementias alike?: Verbal learning and memory in Parkinson's and Huntington's disease patients. *Journal of Clinical and Experimental Neuropsychology, 12,* 729–744.

Mata, M., Fink, D. J., Gainer, H., Smith, C. B., Davidsen, L., Savaki, H., Schwartz, W. J., & Sokoloff, L. (1980). Activity-dependent energy metabolism in rat posterior pituitary primarily reflects sodium pump activity. *Journal of Neurochemistry, 34,* 213–215.

Matison, R., Mayeux, R., Rosen, J., & Fahn, S. (1982). "Tip-of-the-tongue" in Parkinson disease. *Neurology, 32,* 567–570.

Mayes, A., Meudell, P., & Neary, D. (1980). Do amnesics adopt inefficient encoding strategies with faces and random shapes? *Neuropsychologia, 18,* 527–540.

Mazzocchi, F., & Vignolo, L. A. (1979). Localisation of lesions in aphasia: Clinical–CT correlations in stroke patients. *Cortex, 15,* 627–654.

McCarthy, R., & Warrington, E. K. (1984). A two-route model of speech production: Evidence from aphasia. *Brain, 107,* 463–486.

McDuff, T., & Sumi, S. M. (1985). Subcortical degeneration in Alzheimer's disease. *Neurology, 35,* 123–126.

McEntee, W. J., Biber, M. P., Perl, D. P., & Benson, D. F. (1976). Diencephalic amnesia: A reappraisal. *Journal of Neurology, Neurosurgery, and Psychiatry, 39,* 436–441.

McEvoy, J. P. (1987). A double-blind crossover comparison of antiparkinson drug therapy: Amantadine versus anticholinergics in 90 normal volunteers, with an emphasis on differential effects on memory function. *Journal of Clinical Psychiatry, 48*(Suppl. 9), 20–23.

McFarling, D., Rothi, L. J., & Heilman, K. M. (1982). Transcortical aphasia from ischaemic infarcts of the thalamus: A report of two cases. *Journal of Neurology, Neurosurgery, and Psychiatry, 45,* 107–112.

Medalia, A., Isaacs-Glaberman, K., & Scheinberg, H. (1988). Neuropsychological impairment in Wilson's disease. *Archives of Neurology, 45,* 502–504.

Mehler, M. F. (1988). Subcortical aphasia: Specific modulatory functions of the caudate nucleus. *Journal of Clinical and Experimental Neuropsychology, 10,* 26–27.

Mennemeier, M., Fennell, E., & Valenstein, E. (1990). Persistent cognitive deficits following a left intralaminar nuclei lesion: A different perspective on thalamic recruitment and cortical processing. *Journal of Clinical and Experimental Neuropsychology, 12,* 84.

Mennemeier, M., Fennell, E., Valenstein, E., & Heilman, K. M. (1990). *Memory functions of the left intralaminar and medial thalamic nuclei.* Unpublished manuscript.

Mesulam, M.-M., Mufson, E. J., Wainer, B. H., & Levey, A. I. (1983). Central cholinergic pathways in the rat: An overview based on an alternative nomenclature (Ch1-Ch6). *Neuroscience, 10,* 1185–1201.

Metter, E. J., Jackson, D., Kempler, D., Riege, W. H., Hanson, W. R., Mazziotta, J. C., & Phelps, M. E. (1986). Left hemisphere intracerebral hemorrhages studied by (F-18)-fluorodeoxyglucose PET. *Neurology, 36,* 1155–1162.

Metter, E. J., Kempler, D., Jackson, C., Hanson, W. R., Mazziotta, J. C., & Phelps, M. E. (1989). Cerebral glucose metabolism in Wernicke's, Broca's, and conduction aphasia. *Archives of Neurology, 46,* 27–34.

Metter, E. J., Kempler, D., Jackson, C. A., Hanson, W. R., Riege, W. H., Camras, L. R., Mazziotta, J. C., & Phelps, M. E. (1987). Cerebellar glucose metabolism in chronic aphasia. *Neurology, 37,* 1599–1606.

Metter, E. J., Riege, W. H., Hanson, W. R., Camras, L. R., Phelps, M. E., & Kuhl, D. E. (1984). Correlations of glucose metabolism and structural damage to language function in aphasia. *Brain and Language, 21,* 187–207.

Metter, E. J., Riege, W. H., Hanson, W. R., Jackson, C. A., Kempler, D., & van Lancker, D. (1988). Subcortical structures in aphasia: An analysis based on (F-18)-fluorodeoxyglucose, positron emission tomography, and computed tomography. *Archives of Neurology, 45,* 1229–1234.

Metter, E. J., Riege, W. H., Hanson, W. R., Kuhl, D. E., Phelps, M. E., Squire, L. R., Wasterlain, C. G., & Benson, D. F. (1983). Comparison of metabolic rates, language, and memory in subcortical aphasias. *Brain and Language, 19,* 33–47.

Meudell, P. R., Northen, B., Snowden, J. S., & Neary, D. (1980). Long-term memory for famous voices in amnesic and normal subjects. *Neuropsychologia, 18,* 133–139.

Milner, B. (1962). Les troubles de la memoire accompagnant des lesions hippocampiques bilaterales. In P. Passouant (Ed.), *Physiologie de l'hippocampe* (pp. 257–272). Paris: Centre National de la Recherche Scientific.

Milner, G. (1971). Interhemispheric differences in localization of psychological processes in man. *British Medical Bulletin, 127,* 272–277.

Mink, J. W., & Thach, W. T. (1987a). Pallidal ablation: Normal reaction time, muscle cocontraction, and slow movement. *Society of Neuroscience Abstracts, 13,* 982.

Mink, J. W., & Thach, W. T. (1987b). Preferential relation of pallidal neurons to ballistic movements. *Brain Research, 417,* 393–398.

Mishkin, M. (1966). Visual mechanisms beyond the striate cortex. In R. Russell (Ed.), *Frontiers in physiological psychology* (pp. 93–119). New York: Academic Press.

Mishkin, M. (1978). Memory in monkeys severely impaired by combined but not separate removal of amygdala and hippocampus. *Nature, 273,* 297–298.

Mishkin, M. (1982). A memory system in the monkey. *Philosophical Transactions of the Royal Society of London* (Series B, Biolgical Sciences), *298,* 85–95.

Mishkin, M., & Oubre, J. L. (1977). Dissociation of deficits on visual memory tasks after inferior temporal and amygdala lesions in monkeys. *Society for Neuroscience Abstracts, 2,* 1127.

Mitchell, I. J., Jackson, A., Sambrook, M. A., & Crossman, A. R. (1989). The role of the subthalamic nucleus in experimental chorea. *Brain, 112,* 1533–1548.

Mohr, J. P., Watters, W. C., & Duncan, G. W. (1975). Thalamic hemorrhage and aphasia. *Brain and Language, 2,* 3–17.

Montemurro, D. G., & Bruni, J. E. (1988). *The human brain in dissection* (2nd ed.). New York: Oxford University Press.

Mori, E., Yamadori, A., & Mitani, Y. (1986). Left thalamic infarction and disturbance of verbal memory: A clinicoanatomical study with a new method of computed tomographic stereotaxic lesion localization. *Annals of Neurology, 20,* 671–676.

Moscovitch, M. (1982). Multiple dissociations of function in amnesia. In L. S. Cermak (Ed.), *Human memory and amnesia* (pp. 337–370). Hillsdale, NJ: Lawrence Erlbaum.

Moss, M. B., Albert, M. S., Butters, N., & Payne, M. (1986). Differential patterns of memory loss among patients with Alzheimer's disease, Huntington's disease, and alcoholic Korsakoff's syndrome. *Archives of Neurology, 43,* 239–246.

Moutier, F. (1908). *L'Aphasie de Broca.* Unpublished doctoral dissertation, Paris. (Cited by Wallesch & Papagno, 1988)

Murdoch, B. E., Chenery, H. J., & Kennedy, M. (1989). Aphemia associated with bilateral striato-capsular lesions subsequent to cerebral anoxia. *Brain Injury, 3,* 41–49.

Murray, C. L., & Fibiger, H. C. (1985). Learning and memory deficits after lesions of the nucleus basalis magnocellularis: Reversal by physostigmine. *Neuroscience, 14,* 1025–1032.

Murray, C. L., & Fibiger, H. C. (1986). Pilocarpine and physostigmine attenuate spatial memory impairments produced by lesions of the nucleus basalis magnocellularis. *Behavioral Neuroscience, 100,* 23–32.

Nadeau, S. E. (1988). Impaired grammar with normal fluency and phonology: Implications for Broca's aphasia. *Brain, 111,* 1111–1137.

Naeser, M. A., Alexander, M. P., Helm-Estabrooks, N., Levine, H. L., Laughlin, S. A., & Geschwind, N. (1982). Aphasia with predominantly subcortical lesion sites: Description of three capsular/putaminal aphasia syndromes. *Archives of Neurology, 39,* 2–14.

Naeser, M. A., Palumbo, C. L., Helm-Estabrooks, N., Stiassny-Eder, D., & Albert, M. L. (1989). Severe nonfluency in aphasia: Role of the medial subcallosal fasciculus and other white matter pathways in recovery of spontaneous speech. *Brain, 112,* 1–38.

Nauta, W. J. H. (1961). Fiber degeneration following lesions of the amygdaloid complex in the monkey. *Journal of Anatomy, 95,* 515–531.

Nauta, W. J. H. (1962). Neural associations of the amygdaloid complex in the monkey. *Brain, 85,* 505–520.

Nauta, W. J. H., & Feirtag, M. (1986). *Fundamental neuroanatomy.* New York: W. H. Freeman.

Nauta, W. J. H., & Whitlock, D. G. (1954). An anatomical analysis of the nonspecific thalamic projection system. In J. F. Delafresnaye (Ed.), *Brain mechanisms and consciousness* (pp. 81–116). Springfield, IL: Charles C. Thomas.

Netter, F. H. (1972). *The Ciba collection of medical illustrations: Vol. 1. Nervous system.* Summit, NJ: Ciba.

Nichelli, P., Bahmanian-Behbahani, G., Gentilini, M., & Vecchi, A. (1988). Preserved memory abilities in thalamic amnesia. *Brain, 111,* 1337–1353.

Norlen, G., & Lindqvist, G. (1964). The anatomy of memory. *Lancet, 1,* 335.

Norman, D. A. (1973). What have the animal experiments taught us about human memory? In J. A. Deutsch (Ed.), *The physiological basis of memory* (pp. 397–414). New York: Academic Press.

Ojemann, G. A. (1974). Speech and short-term verbal memory: Alterations evoked from stimulation in pulvinar. In I. S. Cooper, M. Riklan, & P. Rakic (Eds.), *The pulvinar-LP complex* (pp. 173–201). Springfield, IL: Charles C. Thomas.

Ojemann, G. A. (1975). Language and the thalamus: Object naming and recall during and after thalamic stimulation. *Brain and Language, 2,* 101–120.

Ojemann, G. A. (1976). Subcortical language mechanisms. In H. Whitaker and H. A. Whitaker (Eds.), *Studies in neurolinguistics* (Vol. 1, pp. 103–138). New York: Academic Press.

Ojemann, G. A. (1977). Asymmetric function of the thalamus in man. *Annals of the New York Academy of Sciences, 299,* 380–396.

Ojemann, G. A. (1983). Brain organization for language from the perspective of electrical stimulation mapping. *Behavioral and Brain Sciences, 2,* 189–230.

Ojemann, G. A. (1985). Enhancement of memory with human ventrolateral thalamic stimulation: Effect evident on a dichotic listening task. *Applied Neurophysiology, 48,* 212–215.

Ojemann, G. A., Blick, K. I., & Ward, A. A. (1971). Improvement and disturbance of short-term verbal memory with human ventrolateral thalamic stimulation. *Brain, 94,* 225–240.

Ojemann, G. A., & Fedio, P. (1968). Effect of stimulation of the human thalamus and parietal and temporal white matter on short-term memory. *Journal of Neurosurgery, 29,* 51–59.

Ojemann, G. A., Fedio, P., & Van Buren, J. M. (1968). Anomia from pulvinar and subcortical parietal stimulation. *Brain, 91,* 99–116.

Ojeman, G. A., Fried, I., & Lettich, E. (1989). Electrocorticographic (ECoG) correlates of language: 1. Desynchroniztion in temporal language cortex during object naming. *Electroencephalography and Clinical Neurophysiology, 73,* 453–463.

Ojemann, G. A., & Ward, A. A. (1971). Speech representation in ventrolateral thalamus. *Brain, 94,* 669–680.

Okawa, M., Maeda, S., Nukui, H., & Kawafuchi, J. (1980). Psychiatric symptoms in ruptured anterior communicating aneurysms: Social prognosis. *Acta Psychiatrica Scandinavica, 61,* 306–312.

Olsen, T. S., Bruhn, P., & Oberg, R. G. E. (1986). Cortical hypoperfusion as a possible cause of "subcortical aphasia". *Brain, 109,* 393–410.

Orsini, A., Fragassi, N. A., Chiacchio, L., Falanga, A. M., Cocchiaro, C., & Grossi, D. (1987). Verbal and spatial memory span in patients with extrapyramidal diseases. *Perceptual and Motor Skills, 65,* 555–558.

Oscar-Berman, M. (1973). Hypothesis testing and focusing behavior during concept formation by amnesic Korsakoff patients. *Neuropsychologia, 11,* 191–198.

Paillard, J. (1982). Apraxia and the neurophysiology of motor control. *Philosophical Transactions of the Royal Society of London* (Series B, Biological Sciences), *298,* 111–134.

Papagno, C., & Guidotti, M. (1983). A case of aphasia following left thalamic hemorrhage. *European Neurology, 22,* 93–95.

Papez, J. W. (1937). A proposed mechanism of emotion. *Archives of Neurology and Psychiatry, 38,* 725–743.

Patterson, T., Spohn, H. E., Bogia, D. P., & Hayes, K. (1986). Thought disorder in schizophrenia: Cognitive and neuroscience approaches. *Schizophrenia Bulletin, 12,* 460–472.

Penfield, W., & Roberts, L. (1959). *Speech and brain mechanisms.* Princeton, NJ: Princeton University Press.

Penney, J. B., Jr., & Young, A. B. (1983). Speculations on the functional anatomy of basal ganglia disorders. *Annual Review of Neuroscience, 6,* 73–94.

Penney, J. B., Jr., & Young, A. B. (1986). Striatal inhomogeneities and basal ganglia function. *Movement Disorders, 1(1),* 3–15.

Percheron, G. (1973). The anatomy of the arterial supply of the human thalamus and its use for the interpretation of the thalamic vascular pathology. *Zeitschrift fur Neurologie, 205,* 1–13.

Percheron, G., & Yelnik, J., & Francois, C. (1984). A Golgi analysis of the primate globus pallidus. 3. Spatial organization of the striato-pallido complex. *The Journal of Comparative Neurology, 227,* 214–227.

Perry, E. K., Tomlinson, B. E., Blessed, G., Bergman, K., Gibson, P. H., & Perry, R. H. (1978). Correlation of cholinergic abnormalities with senile plaques and mental test scores in senile dementia. *British Medical Journal, 2,* 1457–1459.

Perry, T. L., & Hansen, S. (1990). What excitotoxin kills striatal neurons in

Huntington's disease?: Clues from neurochemical studies. *Neurology, 40,* 20–24.

Petersen, S. E., Fox, P. T., Posner, M. I., Mintun, M., & Raichle, M. E. (1988). Positron emission tomographic studies of cortical anatomy of single-word processing. *Nature, 331,* 585–589.

Petersen, S. E., Fox, P.T., Posner, M. I., Mintun, M., & Raichle, M. E. (1989). Positron emision tomographic studies of the processing of single words. *Journal of Cognitive Neuroscience, 1,* 153–170.

Peterson, L. R., & Peterson, J. J. (1959). Short-term retention of individual verbal items. *Journal of Experimental Psychology, 58,* 193–198.

Phillips, S., Sangalang, V., & Sterns, G. (1987). Basal forebrain infarction: A clinicopathologic correlation. *Archives of Neurology, 44,* 1134–1138.

Pillon, G., Dubois, B., Lhermitte, F., & Agid, Y. (1986). Heterogeneity of cognitive impairment in progressive supranuclear palsy, Parkinson's disease, and Alzheimer's disease. *Neurology, 36,* 1179–1185.

Pirozzolo, F. J., Hansch, E. C., Mortimer, J. A., Webster, D. D., & Kuskowski, M. A. (1982). Dementia and Parkinson disease: A neuropsychological analysis. *Brain and Cognition, 1,* 71–83.

Podoll, K., Caspary, P., Lange, H. W., & Notch, J. (1988). Language functions in Huntington's disease. *Brain, 111,* 1475–1503.

Porch, B. E. (1971). *Porch Index of Communicative Ability.* Palo Alto, CA: Consulting Psychologist Press.

Porteus, S. D. (1959). *The maze test and clinical psychology.* Palo Alto, CA: Pacific Books.

Pozzilli, C., Passafiume, D., Bastianello, S., D'Antona, R., & Lenzi, G. L. (1987). Remote effects of caudate hemorrhage: A clinical and functional study. *Cortex, 23,* 341–349.

Preston, R. J., Bishop, G. A., & Kitai, S. T. (1980). Medium spiny neuron projection from the rat striatum: An intracellular horseradish peroxidase study. *Brain Research, 183,* 253–263.

Puel, M., Cardebat, D., Demonet, J.-F., Elghozi, D., Cambier, J., Guiraud-Chaumeil, B., & Rascol, A. (1986). Le role du thalamus dans les aphasies sous-corticales. *Revue Neurologique, 142,* 431–440.

Puel, M., Demonet, J-F., Cardebat, D., Berry, I., & Celsis, P. (1989, September). *Thalamic aphasia revisited. Neuropsychological, NMR, and SPECT study of three cases: One, two or three syndromes?* Paper presented at the Meeting on Neuropsychological Disorders Associated with Subcortical Lesions, Como, Italy.

Puel, M., Demonet, J.-F., Cardebat, D., Bonafe, A., Gazounaud, Y., Guiraud-Chaumeil, B., & Rascol, A. (1984). Aphasies sous-corticales. Etude linguistique avec Scanner X, a propos de 25 observations. *Revue Neurologique, 140,* 695–710.

Rafal, R. D., & Posner, M. I. (1987). Deficits in human visual spatial attention following thalamic lesions. *Proceedings of the National Academy of Science, 84,* 7349–7353.

Ramsberger, G., & Hillman, R. E. (1985). Temporal speech characteristics associated with anterior left hemisphere cortical and subcortical lesions: A preliminary case study report. *Brain and Language, 24,* 59–73.

Ranson, S. W., & Clark, S. L. (1959). *The anatomy of the nervous system: Its development and function*. Philadelphia: W. B. Saunders.

Reep, R. (1984). Relationship between prefrontal and limbic cortex: A comparative anatomical review. *Brain, Behavior, and Evolution, 25*, 5–80.

Reynolds, A. F., Harris, A. B., Ojemann, G. A., & Turner, P. T. (1978). Aphasia and left thalamic hemorrhage. *Journal of Neurosurgery, 48*, 570–574.

Reynolds, A. F., Turner, P. T., Harris, A. G., Ojemann, G. A., & Davis, L. E. (1979). Left thalamic hemorrhage with dysphasia: A report of five cases. *Brain and Language, 7*, 62–73.

Riklan, M., & Cooper, I. S. (1975). Psychometric studies of verbal functions following thalamic lesions in humans. *Brain and Language, 2*, 45–64.

Riklan, M., & Levita, E. (1965). Laterality of subcortical involvement and psychological functions. *Psychological Bulletin, 64*, 217–224.

Riklan, M., Levita, E., Zimmerman, J., & Cooper, I. S. (1969). Thalamic correlates of language and speech. *Journal of the Neurological Sciences, 8*, 307–328.

Rinne, J. O., Rummukainen, J., Paljarvi, L., & Rinne, U. K. (1989). Dementia in Parkinson's disease is related to neuronal loss in the medial substantia nigra. *Annals of Neurology, 26*, 47–50.

Risse, G. L., Rubens, A. B., & Jordan, L. S. (1984). Disturbances of long-term memory in aphasic patients: A comparison of anterior and posterior lesions. *Brain, 107*, 605–617.

Robin, D. A., & Schienberg, S. (1990). Subcortical lesions and aphasia. *Journal of Speech and Hearing Disorders, 55*, 90–100.

Roche, S. W., Lane, R. J. M., & Wade, J. P. H. (1988). Thalamic hemorrhages in Wernicke-Korsakoff syndrome demonstrated by computed tomography. *Neurology, 38*, 312.

Roediger, H. L. (1990). Implicit memory: Retention without remembering. *American Psychologist, 45*, 1043-1056.

Rose, J. E., & Woolsey, C. N. (1948). The orbitofrontal cortex and its connections with the mediodorsal nucleus in rabbit, sheep, and cat. *Association for Research of Nervous and Mental Disease Proceedings, 27*, 210–282.

Russell, E. W. (1975). A multiple scoring method for assessment of complex memory functions. *Journal of Consulting and Clinical Psychology, 43*, 800–809.

Russell, E. W. (1981). The pathology and clinical examination of memory. In S. B. Filskov & T. J. Boll (Eds.), *Handbook of clinical neuropsychology* (pp. 287–319). New York: John Wiley and Sons.

Sagar, H. J., Cohen, N. J., Sullivan, E. V., Corkin, S., & Growdon, J. H. (1988). Remote memory function in Alzheimer's disease and Parkinson's disease. *Brain, 111*, 185–206.

Sagar, H. J., Sullivan, E. V., Gabrieli, J. D. E., Corkin, S., & Growdon, J. H. (1988). Temporal ordering and short-term memory deficits in Parkinson's disease. *Brain, 111*, 525–539.

Sahakian, B. J., Morris, R. G., Evenden, J. L., Heald, A., Levy, R., Philpot, M., & Robbins, T. W. (1988). A comparative study of visuospatial memory and learning in Alzheimer-type dementia and Parkinson's disease. *Brain, 111*, 695–718.

Saint-Cyr, J. A., Taylor, A. E., Lang, A. E., & Trepanier, L. L. (1989, September).

Striatal contributions to frontal lobe function: Evidence from basal ganglia disease. Paper presented at the Meeting on Neuropsychological Disorders Associated with Subcortical Lesions, Como, Italy.

Samra, K., Riklan, M., Levita, E., Simmerman, J., Waltz, J. M., Bergmann, L., & Cooper, I. S. (1969). Language and speech correlates of anatomically verified lesions in thalamic surgery for parkinsonism. *Journal of Speech and Hearing Research, 12,* 510–540.

Samuels, I., Butters, N., Goodglass, H., & Brody, B. (1971). A comparison of subcortical and cortical damage on short-term visual and auditory memory. *Neuropsychologia, 9,* 293–306.

Sax, D. S., O'Donnell, B., Butters, N., Menzer, L., Montgomery, K., & Kayne, H. L. (1983). Computed tomographic, neurologic, and neuropsychological correlates of Huntington's disease. *International Journal of Neuroscience, 18,* 21–36.

Schacter, D. L. (1987). Implicit memory: History and current status. *Journal of Experimental Psychology: Learning, Memory, and Cognition, 13,* 501–518.

Schaltenbrand, G. (1965). The effects of stereotactic electrical stimulation in the depth of the brain. *Brain, 88,* 835–840.

Schaltenbrand, G. (1975). The effects on speech and language of stereotactical stimulation in the thalamus and corpus callosum. *Brain and Language, 2,* 70–77.

Scheibel, M. E., & Scheibel, A. B. (1966). The organization of the ventral anterior nucleus of the thalmus. A Golgi study. *Brain Research, 1,* 250–268.

Schuell, H., Jenkins, J. J., & Jimenez-Pabon, E. (1965). *Aphasia in adults.* New York: Harper and Row.

Schulman, S. (1964). Impaired delayed response from thalamic lesions. *Archives of Neurology, 11,* 477–499.

Schwartz, W. J., Smith, C. B., Davidsen, L., Savaki, H., Sokoloff, L., Mata, M., Fink, D. J., & Gainer, H. (1979). Metabolic mapping of functional activity in the hypothalamo-neurohypophysial system of the rat. *Science, 205,* 723–725.

Scott, W. R., & Miller, B. R. (1985). Intracerebral hemorrhage with rapid recovery. *Archives of Neurology, 42,* 133–136.

Selby, G. (1967). Stereotactic surgery for the relief of Parkinson's disease: 2. An analysis of the results in a series of 303 patients (413 operations). *Journal of the Neurological Sciences, 5,* 343–375.

Selzer, B., & Benson, D. F. (1974). The temporal pattern of retrograde amnesia in Korsakoff's disease. *Neurology, 24,* 527–530.

Sengupta, R. P., Chiu, J. S. P., & Brierly, H. (1975). Quality of survival following direct surgery for anterior communicating artery aneurysms. *Journal of Neurosurgery, 43,* 58–64.

Shallice, T., & Warrington, E. K. (1970). Independent functioning of verbal memory stores: A neuropsychological study. *Quarterly Journal of Experimental Psychology, 22,* 261–273.

Shiffrin, R. M. (1973). Information persistence in short-term memory. *Journal of Experimental Psychology, 100,* 39–49.

Shiffrin, R. M., & Schneider, W. (1977). Controlled and automatic human information processing: 2. Perceptual learning, automatic attending, and a general theory. *Psychological Review, 84,* 127–190.

Shimamura, A. P., Jernigan, T. L., & Squire, L. R. (1988). Korsakoff's syndrome: Radiological (CT) findings and neuropsychological correlates. *Journal of Neuroscience, 8,* 4400–4410.

Shimamura, A. P., Salmon, D. P., Squire, L. R., & Butters, N. (1987). Memory dysfunction and word priming in dementia and amnesia. *Behavioral Neuroscience, 101,* 347–351.

Shimamura, A. P., & Squire, L. R. (1984). Paired-associate learning and priming effects in amnesia: A neuropsychological study. *Journal of Experimental Psychology: General, 113,* 556–570.

Shimamura, A. P., & Squire, L. R. (1986). Korsakoff's syndrome: A study of the relation between anterograde amnesia and remote memory impairment. *Behavioral Neuroscience, 100,* 165–170.

Smith, S., Butters, N., White, R., Lyon, L., & Granholm, E. (1988). Priming semantic relations in patients with Huntington's disease. *Brain and Language, 33,* 27–40.

Somogyi, P., & Smith, A. D. (1979). Projection of neostriatal spiny neurons to the substantia nigra. Application of a combined Golgi-staining and horseradish peroxidase transport procedure at both light and electron microscopic levels. *Brain Research, 178,* 3–15.

Speedie, L. J., & Heilman, K. M. (1982). Amnestic disturbance following infarction of the left dorsomedial nucleus of the thalamus. *Neuropsychologia, 20,* 597–604.

Speedie, L. J., & Heilman, K. M. (1983). Anterograde memory deficits for visuospatial material after infarction of the right thalamus. *Archives of Neurology, 40,* 183–186.

Spencer, H. J. (1976). Antagonism of cortical excitation of striatal neurons by glutamic acid diethyl ester: Evidence for glutamic acid as an excitatory transmitter in the rat striatum. *Brain Research, 102,* 91–101.

Spicer, K. B., Roberts, R. J., & LeWitt, P. A. (1988). Neuropsychological performance in lateralized parkinsonism. *Archives of Neurology, 45,* 429–432.

Sprofkin, B. E., & Sciarra, D. (1952). Korsakoff's psychosis associated with cerebral tumors. *Neurology, 2,* 427–434.

Squire, L. R. (1981). Two forms of human amnesia: An analysis of forgetting. *Journal of Neuroscience, 1,* 635–640.

Squire, L. R. (1982). Comparisons between forms of amnesia: Some deficits are unique to Korsakoff's syndrome. *Journal of Experimental Psychology: Learning, Memory, and Cognition, 8,* 560–571.

Squire, L. R. (1987). *Memory and brain.* New York: Oxford University Press.

Squire, L. R., Amaral, D. G., Zola-Morgan, S., Kritchevsky, M., & Press, G. (1989). Description of brain injury in the amnesic patient N. A. based on magnetic resonance imaging. *Experimental Neurology, 105,* 23–35.

Squire, L. R., Haist, F., & Shimamura, A. P. (1989). The neurology of memory: Quantitative assessment of retrograde amnesia in two groups of amnesic patients. *Journal of Neuroscience, 9,* 828–839.

Squire, L. R., & Moore, R. Y. (1979). Dorsal thalamic lesion in a noted case of human memory dysfunction. *Annals of Neurology, 6,* 503–506.

Squire, L. R., & Shimamura, A. P. (1986). Characterizing amnesic patients for neurobehavioral study. *Behavioral Neuroscience, 100,* 866–877.

Squire, L. R., Shimamura, A. P., & Graf, P. (1987). Strength and duration of priming effects in normal subjects and amnesic patients. *Neuropsychologia, 25,* 195–210.

Starkstein, S., Leiguarda, R., Gershanik, O., & Berthier, M. (1987). Neuropsychological disturbances in hemiparkinson's disease. *Neurology, 37,* 1762–1764.

Steriade, M., & Deschenes, M. (1984). The thalamus as a neuronal oscillator. *Brain Research Reviews, 8,* 1–63.

Stern, Y. (1983). Behavior and the basal ganglia. In R. Mayeux & W. G. Rosen (Eds.), *The dementias* (pp. 195–209). New York: Raven Press.

Stuss, D. T., Guberman, A., Nelson, R., & Larochelle, S. (1988). The neuropsychology of paramedian thalamic infarction. *Brain and Cognition, 8,* 348–378.

Svennilson, E., Torvik, A., Lowe, R., & Leksell, L. (1960). Treatment of parkinsonism by stereotactic thermolesions in the pallidal region. *Acta Psychiatrica et Neurologica Scandinavia, 35,* 358–377.

Swanson, R. A., & Schmidley, J. W. (1985). Amnestic syndrome and vertical gaze palsy: Early detection of bilateral thalamic infarction by CT and NMR. *Stroke, 16,* 823–827.

Swerdlow, N. R., & Koob, G. F. (1987). Dopamine, schizophrenia, mania, and depression: Toward a unified hypothesis of cortico-striato-pallido-thalamic function. *Behavioral and Brain Sciences, 10,* 197–245.

Talland, G. (1965). *Deranged memory.* New York: Academic Press.

Talland, G., Sweet, W. H., & Ballantine, H. T (1967). Amnesic syndrome with anterior communicating artery aneurysm. *Journal of Nervous and Mental Disease, 145,* 179–192.

Tanridag, O. & Kirshner, H. S. (1985). Aphasia and agraphia in lesions of the posterior internal capsule and putamen. *Neurology, 35,* 1797–1801.

Taylor, A. E., Saint-Cyr, J. A., Lang, A. E., & Kenny, F. F. (1986). Frontal lobe dysfunction in Parkinson's disease: The cortical focus of neostriatal outflow. *Brain, 109,* 845–883.

Terry, R. D., & Katzman, R. (1983). Senile dementia of the Alzheimer type. *Annals of Neurology, 14,* 497–506.

Thomson, D. M., & Tulving, E. (1970). Associative encoding and retrieval: Weak and strong cues. *Journal of Experimental Psychology, 86,* 255–262.

Tijssen, C. C., Tavy, D. L. J., Hekster, R. E. M., Bots, G. T. A. M., & Endtz, L. J. (1984). Aphasia with a left frontal interhemispheric hematoma. *Neurology, 34,* 1261–1264.

Tilson, H. A., McLamb, R. L., Shaw, S., Rogers, B. C., Pediaditakis, P., & Cook, L. (1988). Radial-arm maze deficits produced by colchicine administered into the area of the nucleus basalis are ameliorated by cholinergic agents. *Brain Research, 438,* 83–94.

Trojanowski, J. Q., & Jacobson, S. (1974). Medial pulvinar afferents to frontal eye fields in Rhesus monkey demonstrated by horseradish peroxidase. *Brain Research, 80,* 395–411.

Trojanowski, J. Q., & Jacobson, S. (1975). A combined horseradish peroxidase-autoradiographic investigation of reciprocal connections between superior temporal gyrus and pulvinar in squirrel monkey. *Brain Research, 85,* 347–353.

Tulving, E. (1972). Episodic and semantic memory. In E. Tulving & W. Donaldson (Eds.), *Organization of memory* (pp. 381–403). New York: Academic Press.

Tuszynski, M. H., & Petito, C. K. (1988). Ischemic thalamic aphasia with pathologic confirmation. *Neurology, 38,* 800–802.

Umbach, W. (1966). Long-term results of fornicotomy for temporal epilepsy. *Confinia Neurologica, 27,* 121–123.

Valenstein, E., Bowers, D., Verfaellie, M., Watson, R., Day, A., & Heilman, K. M. (1987). Retrosplenial amnesia. *Brain, 110,* 1631–1636.

Van Buren, J. M. (1963). Confusion and disturbance of speech from stimulation in the vicinity of the head of the caudate nucleus. *Journal of Neurosurgery, 20,* 148–157.

Van Buren, J. M. (1966). Evidence regarding a more precise localization of the frontal-caudate arrest response in man. *Journal of Neurosurgery, 24,* 416–417.

Van Buren, J. M. (1975). The question of thalamic participation in speech mechanisms. *Brain and Language, 2,* 31–44.

Van Buren, J. M., & Borke, R. C. (1969). Alterations in speech and the pulvinar: A serial section study of cerebrothalamic relationships in cases of acquired speech disorders. *Brain, 92,* 255–284.

Van Buren, J. M., Li, C. L., & Ojemann, G. A. (1966). The fronto-striatal arrest response in man. *Electroencephalography and Clinical Neurophysiology, 21,* 114–130.

Victor, M., Adams, R. D., & Collins, G. H. (1971). *The Wernicke-Korsakoff syndrome.* Philadelphia: F. A. Davis.

Vilkki, J. (1985). Amnesic syndromes after surgery of anterior communicating artery aneurysms. *Cortex, 21,* 431–444.

Vilkki, J., & Laitinen, L. V. (1974). Differential effects of left and right ventrolateral thalamotomy on some cognitive functions. *Neuropsychologia, 12,* 11–19.

Vilkki, J., & Laitinen, L. V. (1976). Effects of pulvinotomy and ventrolateral thalamotomy on some cognitive functions. *Neuropsychologia, 14,* 67–78.

Volpe, B. T., Herscovitch, P., & Raichle, M. E. (1984). Positron emission tomography defines metabolic abnormality in mesial temporal lobes of two patients with amnesia after rupture and repair of anterior communicating artery aneurysm. *Neurology, 34*(Suppl. 1), 188.

Volpe, B. T., & Hirst, W. (1983). Amnesia following the rupture and repair of an anterior communicating artery aneurysm. *Journal of Neurology, Neurosurgery, and Psychiatry, 46,* 704–709.

Wahoske, P. A., Johnson, M. G., & Rubens, A. B. (1976, November). *Case report: Aphasia and thalamic hemorrhage.* Paper presented at the convention of the American Speech and Hearing Association, Houston.

Wallesch, C.-W. (1985). Two syndromes of aphasia occurring with ischemic lesions involving the left basal ganglia. *Brain and Language, 25,* 357–361.

Wallesch, C.-W., & Fehrenbach, R. A. (1988). On the neurolinguistic nature of language abnormalities in Huntington's disease. *Journal of Neurology, Neurosurgery, and Psychiatry, 51,* 367–373.

Wallesch, C.-W., Henriksen, L., Kornhuber, H. H., & Paulson, O. G. (1985). Observations on regional cerebral blood flow in cortical and subcortical structures during language production in normal man. *Brain and Language, 25,* 224–233.

Wallesch, C.-W., Kornhuber, H. H., Brunner, R. J., Kunz, T., Hollerbach, B., & Suger, G. (1983). Lesions of the basal ganglia, thalamus, and deep white matter: Differential effects on language functions. *Brain and Language, 20,* 286–304.

Wallesch, C.-W., & Papagno, C. (1988). Subcortical aphasia. In F. C. Rose, R. Whurr, & M. A. Wyke (Eds.), *Aphasia* (pp. 256–287). London: Whurr Publishers.

Walshe, T. M., Davis, K. R., & Fisher, C. M. (1977). Thalamic hemorrhage: A computed tomography-clinical correlation. *Neurology, 27,* 217–222.

Waltz, J. M., Riklan, M., Stellar, S., & Cooper, I. S. (1966). Cryothalamectomy for Parkinson's disease: A statistical analysis. *Neurology, 16,* 994–1002, 1021.

Warrington, E. K., & McCarthy, R. A. (1988). The fractionation of retrograde amnesia. *Brain and Cognition, 7,* 184–200.

Warrington, E. K., & Shallice, T. (1969). The selective impairment of auditory verbal short-term memory. *Brain, 92,* 885–896.

Warrington, E. K., & Weiskrantz, L. (1970). Amnesic syndrome: Consolidation or retrieval? *Nature, 228,* 628–630.

Watson, R. T., Miller, B. D., & Heilman, K. M. (1978). Non-sensory neglect. *Annals of Neurology, 3,* 505–508.

Watson, R. T., Valenstein, E., & Heilman, K. M. (1981). Thalamic neglect: Possible role of the medial thalamus and nucleus reticularis in behavior. *Archives of Neurology, 38,* 501–506.

Wechsler, D. (1945). A standardized memory scale for clinical use. *Journal of Psychology, 19,* 87–95.

Weiller, C., Ringlestein, E. B., Reiche, W., Thron, A., & Buell, U. (1990). The large striatocapsular infarct: A clinical and pathophysiological entity. *Archives of Neurology, 47,* 1085–1091.

Weinberger, D. R., Berman, K. R., & Zec, R. F. (1986). Physiologic dysfunction of dorsalateral prefrontal cortex in schizophrenia: 1. Regional cerebral blood flow evidence. *Archives of General Psychiatry, 43,* 114–124.

Weingartner, H., Caine, E. D., & Ebert, M. H. (1979). Imagery, encoding, and retrieval of information from memory: Some specific encoding-retrieval changes in Huntington's disease. *Journal of Abnormal Psychology, 88,* 52–58.

Weiskrantz, L., & Warrington, E. K. (1970). A study of forgetting in amnesic patients. *Neuropsychologia, 8,* 281–288.

Wernicke, C. (1874). *Der Aphasische Symptomencomplex.* Breslau: Cohn and Weigert. [Cited in Wallesch & Papagno, 1988].

Wetzel, C. D., & Squire, L. R. (1980). Encoding in anterograde amnesia. *Neuropsychologia, 18,* 177–184.

Whitehouse, P. J., Price, D. L., Clark, A. W., Coyle, J. T., & Delong, M. R. (1981). Alzheimer disease: Evidence for selective loss of cholinergic neurons in the nucleus basalis. *Annals of Neurology, 10,* 122–126.

Whitehouse, P. J., Price, D. L., Struble, R. G., Clark, A. W., Coyle, J. T., & DeLong, M. R. (1982). Alzheimer's disease and senile dementia: Loss of neurons in the basal forebrain. *Science, 215,* 1237–1239.

Williams, M., & Pennybacker, J. (1954). Memory disturbances in third ventricle tumors. *Journal of Neurology, Neurosurgery, and Psychiatry, 17,* 115–123.

Wilson, C. J., & Groves, P. M. (1980). Fine structure and synaptic connections of the common spiny neuron of the rat neostriatum: A study employing intracellular injection of horseradish peroxidase. *Journal of Comparative Neurology, 194,* 599–615.

Wilson, F. A. W., & Rolls, E. T. (1990). Learning and memory is reflected in the responses of reinforcement-related neurons in the primate basal forebrain. *Journal of Neuroscience, 10,* 1254–1267.

Wing, A., & Miller, E. (1984). Basal ganglia lesions and psychological analyses of the control of voluntary movement. In D. Evered & M. O'Connor (Eds.), *Functions of the basal ganglia. Ciba Foundation Symposium 107* (pp. 242–257). Summit, NJ: Ciba.

Winocur, G., & Kinsbourne, M. (1978). Contextual cueing as an aid to Korsakoff amnesics. *Neuropsychologia, 16,* 671–682.

Winocur, G., Oxbury, S., Roberts, R., Agnetti, V., & Davis, C. (1984). Amnesia in a patient with bilateral lesions to the thalamus. *Neuropsychologia, 22,* 123–143.

Woolsey, R. M., & Nelson, J. S. (1975). Asymptomatic destruction of the fornix in man. *Archives of Neurology, 32,* 566–568.

Yakovlev, P. I. (1948). Motility, behavior and the brain: Stereodynamic organization and neural coordinates of behavior. *Journal of Nervous and Mental Disease, 107,* 313–335.

Yamadori, A., Ohira, T., Seriu, M., & Ogura, J. (1984). Transcortical sensory aphasia produced by lesions of the anterior basal ganglia area. *Brain and Nerve, 36,* 261–266.

Yelnik, J., Percheron, G., & Francois, C. (1984). A golgi analysis of the primate globus pallidus. 2. Quantitative morphology and spatial orientation of dendritic aborizations. *Journal of Comparative Neurology, 227,* 200–213.

Yeterian, E. H., & Van Hoesen, G. W. (1978). Cortico-striate projections in the rhesus monkey: The organization of certain cortico-caudate connections. *Brain Research, 139,* 43–63.

Zola-Morgan, S., Cohen, N. J., & Squire, L. R. (1983). Recall of remote episodic memory in amnesia. *Neuropsychologia, 21,* 487–500.

Zola-Morgan, S., & Squire, L. R. (1985). Amnesia in monkeys after lesions of the mediodorsal nucleus of the thalamus. *Annals of Neurology, 17,* 558–564.

Index

Acetylcholine
  in striatum, 14
  in basal forebrain, 244–246, 255–256
Agrammatism, 122
Agraphia
  with lesions of basal ganglia and
    subcortical white matter, 61–63
  with thalamic lesion, 100–101
Akinesia
  and basal ganglia, 116, 309, 310
  endo- vs. exo-evoked, 309–310
  and memory vs. language, 318
Alcoholic Korsakoff's syndrome.
    See Korsakoff's syndrome, alco-
    holic
Alzheimer's disease. *See also entries
    under* Huntington's disease, Kor-
    sakoff's syndrome, Parkinson's
    disease
  vs. alcoholic Korsakoff's syndrome,
    203, 204, 212, 220
  basal forebrain cholinergic cells in,
    243, 245, 246
  vs. Huntington's disease, 261–263,
    266–268, 272, 275
  implicit memory, 220, 272
  vs. Parkinson's disease, 277–278,
    279–281, 282
  proactive interference, 212
Amnesia. *See also* Memory disorder
  defined, 183

bitemporal
  vs. alcoholic Korsakoff's syn-
    drome, 203–205, 306
  vs. basal forebrain amnesia, 307,
    314
  vs. diencephalic amnesia, 306,
    314
  retrograde, temporal gradient in
    and alcoholic Korsakoff's syn-
      drome, 224–228, 274
    explanation of, 224
    and Huntington's disease, 226,
      274–275
    hypothetical experiment, graph,
      225
    and other diencephalic lesion,
      232, 235, 236
Amphetamine, 256
Amygdala
  and basal forebrain, 156–158, 160
  and basal ganglia, 13, 313
  and dorsal medial nucleus, 27, 32,
    168, 183–184
  and memory systems, 167–169
  surgical removals of, 189
  and ventral amygdalofugal path-
    way, 163–164
Aneurysm, anterior communicating
    artery
  effects of, 246–254
  surgical treatment, procedures, 249